Editors
Filippo Familiari
Department of Orthopaedic and Trauma Surgery
Magna Graecia University
Catanzaro, Italy

Olimpio Galasso
Department of Orthopaedic and Trauma Surgery
University of Salerno
Salerno, Italy

Giorgio Gasparini
Department of Orthopaedic and Trauma Surgery
Magna Graecia University
Catanzaro, Italy

ISBN 978-3-031-70309-6 ISBN 978-3-031-70310-2 (eBook)
https://doi.org/10.1007/978-3-031-70310-2

This Springer imprint is published by the registered company Springer Nature Switzerland AG
The registered company address is: Gewerbestrasse 11, 6330 Cham, Switzerland

Foreword

Late in the year 2022 artificial intelligence became the topic of discussion worldwide. This event was not related to AI being new by any means. The triggering event was the advancement of microchip technology hitting new heights in capabilities. This allowed Large Language Model AI platforms to become available to the public through all the major technology players. The discussions regarding the wonderful potential of these tools rapidly became equated with alarm regarding the use of these tools in educational and research environments. The impact of the use of these tools in scholarly publication shortly followed. The upsides of the use of AI to improve manuscript submissions from non-primary English-speaking authors to produce drafts of test items and case summaries were equaled by concerns for fabricated data, manuscripts, reviews, and analyses. Journals were subject to large numbers of manuscript submissions regarding the use of these tools to aid in patient care, informed consent, treatment algorithms, outcomes assessment, and test taking. The major orthopaedic journals collaborated to establish basic policies for the use of LLMAI tools in scholarly publication 1.

This explosion of interest comes on top of a decade of increasing interest in AI-driven tool use in arthroplasty, machine learning image and risk assessment, image-guided surgical procedures of all types, and so on. The need for a comprehensive book on AI in orthopaedic surgery is thereby firmly established.

Familari, Galasso, and Gasparini have assembled an experience and knowledgeable author panel to provide this resource. The chapter on the history of AI by Guizzi et al. is valuable for any physician to understand that AI is nothing new and that we have been working on the expanding portfolio of AI-based tools for a century or more. This chapter alone is worth whatever is required to gain access. AI touches our individual lives hundreds of times every day on our smart phones, at the airport, and in commerce and personal lives to the point where we do not even have conscious awareness of the mechanics of AI techniques. This same phenomenon is in play within our lives as orthopaedic practitioners. EMR, OR scheduling and processing, and supply chain interactions all perform without us thinking about how these functions are driven by AI approaches. The comprehensive nature of the chapter outline across all aspects of patient care in our specialty inclusive of the nuances of every subspecialty is wise. The tools are all the same but the application in sports is different than in arthroplasty or spine. The book is a most welcome and valuable addition to our understanding of the current situation of AI as it aids our research and practice in the field of orthopaedic surgery. The use of AI tools in orthopaedic surgery is evolving so rapidly that frequent updates will be required. Of course, when discussing AI as a broad topic, one is inclined to ask the question about the future of books writ large in medicine—but that discussion will be nicely supported by AI based tools !!!

University of Minnesota
Minneapolis, MN, USA

Marc Swiontkowski

Foreword

Data Is the New Gold

The only constant in life is change. In recent years, there seems to be an acceleration in major and impactful changes which transform our world. More than ever, the world is transforming itself to create a more healthy and livable future and that happens at unexpected speeds and impact. Changes due to geopolitical tensions but also climate change have a great impact on human beings and society. Autonomous trends continue, such as the aging of the population and the availability of more technical options, especially in the field of digitalization. In particular, concepts such as AI and robotization seem to be taking off to have a major influence on the medical field.

Starting with simple rule-based systems in the 1950s and 1960s, with digitization of data and the creation of resources like the Medical Literature Analysis and the PubMed search engine, AI has now grown from its infancy. Clinical decision support systems and imaging analysis are two important areas where AI has proven its potential.

Unprecedented amounts are currently invested in the development of AI technology, such as Copilot and ChatGPT. These applications have resulted in all kinds of positive as well as negative implications.

For that reason it is important to be aware of the current situation and future developments.

For some this book will serve as an introduction to the field; for others it will serve as a guide and a glimpse into the future.

Arthroscopy and Sports Medicine

Several chapters in this book cover the use of AI-driven systems in the field of arthroscopy and orthopaedic sports medicine. AI-driven models have already been shown to provide highly personalized treatment plans to individual patients. But they can also forecast the progression from silent to clinical OA (osteoarthritis). Augmented reality overlays can provide surgeons with the ability to place virtual information onto their (arthroscopic) surgical field, to provide intuitive guidance while still having vision of the real world.

AI algorithm models can accurately predict postoperative functional outcomes and predict complications after surgery. In the near future, surgeons will be able to utilize AI algorithm models to provide their patients with a full personalized picture of their expected recovery timeline, likely complications and postoperative outcomes, allowing patients to make an informed decision and hold realistic expectations postoperatively. AI models will be used to optimize intraoperative ACL or meniscal repairs. For instance, the use of a head-up display could enable AI-generated guidance on precise locations for re-inserting the ACL or repairing the meniscus.

AI will also play a role in the future of arthroscopy, through virtual reality surgical training and augmented reality intraoperative overlays, real-time image and acoustic processing, and intelligent instruments. I specifically recommend to read Chap. 11 *(=chapter on shoulder arthroscopy).*

A chapter on rehabilitation mentions the use of a virtual assistant which provides a personalized exercise plan, monitors progress, offers real-time feedback, and adapts the rehabilitation program based on individual needs and progress.

Arthroplasty

Several chapters cover the use of AI-driven systems in the field of arthroplasty. AI algorithm models are primarily employed in preoperative templating, implant selection, determination of the position of the implant to be applied, and risk assessment.

Nearly two decades ago, the concept of AI use in the operating room was applied to navigation-assisted arthroplasties. Currently by means of semi-active technology, the model provides feedback to the practitioner about its actions, such as with robotic arm-assisted total knee surgery. The robotic systems aim not to replace the surgeon but to be an accurate and consistent delivery tool. The major benefit of robotic systems is accurate and reproducible bone preparation. Current use of AI technology in arthroplasty has a role in surgical planning, optimizing implant selection, enhancing the validity of alignment (for the lower extremity) positioning of implants, and calculating soft tissue balance.

Analysis of clinical and radiological data from previous patients is used to predict postoperative outcomes and to monitor patients postoperatively by remotely examining data such as gait, knee flexion angle, and recovery progress.

There are several limitations associated with robotic-assisted arthroplasty. These include the need for significant capital investment and ongoing expenses for operating room consumables. Additionally, surgeons and staff require extensive education and robotic-assisted implants often require longer operative times and necessitate a learning curve for the surgical team.

Nevertheless, the marriage of AI and robotics in orthopaedic surgery is not merely a futuristic concept but a clinical necessity that is already reshaping the healthcare industry.

Organization of Practice

As is highlighted in several chapters, AI shows great promise in automating pre-visit chart review, documentation, coding, and billing, decreasing physician workload and improving clinical efficiency.

Limitations, Potential Risks, and Ethical Issues with AI in Orthopaedics

Medical AI faces some challenges which are mentioned in several chapters. I specifically recommend to read Chap. 20 (*Toyooka etal Potential Risks and Ethical Issues with Intelligent Technologies in Orthopedics).*

AI does not possess traits that are uniquely human like morality and intuition and is liable to make mistakes that seem absurd to humans.

In the future, legislation needs to be constructed to clearly address who is liable for medical errors that are a result of using AI algorithms, and/or liability could be inferred on third parties such as insurers. In the meantime, physicians can and should be held accountable for any medical errors made in their practice and thus should have a sound understanding of any algorithm they use to treat patients.

However, this is complicated by the "black box" effect, the idea that it is difficult to know precisely how an AI algorithm arrives at a particular conclusion. AI algorithms often take a vast amount of data into account when coming to a treatment decision, but it is often unclear how different pieces of information are weighed in the decision-making process.

The expertise and professional competence (knowledge and skills) is the human capital of the medical profession; building databases of actions and instructions in a context that matches best practices would be the ideal situation. Unfortunately, this is not how it works.

Much of the available historic medical data is based on retrospective level IV studies. These results are used to feed the algorithms and guide care decisions. Results from historic studies can contain unknown bias. An algorithm trained on studies based on medical records of white men may make less accurate predictions about women, other races and ethnicities, or any other underrepresented group in the dataset. In the case of skin cancer, the likely site and appearance of the disease changes slightly depending on skin colour and age.

AI-based algorithm creators should provide a substantiation of how they came to their conclusions and how much weight was given to each component. This is a process which is currently under development.

Data transfer laws and regulations may pose a barrier to data sharing.

Several governing bodies such as the GDPR enforced by the EU now exist and impose strict rules on how personal data is used. Currently, four laws are being developed that will set the standard for Europe (Data Act, Data Governance Act, Digital Services Act, Digital Markets Act). These are expected to be active from September 2025 (*CoE Data sharing & Cloud: An overview of relevant European legislation for MSMEs engaged in Data*

Sharing (Centre of Excellence for Data Sharing & Cloud (coe-dsc.nl) (TNO 2024: R12799).

These laws and regulations will also apply for the USA and China entering the European market. There is a saying that America invents, Asia implements, and Europe sets rules and regulates. These EU guidelines classify the risk for application of AI into three categories: unacceptable risk (forbidden by EU act), high risk (needs to fulfil a series of assessments, litigation, etc.), and low risk. Medical application of AI falls into this last category.

Medical AI is more powerful for diseases with a large number of cases that can serve as training data. To this end, AI applications in medical imaging focus on the diagnosis of the most common diseases. It is difficult for AI to be powerful against rare diseases for which little data exists, much less against unknown diseases for which no data exists, and AI may not be able to accurately diagnose these rare diseases. This means that physicians need to be cautious and not rely solely on AI tools, because these models may not work well in all situations.

Since ultimately a physician can be held liable for any medical errors in their care, physicians should have at minimum an understanding of the workings of any AI algorithm they plan to use to assist in their medical decision-making.

For clinicians who are involved with research and publishing, it is important to realize that data entered into ChatGPT and other tools is automatically owned or co-owned by the creators of the program. ChatGPT is often used to further analyse data or to linguistically clean up a manuscript. At the moment you enter your—research—data into ChatGPT; they are directly available to the world.

Conclusion and Future Perspective

The current acceleration in the development of AI technology is seen as revolutionary, comparable to the invention of the personal computer. Data is the new gold! Various tasks are expected to be performed better by AI than by a hospital employee such as planning work, work preparation, and simple customer contacts. It can be expected that very soon at all levels in the hospital organization employees will be using task-oriented AI tools and our work will be facilitated by making use of a personal AI assistant.

Implementation of AI into your practice will increase clinical efficiency and patient outcomes while reducing physician workloads and burnout.

In the future, AI will not replace the surgeon, nor the radiologist or the emergency practitioner. Instead, some time-consuming tasks might be done more efficiently, and some tasks might be done more accurately. It will improve diagnostic accuracy, realize some better predictions based on the patient's personal information, and perform highly precise surgery. It is time to get on board!

University of Minho
Braga, Portugal

C. Niek van Dijk

Foreword

Suddenly, artificial intelligence seems to be everywhere in our lives. Its potential can be exciting or disconcerting. When we surf the Internet, algorithms track our path and constantly remind us where we have been or offer us personally curated menus of places we might like to go. Computer applications are able to modify our existing images or generate entirely new ones based upon our ideas. Large language models can refine our writing style or write entire new works for us, even fabricating research that was never actually conducted.

However, the possibilities created by artificial intelligence go far beyond these most mundane uses. In this book, Familiari and his colleagues exhaustively explain the vast potential of artificial intelligence to help us in almost every aspect of orthopaedic practice. They start at the very beginning, explaining the history and diverse capabilities of artificial intelligence. Then, in a series of chapters written by world-renowned experts, they delve into the potential uses of artificial intelligence to enhance virtually every orthopaedic subspecialty interest, from the hand to the foot, from arthroplasty to arthroscopy, and from elective surgery to acute trauma. Responsibly, the volume ends with a thoughtful consideration of the potential risks and ethical pitfalls of the use of artificial intelligence in orthopaedics.

I congratulate the authors on producing a book that will edify and fascinate any practising orthopaedic surgeon.

Chicago, IL, USA Bruce Reider

Preface

Dear Reader,

Welcome to *Artificial Intelligence in Orthopaedic Surgery (Made Easy)*, a comprehensive exploration of the transformative impact of artificial intelligence (AI) on the field of orthopaedics. As the editors of this volume, it is our pleasure to introduce you to a collection of cutting-edge research, innovative applications, and insightful perspectives that collectively underscore the remarkable potential of AI in revolutionizing orthopaedic surgery.

Orthopaedic surgery is a discipline where precision, accuracy, and patient well-being are paramount. In recent years, AI has emerged as a powerful tool that can enhance every aspect of orthopaedic care, from diagnosis and treatment planning to surgical execution and post-operative management. The integration of AI technologies into orthopaedic practice promises to improve patient outcomes, streamline clinical workflows, and expand the boundaries of what is possible in the field.

This book is a testament to the collaborative efforts of leading experts in orthopaedic surgery and AI from around the world. It brings together a diverse range of perspectives, methodologies, and real-world applications to provide readers with a comprehensive overview of this exciting frontier in healthcare.

In the pages that follow, you will find:

- Foundations of AI in orthopaedics: We begin by laying the groundwork, exploring the fundamental principles of artificial intelligence and machine learning as they apply to orthopaedic surgery. This section is designed to make AI accessible and understandable to readers with varying levels of expertise.
- AI in diagnosis and imaging: AI has revolutionized the way orthopaedic conditions are diagnosed, with computer vision and image analysis algorithms aiding in the interpretation of medical images, such as X-rays, MRIs, and CT scans. You will delve into the latest advancements in AI-assisted diagnosis and discover how these tools are enhancing clinical decision-making.
- Surgical planning and navigation: AI-driven surgical planning and navigation systems are transforming the way orthopaedic procedures are performed. Explore how these technologies are enabling surgeons to achieve greater precision and accuracy, resulting in improved patient outcomes and reduced surgical risks.

- Rehabilitation and post-operative care: Beyond the operating room, AI plays a pivotal role in optimizing rehabilitation protocols and monitoring patient progress. Learn how AI-powered devices and wearable technologies are enhancing the recovery process for orthopaedic patients.
- Future horizons: The final section of this book offers a glimpse into the future of AI in orthopaedic surgery. From the development of personalized treatment plans to the potential for autonomous surgical robots, the possibilities are boundless, and this section explores the exciting avenues that lie ahead.

Throughout this journey, you will gain insights from leading researchers, clinicians, and technologists who are at the forefront of this rapidly evolving field. Whether you are a healthcare professional, a researcher, a student, or simply curious about the intersection of AI and orthopaedic surgery, this book provides a valuable resource for understanding the present and envisioning the future.

We extend our deepest gratitude to all the contributors who have dedicated their expertise and passion to this project. Their collective efforts have made *Artificial Intelligence in Orthopaedic Surgery (Made Easy)* a significant contribution to the ongoing dialogue about the role of AI in reshaping the landscape of orthopaedic care.

We hope that you find this book informative, inspiring, and thought-provoking. As you embark on this journey through the world of AI in orthopaedic surgery, we encourage you to engage with the content, question the possibilities, and join the conversation that will shape the future of orthopaedic care.

Thank you for choosing to explore this exciting field with us.

Catanzaro, Italy — Filippo Familiari
Salerno, Italy — Olimpio Galasso
Catanzaro, Italy — Giorgio Gasparini

Contents

1 **History of Artificial Intelligence** 1
Alberto Guizzi, Patrick J. Denard, Philippe Collin, and Alexandre Lädermann

2 **Artificial Intelligence** 11
Lorella Bottino, Marzia Settino, and Mario Cannataro

3 **Machine Learning** 25
Emin Suha Dedeogullari, Ataberk Beydemir, Zeynep Beyza Arik, Mahmut Nedim Doral, and Gazi Huri

4 **Deep Learning** 33
Ataberk Beydemir, Emin Suha Dedeogullari, Zeynep Beyza Arik, Erdi Özdemir, and Gazi Huri

5 **Artificial Intelligence in Hip Arthroplasty** 43
Biagio Zampogna, Francesco Rosario Parisi, Andrea Zampoli, and Rocco Papalia

6 **Artificial Intelligence in Knee Arthroplasty** 55
Enrico Bertugli, Sébastien Lustig, Sébastien Parratte, Fabio Catani, and Cécile Batailler

7 **Artificial Intelligence in Shoulder Arthroplasty** 65
Edward G. McFarland, Piotr Łukasiewicz, and Sarah I. Goldfarb

8 **Artificial Intelligence in Surgical Robotics** 73
Filippo Calanna, Joil Ramazzotti, Pierrenzo Pozzi, Riccardo Compagnoni, Paolo Ferrua, and Pietro Simone Randelli

9 **Artificial Intelligence in Hip Arthroscopy** 83
Kyle N. Kunze, Benedict U. Nwachukwu, Shane J. Nho, and Jorge Chahla

10 **Artificial Intelligence in Knee Arthroscopy** 93
Luke V. Tollefson, Evan P. Shoemaker, Nicholas I. Kennedy, and Robert F. LaPrade

11 Artificial Intelligence in Shoulder Arthroscopy 105
Marco-Christopher Rupp, Annabel R. Geissbuhler, Grant Dornan, Jonas Pogorzelski, and Peter J. Millett

12 Artificial Intelligence in Sports Medicine 119
Mohamad Y. Fares, Peter Boufadel, Amar S. Vadhera, and Joseph A. Abboud

13 Artificial Intelligence in Hand Surgery 129
Niyathi Prasad, Giorgio Pajardi, Raffaella Russo, and Dawn LaPorte

14 Artificial Intelligence in Foot and Ankle Surgery 135
Emanuel Cortesão Seiça, Daniel Mendes, Manuel Resende Sousa, and João Vide

15 Artificial Intelligence in Trauma Surgery 155
Corentin Pangaud and Matthieu Ollivier

16 Artificial Intelligence in Musculoskeletal Oncology 173
Raffaele Vitiello, Antonio Ziranu, and Giulio Maccauro

17 Artificial Intelligence in Spine Surgery 179
Lukas Jud, Mazda Farshad, José Miguel Spirig, Jonas Widmer, Reto Sutter, and Philipp Fürnstahl

18 Artificial Intelligence in Osteoporosis 189
Efstathios Chronopoulos, Angelos Kaspiris, Laurence Okeke, Raffaella Russo, Tiziana Montalcini, Arturo Pujia, and Edward G. McFarland

19 Artificial Intelligence in Rehabilitation 197
Emily R. McDermott, Mikalyn T. DeFoor, Travis J. Dekker, and Nicholas N. DePhillipo

20 Potential Risks and Ethical Issues with Intelligent Technologies in Orthopedics 205
Seikai Toyooka, R. Kyle Martin, Lars Engebretsen, and Gilbert Moatshe

History of Artificial Intelligence

1

Alberto Guizzi, Patrick J. Denard, Philippe Collin, and Alexandre Lädermann

1.1 Introduction

Artificial intelligence (AI) refers to a scientific and engineering discipline concerned with developing computer systems that can perform tasks that usually require human intelligence, such as natural language processing, machine vision, robotics, and diagnostics [1, 2]. The definition of AI dates back to the ancient Greek philosopher Aristotle, who attempted to formalize logical reasoning through his syllogisms. The study of human mind functionality has helped establish modern logical thinking and has inspired much of the work in the field of AI. However, in the twentieth century, researchers began to seriously explore the idea of creating intelligent machines.

This chapter will provide a brief overview of the history of AI, including its early origins, significant breakthroughs, and current developments.

1.2 History

The preoccupation with developing practical methods for making intelligent machines has a long history. For instance, already in 1308, poet and theologian Ramon Llull (1232–1316) published Ars generalis ultima (The Ultimate General Art) [3], further perfecting a method to create new knowledge from combinations of concepts. However, it was not until the 1950s that computer scientists began developing algorithms and models to simulate decision-making. The actual beginnings of modern AI can be dated to the Dartmouth conference in 1956, where a group of researchers (Marvin Minsky, John McCarthy, Claude Shannon, and Nathan Rochester) convened to discuss the possibility of creating intelligent machines [4], asserting that any step and feature of intelligence and learning could be so precisely described that a machine could be designed to simulate this process. This conference marked the birth of AI as a formal academic

A. Guizzi
Department of Medical and Surgical Specialties, Radiological Sciences, and Public Health, University of Brescia, Brescia (BS), Italy

P. J. Denard
Oregon Shoulder Institute, Medford, OR, USA

P. Collin
CHP Saint-Gregoire, Saint-Grégoire, France

Clinique Victor Hugo, Paris, France

American Hospital of Paris, Neuilly-sur-Seine, France

A. Lädermann (✉)
Division of Orthopaedics and Trauma Surgery, Hôpital de La Tour, Meyrin, Switzerland

Division of Orthopaedics and Trauma Surgery, Department of Surgery, Geneva University, Hospitals, Geneva, Switzerland

Faculty of Medicine, University of Geneva, Geneva, Switzerland

F. Familiari et al. (eds.), *Artificial Intelligence in Orthopaedic Surgery Made Easy*, https://doi.org/10.1007/978-3-031-70310-2_1

discipline and allowed the participants to dream of creating machines that could "reason, learn, and create." Historically, AI research developed in two main directions: symbolic AI and connectionist AI.

1.2.1 Symbolic AI

Symbolic AI, also known as rule-based AI, uses algorithms and logical reasoning to simulate human thinking. It relies on logic, rules, and symbolic representations of knowledge to perform tasks such as natural language processing, expert systems, and automated reasoning. The approach involves representing knowledge in a formal language and using algorithms to manipulate and reason with these symbols. The main advantage of symbolic AI is its ability to provide explainable reasoning and decision-making. However, it also has limitations, such as difficulties handling uncertainty, real-world complexity, and the need for expert knowledge to develop knowledge representations and rules. One of the first programs that demonstrated that a computer could perform tasks that required intelligence rather than just simple calculations was the Logic Theorist. Developed by Allen Newell, Herbert Simon, and John Clifford Shaw at the RAND Corporation in the late 1950s [5], the program was designed to prove mathematical theorems by constructing proofs in first-order logic. The Logic Theorist was based on a set of rules for manipulating symbols, which represented logical statements and propositions. The program would take as input a statement to be proved and then apply these rules to generate proof of the statement. One of the most famous examples of the Logic Theorist's capabilities was its proof of the "principle of mathematical induction." Humans had previously shown this proof, but the Logic Theorist was able to generate a shred of evidence that was much simpler and more elegant.

Another significant tile in symbolic AI systems was the General Problem Solver (GPS), developed as a joint project between the RAND Corporation and the Massachusetts Institute of Technology AI Laboratory. The GPS was designed to be a program capable of solving problems in various domains, such as puzzle-solving, geometry, algebra, and planning [6]. It used a set of problem-solving heuristics and created plans to achieve goals, and it was written in the Lisp programming language. One of the critical features of the GPS was its ability to generate and modify plans as necessary. It also learned from its experiences and adapted its problem-solving strategies accordingly. The GPS demonstrated the potential of a general problem-solving approach to AI and provided a foundation for the development of future intelligent systems. However, the GPS could not solve problems requiring extensive domain knowledge, and its performance deteriorated rapidly as the complexity of the problem increased. Despite its limitations, it was an essential milestone in the development of AI, and many of its techniques are still used in modern systems.

1.2.2 Connectionist AI

Connectionist AI [7], also known as Artificial Neural Networks, is a subfield of AI that aims to model the human brain's ability to learn and process information. The field of neuroscience-inspired this approach, and it is based on the idea that the brain is composed of interconnected networks of neurons that work together to process information, and so is connectionist AI, which is composed of layers of interconnected nodes, each of which emulates neurons in the brain. The network is trained using a dataset, and the weights between the nodes are adjusted to minimize the error between the actual output and the desired output. Once trained, the network can make predictions on new data. One of the most significant early connectionist AI systems was the perceptron (or McCulloch-Pitts neuron), developed in 1943 by Warren McCulloch and Walter Pitts [8] and first implemented by Frank Rosenblatt in 1958 [9]. This was an artificial single-layer neural network that could be used for binary classification problems. The perceptron received input

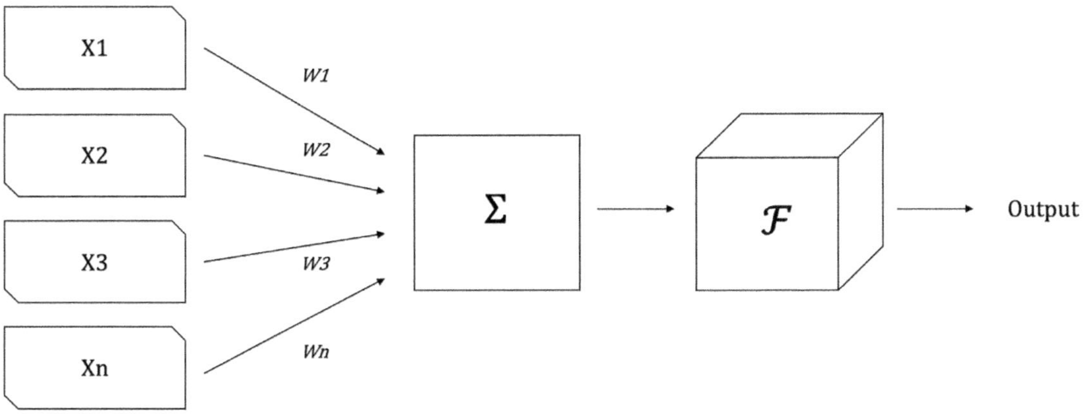

Fig. 1.1 Visualization of the perceptron: it receives input values (X1, X2, X3, Xn) and weight values (W1, W2, W3, Wn); every input value is multiplied by its corresponding weight value. The sum of the resulting values is calculated in order to have a single value; this value is then added to an activation function ($\mathcal{F}$) to obtain the final output

signals, performed a weighted sum of these inputs, applied an activation function to this sum, and produced an output (Fig. 1.1). It was trained using a supervised learning algorithm called the perceptron learning rule. During training, the perceptron weights were adjusted to minimize the error between the predicted and actual outputs. The perceptron learning rule was based on gradient descent, where the weights were updated in the direction that minimizes the error. For these reasons, there has been a significant development in this field as well as the GPS.

As AI models continued to advance, there was a need for a systematic approach to evaluating their intelligence and reliability. Alan Turing's work on Computing Machinery and Intelligence, published in 1950 [10], introduced the concept of assessing the intelligence of AI models. Turing proposed a test, which involved a human interviewer communicating with a human and a machine respondent without knowing which was which. If the interviewer was unable to distinguish the machine's answers from the human's answers, then the machine was considered to have passed the Turing test. The Turing test actually achieved one of the highest goals in the field of AI, creating high expectations. These expectations were so high that it took much work to meet them in the next steps of scientific advancement [11].

1.2.3 Winter Is Coming

During this period, indeed, media and population excitement toward AI was very high due to the achievement of significant milestones that had never been reached before and, consequently, the hope to conquer many more. However, the technological progress and knowledge of that time did not meet those expectations, resulting in discontent and disappointment among the scientific community. This period can be thus identified as the first winter of AI. The latter occurred between 1974 and 1980 [12]. Perceptron had gathered much hype and was shown to be capable of modeling simple systems. However, Minsky and Papert [13] published a book in 1969 that criticized the perceptron algorithm. The book describes the limitations of single-layer neural networks (specifically perceptrons) in solving certain types of problems. The authors argued that perceptrons are limited in their ability to classify patterns that are not linearly separable. In other words, if the patterns cannot be separated by a single straight line, a perceptron will not be able to learn how to classify them correctly. Moreover, in 1973, Lighthill [14] published a report summarizing the slow progress in the field. The report criticized AI research for its overhyped promises, lack of practical results, and insufficient theoretical understanding. It argued that the approach of symbolic AI was too limited and could not capture the complexity and nuances of human intelligence. The report also questioned the feasibility of creating intelligent machines. It argued that AI research should focus on more practical applications, such as language translation and robotics, rather than trying to mimic human cognition. Additionally, it criticized the lack of collaboration between AI researchers and other fields, such as psychology and linguistics. The Lighthill report further contributed to decreased interest and funding in AI research: less money, less research, less progress. As a result, many governmental organizations stopped or significantly decreased AI research grants and changed their investment front. During those years, many AI researchers shifted their focus from trying to develop AI algorithms that could learn and represent knowledge from data toward expert rule-based systems (ERBS).

An ERBS is a computer program that provides expert-level solutions to important problems; it is characterized by being heuristic, transparent, and flexible [15]. These systems were based on the idea of encoding human knowledge in a particular field in the form of a set of rules that could be used to reach a conclusion or make decisions [16]. ERBS uses an inference engine to apply a set of logical rules to a specific problem or situation. The system first gathers data from the problem domain and applies it to the knowledge base, which contains a set of rules. The inference engine then evaluates these rules and determines the best course of action or decision based on the information provided. One of the main advantages of ERBS is its ability to capture the expertise of human experts in a particular domain and use that knowledge to make informed decisions. However, ERBS also had limitations. They relied heavily on the quality and completeness of the knowledge base and the rules contained within it. Additionally, ERBS may struggle with problems that do not have explicit, well-defined solutions or require the system to handle uncertain or incomplete information. However, even if these systems had some success and have played an important role in modern intelligent structures, by the mid-1980s, researchers began to realize that they were not a viable long-term solution. Therefore, the lack of progress in representation learning was one of the main factors that led to the previously mentioned AI winter. As a result, disappointment and discontent became the main feeling toward the field of AI.

In 1985, Rumelhart et al. [17] published a paper introducing the backpropagation algorithm, a method for training multi-layer neural networks. They described how the algorithm works by computing the error in the network's output and then propagating it backward through the layers to adjust the weights of the connections between the neurons to reduce the mistake. This process is repeated iteratively until the error is minimized, allowing the network to learn to map inputs to outputs. This work helped end the first AI winter by demonstrating that neural networks could be used not only for simple problems but also for various tasks, including pattern recognition (image and speech recognition) and function approximation. Through this article, the authors restored credibility and trust in AI, demonstrating that the backpropagation algorithm could ensure the development of increasingly powerful neural networks.

However, it became evident in the early 1990s that the lack of computing power made these networks not improvable, and the awareness of those limits led to another dark period: the second AI winter. It occurred when it became clear that the capabilities of neural networks were being overhyped, and the lack of advancement in computing power made it difficult for these networks to upgrade. As a result, researchers shifted their focus to simpler and more practical algorithms. One such algorithm was the Support Vector Machine, which was introduced in 1963, but not widely used until the early 1990s when researchers realized that it could solve for nonlinear hyperplanes without significantly increasing the computational requirements of the algorithm [18]. This was possible thanks to the implementation of nonlinear kernels in 1992, which allowed the Support Vector Machine algorithm to capitalize on the low computational power available at the time.

1.2.4 After the Rain Comes the Sunshine

The 1990s were a decade of rapid technological evolution, especially in the field of computing and communication technologies. The widespread availability of personal computers and the Internet fueled an explosion in the development of new software and hardware products. With this technological explosion, the power of computers increased exponentially, providing the basis for AI to reach heights previously missed due to technical limitations. This is how scientists rediscovered interest in AI during those years.

A great example of the achievements that occurred with these new computing capabilities was the development of Deep Blue. Deep Blue was a chess-playing computer developed by IBM. It was explicitly designed to play chess and competed against the world champion Garry Kasparov in 1996 and 1997. The 1997 match was the first time a computer had beaten a human world champion in a six-game match [19]. The machine was composed of a custom-designed chess processor, a disk array for storing game trees, and a parallel search algorithm [20]. That allowed it to search up to 200 million positions per second. Deep Blue used a brute-force approach to chess, selecting the best move based on its evaluation function. Deep Blue's success demonstrated AI's potential to compete and even overcome human intelligence in certain domains.

Attempts to advance AI technology progressed further when the concept of convolutional neural network (CNN) was introduced. A CNN is a type of deep learning algorithm commonly used for image recognition and classification. CNNs are designed to process inputs such as images and extract features from them through convolutional layers, which apply a set of filters to the input image. The filters are designed to detect specific features, such as edges or corners. The resulting feature maps are then passed through pooling layers, which reduce the size of the feature maps while preserving their important features [21]. The first successful application of CNNs was LeNet-5 network, which was developed in 1998 by Ann LeCun, Leon Bottou, Yoshua Bengio, and Patrick Haffner [22]. It is a CNN that was designed for the purpose of recognizing handwritten digits in images. The network consists of seven layers, including two convolutional layers, two subsampling (pooling) layers, and three fully connected layers. The first two layers apply filters to the input image to extract features; after each convolutional layer, there is a subsampling layer (pooling layer) which downsamples the feature maps produced by the convolutional layers, reducing their size while retaining important information; the final three layers of the network are fully connected layers that take the output from the subsampling layers and use it to classify the input image. The output layer of the network produces a probability distribution over the possible digits (0–9), and the digit with the highest probability is chosen as the classification for the input image. Although this network represented a revolution in its field, it had to contend with issues concerning once again the limited capacity of the hardware and data constraints, problems that will be a constant in the evolutionary history of AI for some years to come. Besides its issues, LeNet-5 was groundbreaking in its time, and its success inspired the development of many other CNN architectures. It is considered to be one of the foundational models in the field of deep learning.

1.2.5 Machine Learning

The aforementioned developments led to the creation of what we can define as Machine Learning (ML), a subfield of AI that involves developing algorithms and statistical models that enable computers to learn and improve from their experience (Fig. 1.2). In the past, its use was severely constrained by the intrinsic limitations of Central Processing Units (CPUs) and the limited ability of computers to store large amounts of data. However, with the arrival of the new millennium, the era of Big Data was introduced, and the first Graphical Processing Units (GPUs) were created, two key elements in the evolution of AI.

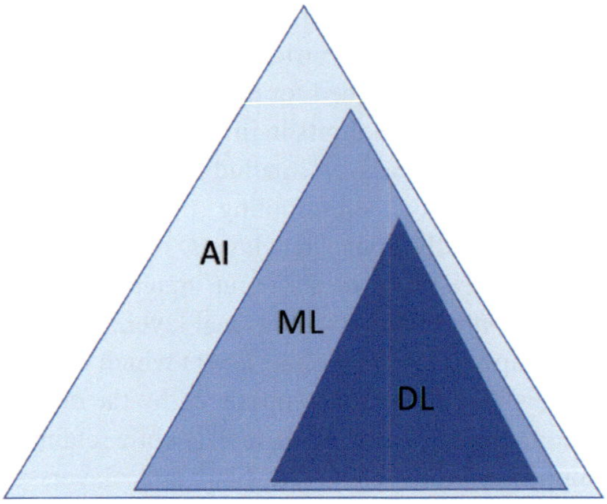

Fig. 1.2 Artificial Intelligence (AI), a scientific discipline whose goal is to simulate human intelligence, embraces Machine Learning (ML), which gains new experience from data given by experts. Deep Learning (DL), is a subfield of ML that improves thanks to auto data processing

The era of Big Data refers to a period in recent history when the volume, velocity, and variety of data being generated grew exponentially [23]. It is characterized by the explosion of data generated from a wide variety of sources, including social media, mobile devices, sensors, and other digital platforms. As the amount of data being generated grew, it was no longer easy to handle them using traditional tools and technologies. It, therefore, became increasingly important to develop new technologies and instruments to process, analyze, and derive insights from this data. A GPU is a specialized electronic circuit designed to rapidly process and manipulate memory-intensive tasks like computer graphics, video processing, and machine learning algorithms. Unlike a CPU, which is designed to perform a wide range of functions, a GPU is designed to achieve a smaller set of highly specialized tasks exceptionally quickly and efficiently. The massively parallel processing power of a GPU makes it well-suited for speeding up computation tasks. It allows it to process large amounts of data much faster than traditional CPUs. As data storage capacity and data handling speed have increased, ML's power and performance have grown increasingly. In fact, the more data administered to computers, the more examples will be available to the machine to build models or systems that can improve their performance.

1.2.6 Deep Learning

The power evolution in machine learning thus led to the development of deep learning, officially introduced to the public in 2006 by Hinton et al. [24]. While in traditional machine learning human experts typically manually select or engineer a set of features that are expected to be informative for a given task (feature engineering), in deep learning the general characteristics are automatically learned from data in neural networks. These networks comprise many layers of interconnected processing nodes that work together to analyze and learn from large amounts of data. Deep learning has revolutionized fields such as computer vision, natural language processing, and speech recognition, leading to advances in areas such as autonomous vehicles, medical imaging, and more. In 2012, Alex Krizhevsky, Ilya Sutskever, and Geoffrey Hinton [25] introduced AlexNet, which was the first deep neural network to win the ImageNet Large Scale Visual Recognition Challenge with a significant margin over the second place model: it was able to achieve an error rate of 15.3% on the dataset, which was 10.9% lower than the runner-up. This breakthrough demonstrated the potential of deep learning, specifically CNNs, in the field of computer vision and marked a shift from traditional machine learning methods to deep learning. AlexNet's success was partly due to its innovative architecture, which included several novel techniques such as rectified linear unit activation functions, overlapping pooling, and dropout regularization. Its impact on the field of AI was significant, inspiring many subsequent developments in deep learning and contributing to the area's explosive growth.

1.2.7 History of AI in Medicine

In the early stages of AI in medicine, progress was made in engineering and digitizing data.

However, the adoption of AI by the medical industry was slow at this time. Obviously, in the first period, AI technology was not ready to be applied to medicine; thus, the only practice that could be performed was data storage, which could have been used in the future by AI. The digitization of data during this period, including the creation of resources like the Medical Literature Analysis and Retrieval System and the PubMed search engine, laid the groundwork for future advancements in biomedicine. Additionally, the development of clinical informatics databases and medical record systems helped establish the foundation for future AI developments in medicine [26].

During the period from the 1970s to the early 1990s, as previously mentioned in this chapter, there was reduced funding and interest in AI, known as the AI winter. This period also saw limited developments in AI in medicine, with only a few collaborations among pioneers in the field. Nevertheless, some significant events took place, including establishing the first National Institutes of Health-sponsored AI workshop in 1975 [27] and creating several programs and databases that demonstrated the feasibility of applying AI to medicine. These programs included the CASNET model and MYCIN. The CASNET model was developed in 1976 at Rutgers University and shown at a meeting of ophthalmologists in Las Vegas. It was one of the first examples of AI being used in medicine. It was designed to help manage glaucoma patients by using a network of programs to analyze patient data and provide doctors with advice on patient management [28]. The MYCIN system [29], developed in the 1970s, was an early example of a "backward chaining" AI system used to provide recommendations for antibiotic treatment based on patient information and a knowledge base of rules. It later became the basis for rule-based systems such as EMYCIN and INTERNIST-1 [27], developed to assist with medical diagnosis.

The DXplain decision support system, developed in 1986 by the University of Massachusetts, uses inputted symptoms to generate a differential diagnosis and provide detailed descriptions of diseases and references [30]. It has expanded over the years to cover more than 2400 diseases. Its development, along with the renewed interest in machine learning in the late 1990s, set the stage for the modern era of AI in medicine.

In 2011, IBM's open-domain question-answering system named Watson won first place on the television show *Jeopardy!* by using natural language processing and various searches to analyze data over unstructured content to generate probable answers. This technology, called DeepQA, used a different approach than traditional AI systems that used forward reasoning, backward reasoning, or hand-crafted rules. This system was more readily available for use, easier to maintain, and more cost-effective [31]. The use of DeepQA technology by IBM can be applied to provide evidence-based medicine responses by drawing information from a patient's electronic medical record and other electronic resources, thereby opening new possibilities in evidence-based clinical decision-making [31]. In 2017, IBM Watson was used successfully to identify new RNA-binding proteins altered in amyotrophic lateral sclerosis. The availability of digitalized medicine, improved hardware, and software programs have led to the rapid growth of AI. Natural language processing has transformed chatbots from superficial communication to meaningful conversation-based interfaces, and this technology has been applied to virtual assistants like Siri and Alexa. Chatbots like Pharmabot have been developed to assist in medication education for pediatric patients, while Mandy was created as an automated patient intake process for a primary care practice [32]. The development of deep learning was a significant advancement in AI. It can be trained to classify data independently, while machine learning requires human input.

One of the most exciting applications of deep learning in medicine is in the field of medical imaging. Deep learning algorithms can analyze medical images with incredible accuracy, allowing for more precise diagnoses and treatment planning. For example, deep learning algorithms have been used to develop computer-aided diagnosis systems for breast cancer that can identify cancerous lesions with high accuracy [33].

Another area where deep learning has shown promise is in drug discovery. Deep learning algorithms can analyze large databases of molecular structures to identify potential drug candidates. This can help researchers identify new drug targets and accelerate the drug discovery process [34].

1.3 Conclusion

The history of AI has been a journey of reflection, innovation, and progress over the last millennium, with an unbelievable acceleration during the last decades. Starting with simple rule-based systems in the 1950s and 1960s, AI has grown to encompass more complex models such as decision support systems, chatbots, and deep learning algorithms. These advancements have revolutionized the way we approach various fields, especially in healthcare, where AI has become a critical tool for improving patient outcomes and streamlining clinical workflows. Although AI still faces challenges, such as ethical concerns and data privacy issues, its potential to transform our society and solve some of our most pressing problems is undeniable. As we continue to invest in research and development, AI will undoubtedly continue to evolve and shape the future of our world in exciting and unexpected ways. This is what you will discover in the following chapters.

Conflicts of Interest Alberto Guizzi: nothing to declare.

Patrick J. Denard receives royalties from and is a consultant and paid speaker for Arthrex. He is the co-founder of Med4Cast.

Philippe Collin has received personal fees from Advanced Medical Applications, ConMed, Smith & Nephew, Stortz, and Stryker. He is the co-founder of Med4Cast.

Alexandre Lädermann is a paid consultant for Arthrex, Stryker, Medacta, and Enovis. He received royalties from Stryker and Medacta. He is the co-founder of FORE, Med4Cast, and BeeMed. He owns stock options in Medacta and Follow Health.

Funding FORE (Foundation for Research and Teaching in Orthopedics, Sports Medicine, Trauma, and Imaging in the Musculoskeletal System). Grant # 2023-58.

References

1. Ren S, He K, Girshick R, Sun J. Faster R-CNN: towards real-time object detection with region proposal networks. Advances in neural information processing Systems [Internet]. Curran Associates, Inc.; 2015 [cited 2023 May 1]. Available from https://papers.nips.cc/paper_files/paper/2015/hash/14bfa6bb14875e45bba028a21ed38046-Abstract.html
2. Devlin J, Chang M-W, Lee K, Toutanova K. BERT: pre-training of deep bidirectional transformers for language understanding [Internet]. arXiv; 2019 [cited 2023 May 1]. Available from http://arxiv.org/abs/1810.04805
3. Lullus R. Ars magna, generalis et ultima. Sutor; 1596.
4. Stone P, Brooks R, Brynjolfsson E, Calo R, Etzioni O, Hager G, et al. Artificial intelligence and life in 2030: The one hundred year study on artificial intelligence [Internet]. arXiv; 2022 [cited 2023 May 1]. Available from http://arxiv.org/abs/2211.06318
5. Gugerty L. Newell and Simon's logic theorist: historical background and impact on cognitive modeling. Proc Hum Factors Ergonomics Soc Annu Meet. 2006;50:880–4.
6. GPS, A program that simulates human thought [Internet]. Available from https://apps.dtic.mil/sti/citations/AD0294731
7. Bechtel W. Connectionism and the philosophy of mind: an overview. In: Horgan T, Tienson J, editors. Connectionism and the philosophy of mind [Internet]. Dordrecht: Springer; 1991 [cited 2023 May 1]. p. 30–59. https://doi.org/10.1007/978-94-011-3524-5_2.
8. McCulloch WS, Pitts W. A logical calculus of the ideas immanent in nervous activity. Bull Math Biophys. 1943;5:115–33.
9. Rosenblatt F. The perceptron: a probabilistic model for information storage and organization in the brain. Psychol Rev. 1958;65:386–408.
10. Turing AM. Computing machinery and intelligence. Mind Oxford University Press. 1950;59:433–60.
11. Saygin AP, Cicekli I, Akman V. Turing test: 50 years later. Minds Mach. 2000;10:463–518.
12. Muthukrishnan N, Maleki F, Ovens K, Reinhold C, Forghani B, Forghani R. Brief history of artificial Intelligence. Neuroimaging Clin N Am. 2020;30:393–9.
13. Minsky M, Papert S. Perceptrons; an introduction to computational geometry. MIT Press; 1969.
14. Artificial Intelligence: A General Survey (The Lighthill Report) | AITopics [Internet]. [cited 2023 May 1]. Available from https://aitopics.org/doc/classics:D8235CF9/
15. Buchanan BG, Duda RO. Principles of rule-based expert systems. In: Yovits MC, editor. Advances in computers [Internet]. Elsevier; 1983. p. 163–216. https://www.sciencedirect.com/science/article/pii/S0065245808601291.

16. Abraham A. Rule-based expert systems. Handbook of measuring system design [Internet]. Wiley; 2005 [cited 2023 May 2]. https://doi.org/10.1002/0471497398.mm422
17. Rumelhart DE, Hinton GE, Williams RJ. Learning representations by back-propagating errors. Nature. 1986;323:533–6.
18. Boser BE, Guyon IM, Vapnik VN. A training algorithm for optimal margin classifiers. Proceedings of the fifth annual workshop on Computational learning theory [Internet]. New York: Association for Computing Machinery; 1992 [cited 2023 May 2]. p. 144–52. https://doi.org/10.1145/130385.130401
19. Schaeffer J, Plaat A. Kasparov versus Deep Blue: the rematch. ICG. 1997;20:95–101.
20. Campbell M, Hoane AJ, Hsu F. Deep Blue. Artif Intell. 2002;134:57–83.
21. O'Shea K, Nash R. An introduction to convolutional neural networks [Internet]. arXiv; 2015 [cited 2023 May 2]. Available from: http://arxiv.org/abs/1511.08458
22. Lecun Y, Bottou L, Bengio Y, Haffner P. Gradient-based learning applied to document recognition. Proc IEEE. 1998;86:2278–324.
23. Elgendy N, Elragal A. Big data analytics: a literature review paper. 2014. p. 214–27.
24. Hinton GE, Osindero S, Teh Y-W. A fast learning algorithm for deep belief nets. Neural Comput. 2006;18:1527–54.
25. Krizhevsky A, Sutskever I, Hinton GE. ImageNet classification with deep convolutional neural networks. Advances in neural information processing Systems [Internet]. Curran Associates, Inc.; 2012 [cited 2023 Apr 30]. Available from https://proceedings.neurips.cc/paper_files/paper/2012/hash/c399862d3b9d6b76c8436e924a68c45b-Abstract.html
26. Kaul V, Enslin S, Gross SA. History of artificial intelligence in medicine. Gastrointest Endosc. 2020;92:807–12.
27. Kulikowski CA. Beginnings of artificial Intelligence in medicine (AIM): computational artifice assisting scientific inquiry and clinical art - with reflections on present AIM challenges. Yearb Med Inform. 2019;28:249–56.
28. Weiss S, Kulikowski CA, Safir A. Glaucoma consultation by computer. Comput Biol Med. 1978;8:25–40.
29. Shortliffe EH, Davis R, Axline SG, Buchanan BG, Green CC, Cohen SN. Computer-based consultations in clinical therapeutics: explanation and rule acquisition capabilities of the MYCIN system. Comput Biomed Res. 1975;8:303–20.
30. Amisha MP, Pathania M, Rathaur VK. Overview of artificial intelligence in medicine. J Family Med Prim Care. 2019;8:2328–31.
31. Ferrucci D, Levas A, Bagchi S, Gondek D, Mueller ET. Watson: beyond jeopardy! Artif Intell. 2013;199–200:93–105.
32. Ni L, Lu C, Liu N, Liu J. In: Chen J, Theeramunkong T, Supnithi T, Tang X, editors. MANDY: Towards a smart primary care Chatbot application. Singapore: Springer Singapore; 2017. p. 38–52. https://doi.org/10.1007/978-981-10-6989-5_4.
33. Anaya-Isaza A, Mera-Jiménez L, Zequera-Diaz M. An overview of deep learning in medical imaging. Informat Med Unlocked. 2021;26:100723.
34. Askr H, Elgeldawi E, Aboul Ella H, Elshaier YAMM, Gomaa MM, Hassanien AE. Deep learning in drug discovery: an integrative review and future challenges. Artif Intell Rev [Internet]. 2022 [cited 2023 May 13]. Available from https://doi.org/10.1007/s10462-022-10306-1

2 Artificial Intelligence

Lorella Bottino, Marzia Settino, and Mario Cannataro

2.1 What's Artificial Intelligence?

AI, sometimes called machine intelligence, is a branch of computer science concerned with building machines that are able to simulate human intelligence [1]. AI-based systems are equipped with cognitive functions usually associated with human intelligence, such as pattern recognition, learning from data, decision-making (e.g., expert systems) and problem-solving, and even the ability to make decisions with minimal human intervention. Furthermore, AI enables machines to learn from experience, process massive amounts of data and identify patterns in data to support the decision-making process.

Machine learning (ML) is a subfield of AI that uses statistical techniques to enable machines to learn and improve from experience without being explicitly programmed.

Deep learning (DL) is a class of machine learning methods that leverage artificial neural networks (ANNs) to extract higher-level features from the input data. The ANN is a computational model inspired by the neural structure of the human brain. A convolutional neural network (CNN) is a kind of artificial neural network architecture best suited for solving Computer Vision-related problems. An overview of the AI subfields is shown in Fig. 2.1.

L. Bottino · M. Settino · M. Cannataro (✉)
Department of Medical and Surgical Sciences, Data Analytics Research Center, University Magna Graecia of Catanzaro, Catanzaro, Italy
e-mail: lorella.bottino@unicz.it; marzia.settino@unicz.it; cannataro@unicz.it

2.1.1 Principles of Machine Learning

Arthur Samuel, a pioneer in the AI field, coined the term "Machine Learning" as—"Field of study that gives computers the capability to learn without being explicitly programmed" (i.e., without any human assistance) [2].

ML applications are used in many different fields such as image and speech recognition, natural language processing, recommendation systems, fraud detection, automated tasks, and so on. For example, ML is used for self-driving cars, drones, and robots, making them more adaptable to changing environments. ML techniques rely on the following main approaches:

- *Supervised approaches* use labeled datasets to build a model that predicts the labels for new observations. There are two main subcategories of supervised learning (SL) problems: (1) *classification*, which identifies which category a set of data items belongs to (i.e. predicting a class label) to produce a discrete output value; and (2) *regression*, which tries to predict the output values on the basis of the input variables to produce a continuous output value.

F. Familiari et al. (eds.), *Artificial Intelligence in Orthopaedic Surgery Made Easy*,
https://doi.org/10.1007/978-3-031-70310-2_2

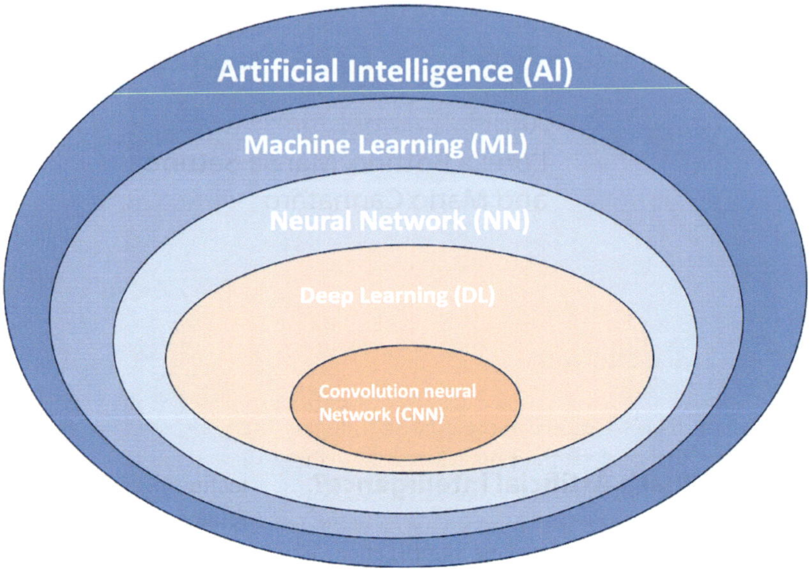

Fig. 2.1 An overview of the different logical levels that form artificial intelligence

An example of classification problem in the medical field is to detect the presence of a bone fracture by the X-ray images or to detect cancer features by histopathological images (e.g., to detect alterations of the color in image areas) [3, 4]. An example of a regression problem is to predict how long surgery patients will stay in the hospital based on their age, height and weight [5].

- *Unsupervised approaches* try to identify patterns from unlabeled datasets. The goal is to group samples according to their similarities [6]. *Clustering* is an unsupervised method that deals with datasets in which the outcome (target) variable is not provided nor any relationship between the observations is known. Clustering assigns unlabeled items to different groups by their uncovered similarities. For instance, this technique has been used for stratifying patients with osteoporotic vertebral fractures (OVF) on the basis of their increasing pain [7] and also for improving risk stratification in patient with multiple myeloma [8].
- *Semi-supervised approaches* combine a small amount of labeled data with a large amount of unlabeled data to train a predictive model. A semisupervised learning approach has been used in [9] for the scoliosis curve type prediction.
- *Reinforcement learning approaches* use feedback-based techniques for rewarding desired behaviors and/or punishing undesired ones with the goal of maximizing the total reward. More specifically, for a good action, an agent gets positive feedback; otherwise, for a bad action, the agent gets negative feedback or a penalty. There are no labeled datasets, therefore the agent learns by its experience only [10].

2.1.2 Deep Learning

Deep learning (DL) is a subset of ML based on the concept of Artificial Neural Networks. It is widely applied in various areas such as healthcare, visual recognition, cybersecurity, etc., for its great ability to find complex patterns in huge datasets [11, 12].

The adjective "deep" in deep learning refers to the use of multiple layers in the network, i.e., neural networks with more than three layers (including input and output).

Figure 2.2 shows the structure of a DL network that consists of a collection of interconnected processing nodes (i.e., neurons) organized into layers that work together. Circles represent the neurons while the arrows represent the

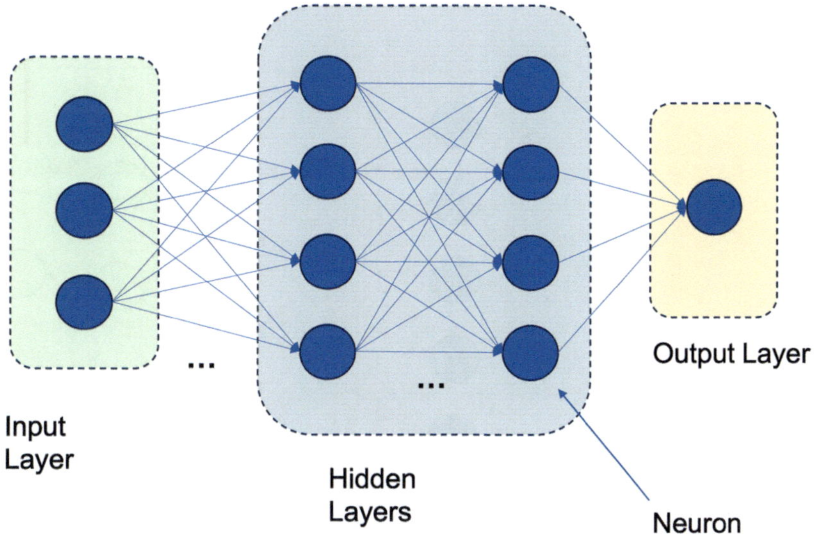

Fig. 2.2 Structure of a deep neural network

weighted connections between neurons. The input layer receives data as input and it passes them to the next intermediate layers, i.e., hidden layers. Input layers do not apply any operations to the input data.

The multiple hidden layers contain several neurons that apply non-linear transformations to the data to learn complex patterns. Weights represent the strength of the connections between two neurons and they establish how much influence the input will have on the output. The output layer produces the final result. Training a DL model consists of learning (i.e., calculate) the optimal values for all the weights from labeled examples [13].

Convolutional Neural Networks (CNNs) are a class of ANNs that have at least one convolution layer. The convolution layer applies a filter to the input to create a feature map that summarizes the detected features. CNNs are specialized in processing data that have a grid-like topology such as images and therefore they are well-suited to be applied in the medical domain [14, 15]. Like the traditional ANNs, the CNN structure consists of neurons, layers, and weights. However, CNNs are distinguished from the ANNs because CNNs have three types of layers: convolution, pooling, and fully connected layers. Each layer performs a specific task, such as detecting edges or patterns in the input image. The convolution layer applies a mathematical operation called convolution[1] to the input and then it passes the obtained result to the next layer.

CNNs demonstrated widely superior performance in object recognition and classification from images, with respect to the traditional ANNs thanks to their ability to detect different features of an input image through back-propagation and multiple layers [16–18].

U-net is the most famous CNN architecture for the automatic segmentation of biomedical images [19]. Several variants of U-net, such as UNet++ [20], MQANet [21], MAnet [22], and X-Net [23] have been further developed for dealing with medical images.

Recurrent Neural Networks (RNNs) are a class of ANNs in which the information cycle in the network through the loops. This makes the output determined by the current input as well as the previously received inputs. Due to the use of the feedback loops, RNNs introduce the concept of "memory" that allows them to store past computations and to act assuming a dynamic temporal behavior (i.e., each state is influenced by its previous ones). RNNs are an extension of the feed-forward neural networks (FFNNs) in which, unlike RNNs, the information moves from layer

[1] Convolution combines two functions $f(x)$ and $h(x)$ to generate a third function $g(x)$ that represents how much the areas of $f(x)$ and $h(x)$ overlap between them.

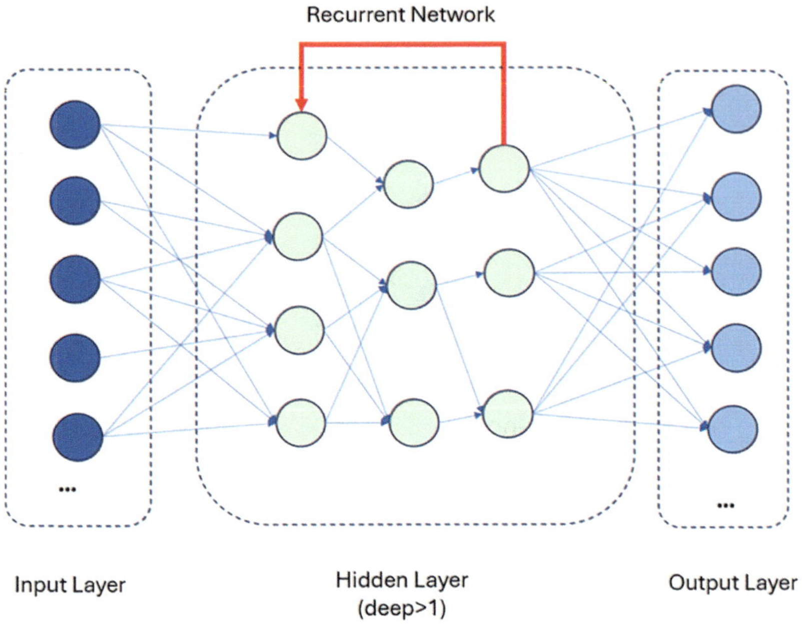

Fig. 2.3 General architecture of the RNNs

to layer in the network in only one direction (i.e., forward) from the input nodes to the output nodes and they have no loops [24]. The general architecture of the RNNs is shown in Fig. 2.3.

2.1.3 Generative Artificial Intelligence

Generative artificial intelligence is a subfield of AI that focuses on computational techniques able to generate novel and meaningful outputs based on learned patterns (e.g., images, audio, text, and more). In particular, Generative AI models leverage the DL techniques to produce autonomously contents that are similar to human-generated creations [25, 26]. Generative models are able to learn the data distribution of the training set to generate new data points with some variations (i.e., similar as possible to the original data distribution). The most popular approaches of the Generative models are discussed below:

- *Generative Adversarial Networks* (GANs) are a powerful class of ANNs used for unsupervised learning. They combine two neural networks competing against each other in a zero-sum game scenario.[2] GANs have two primary components: Generator and Discriminator. The first produces fake samples of data (e.g., image, audio, etc.) and tries to fool the Discriminator. For instance, the Generator tries to make fake images in such a way that they result sufficiently realistic. The Discriminator, on the other hand, tries to distinguish the real from the fake samples. The Generator and the Discriminator are both based on the ANNs architecture and they are continuously engaged in a "learning loop" in which the Generator tries to minimize a loss function while the Discriminator tries to maximize it [27]. The general architecture of the GANs is shown in Fig. 2.4.
- *Variational Autoencoders* (VAEs) are a type of ANNs for unsupervised learning able to compress and reconstruct the input dataset to make it easier to visualize, analyze, and interpret.

[2] The zero-sum game scenario is a mathematical representation in the game theory in which the amount won by the winning player equals the combined losses of the losing players.

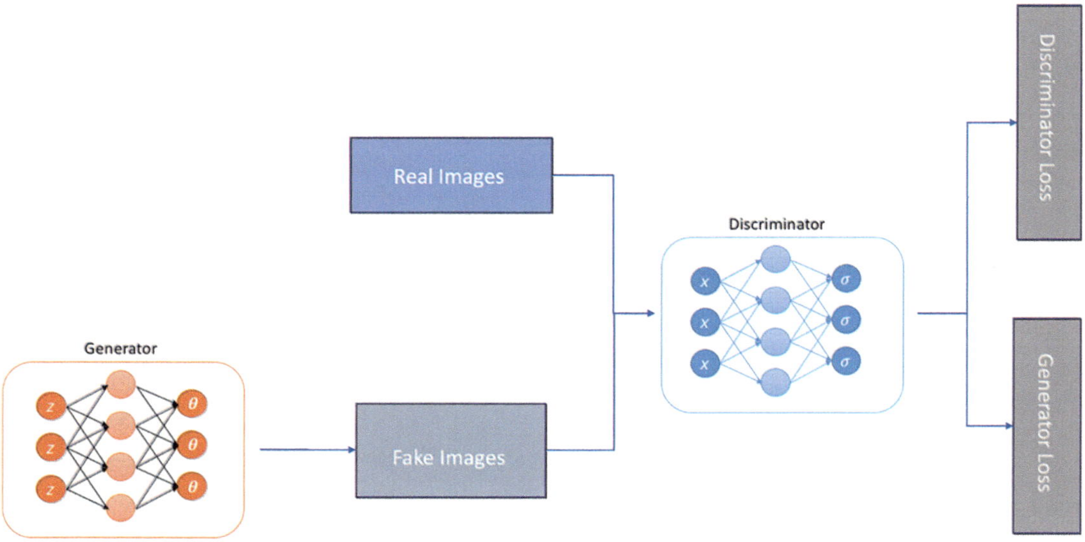

Fig. 2.4 General architecture of the GANs

VAEs are enhanced Autoencoders where a statistical approach is used to learn the probability distribution of the input dataset [28]. Classical autoencoders are ANNs that learn to change the input into a compressed form and then rebuild again the input. Autoencoders have two components: an Encoder and a Decoder. The Encoder transforms the input dataset into a lower-dimensional representation (called latent space or bottleneck). The Decoder gets the latent space and tries to reconstruct the original input dataset as accurately as possible. The latent space captures the most important features in the input dataset discarding redundancy and noise. Reconstruction error is the error between the original dataset and its low-dimensional reconstruction. The entire encoder–decoder architecture works by minimizing the reconstruction error. While classical autoencoders provide a representation of the input dataset in a lower-dimensional form, VAEs describe the observations in the latent space in a probabilistic manner. More specifically, VAEs describe a probability distribution for each latent attribute to build a continuous latent space able to generate new datasets that are similar to those observed during training [29]. The general architecture of the VAEs is shown in Fig. 2.5.

– *Transformer* is based on the ANNs architecture, and it relies on the mechanisms of *cross-attention* and *self-attention* in a stack of encoders and decoders. The concept of Transformer was proposed in 2017 by Vaswani and team in the article titled "Attention is all you need" and it is nowadays a state-of-the-art technique in the field of Natural Language Processing (NLP) [30]. NLP is a branch of AI that enables computers to understand, manipulate, and generate human language [31]. Over the years, different ANN architectures, such as RNNs and CNNs, have been used to address the NLP tasks until recently transformers came out as a novel and more powerful approach.

The *self-attention* mechanism has been defined by Vaswani as "Self-attention, sometimes called intra-attention, is an attention mechanism relating different positions of a single sequence in order to compute a representation of the sequence". Self-attention makes the model able to capture the relation-

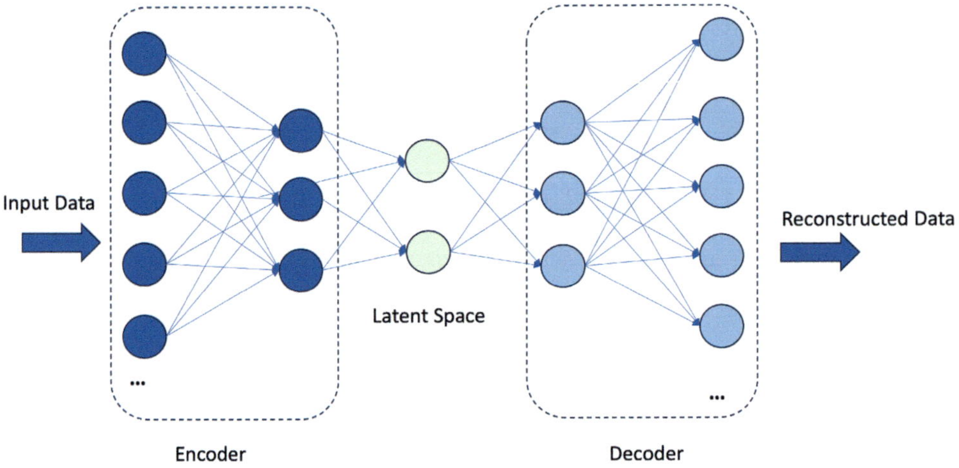

Fig. 2.5 General architecture of the VAEs

ships between different words or phrases in a sentence. Using self-attention, the model focuses on important input elements and it assigns weights to each element on the basis of its relevance in the context. The cross-attention mechanism enable the model to identify the significant parts of an input text that are useful for accurately predicting the next word in the generated output text.

Large Language Models (LLMs) have recently achieved great success in the field of NLP due to their ability to process huge amounts of text and generate accurate results. The LLMs are a class of DL models designed to process, understand, and generate text in a human-like fashion (see Fig. 2.6). More specifically, LLMs rely on complex algorithms that leverage transformer-based architectures to capture complex language patterns and relationships between words or phrases in sentences. There are three main types of LLMs based on the transformer architecture [32]:

- *Autoregressive Language Models* (ALMs) use autoregressive[3] techniques to generate text by predicting the next word in a sequence, given a set of words in a given context. The most popular examples of ALMs are the OpenAI Generative Pre-trained Transformers (GPTs) and ChatGPT which is its variant designed for chatbot applications. They both have a transformer-based architecture that is trained in an unsupervised manner on a large amount of text data [33]. Recently, Google launched Bard to compete with ChatGPT which is a bidirectional autoregressive decoder. Bidirectional means that it can process words and phrases in both forward and backward directions to achieve a better understanding of the text and to produce high-quality outputs by anticipating the next word in a context.
- *Autoencoding Language Models* learn to generate a vector space representation of the text provided in input (called embeddings) by a

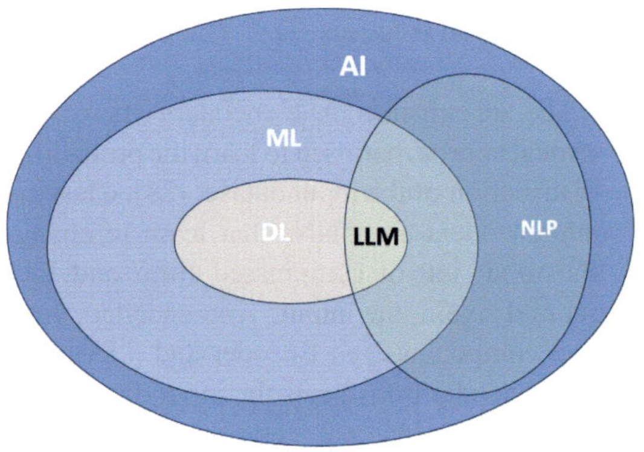

Fig. 2.6 Overview of LLMs context with respect to the other AI subfields

[3]Autoregressive models predict future values based on past values.

dimensionality reduction of the input. The purpose is to reconstruct the original input from the embedded version of it. These models are pre-trained by corrupting the input tokens (e.g., the original sentence) that must be reconstructed more accurately as possible. These models are able to build a bidirectional representation of the whole sentence and achieve great results in text generation and token classification. A typical example of such models is the Bidirectional Encoder Representations from Transformers (BERT). BERT is a deep learning-based language model that uses a pre-trained Transformer encoder to provide precision results in word processing tasks such as conversational bots, machine translation to voice assistants, and language translation [34, 35]. BERT uses deep bidirectional representations meaning that the model learns from both left and right context. Differently, OpenAI GPT is unidirectional meaning that it only considers the context of text provided as input from left to right.

- the third type of LLM is the combination of the previous two models, i.e., autoencoding and autoregressive. An example is the T5 Text-to-Text Transformer model.

Figure 2.6 shows an overview of the LLMs subfield with respect to the other AI subfields; Table 2.1 lists the most popular applications based on Large Language Models.

Table 2.1 Most popular examples of large language models

LL model	Vendor/Creator	References	Open source
GPT-4	OpenAI	[33]	No
BERT	Google	[34, 35]	Yes
LaMDA	Google	[36]	Yes
PaLM	Google	[37]	Yes
BLOOM	Hugging Face	[38]	Yes
LLaMA	Meta	[39]	Yes
T5	Google	[40]	Yes
BARD	Google	[41]	Yes

2.2 Artificial Intelligence in Medicine

Nowadays, AI is used extensively in medical settings. Clinical decision support systems (CDSS) and imaging analysis are two important areas where AI has already proven its potential. CDSS tools help physicians enhance the decision-making process in the clinical workflow to improve patient care and the clinical performance. Regarding medical imaging, AI is successfully used for diagnosis and pathological classification [42]. For instance, lesion detection, disease classification and staging, treatment planning, and assessing response to treatment are common tasks performed through AI-based tools.

Other common AI applications in the medical settings include identifying outbreaks of infectious diseases, combining clinical with genetic data, aiding in hospital business operations [43].

AI has the potential to revolutionize the practice of medicine by enhancing the clinicians abilities, AI-driven systems are inevitably prone to errors. Therefore, they require the supervision of the clinician. Furthermore, AI-driven mechanisms are often unclear due to their intrinsic opacity that the clinician must clarify. A structured and comprehensible description of the generated models must accompany AI-driven systems to help the clinician use the system appropriately.

In particular, providing a detailed description of AI application's intended use (i.e. the purpose for which the AI application is intended according to the data supplied by the manufacturer) and the intended users (i.e. the users that are intended to use the AI application, for example health-care professionals or patients) is a clinical challenge that helps to ensure transparency and hold a standard approach [44].

Moreover, having a standardized protocol allows to validate the performance of the AI system and make an accurate clinical evaluation.

2.3 Key Challenges of Artificial Intelligence

Thanks to the availability of a large amount of labeled data and greatly improved computational power, AI is used in various medical applications, such as disease diagnosis, surgery, and many more. For example, AI is applied in the medical setting for the detection of skin tumors in dermatology or the classification of pathology by X-rays. Furthermore, AI models may be used to overcame the limits of the traditional surgical decision-making systems in all its phases (i.e., preoperative, intraoperative, and postoperative phases of patient care). However, AI-based tools have some significant barriers that hinder their successful adoption in the medical domain. The following section will discuss the main challenges to address for a widespread adoption of the AI in the medical domain.

2.3.1 Explainable Artificial Intelligence

AI has been applied in a variety of domains such as recommendation systems, NLP, classification of text, images, speech, etc. [45]. Despite the successes, a key impediment to the spread of the AI systems in the real-world is related to the lack of transparency behind their behaviors which does not allow to understand how the AI-based models take certain decisions. Indeed, most AI-based systems behave as black-boxes meaning that they provide results without explanation of how they are achieved. For instance, this lack of transparency have hampered the application of AI in our society especially in critical decision-making domains such as self-driving cars, autonomous weapons and medical diagnostic tools.

Applications of AI in the medical field offer exciting opportunities for providing new insights and more precise diagnosis and treatment. However, also in this area the lack of transparency has a negative impact on trust in AI systems limiting their adoption in the clinical practice even when they could clearly provide a great benefit. For instance, ML can be used to optimize costs by managing patients by making prediction on the probability of the death of patients affected by pneumonia so that the high-risk patients are admitted to the hospital while low-risk patients are treated as outpatients [46]. In all critical decision-making processes, physicians must be able to understand why a computer program makes a certain prediction or recommendation in such a way as to judge whether that decision is reliable.

Moreover, since ML algorithms are generally trained on large amount of data that may contain prejudice or biases, this may lead to discriminative predictions [47, 48]. For instance, the popular Criminal Risk Assessment tool (COMPAS), used by U.S. courts to evaluate the potential recidivism risk in crime, has been highly criticized because it discriminates against blacks people. The algorithm used by COMPAS produces much higher risk scores for black people than white ones, even though data do not include information about race. This leads to overpredict high risk of reoffending for blacks with respect to whites [48].

Generally, there are two main issues related to transparency. The first is related to the public perception and understanding of how AI-based systems work while the latter is related to how much the developers understand about their own AI-based systems. Explainable artificial intelligence (XAI) can effectively mitigate these issues [49, 50].

Explainability is the ability to provide an explanation, in user-friendly terms, that justifies system decisions and/or actions, in order to increase the trasparency and gain trust by all users. The growing demand for explainable AI has been also transposed by the General Data Protection Regulation (GDPR), a noteworthy law within the European Union that became enforceable on May 25, 2018. GDPR provides a legal framework that regulates the collection, storage, and use of personal information (i.e., it aims to guarantee the protection of personal data). The GDPR opened the extensive debate over the "right to explanation" concerning the decisions made by algorithms highlighting the need of XAI especially in the critical real-life applications

[51]. Therefore, a multitude of XAI approaches have been proposed that can be grouped into the following two main categories [52]:

- *local explanations* tries to explain the reasoning behind individual predictions of ML models;
- *global explanations* relies on a holistic approach to uncover the overall functioning mechanism of a ML model by examining its structure and parameters.

Another classification of the XAI approaches identifies the following two categories:

- *post-hoc explainability* is based on the application of the explainability techniques after the model training. Generally, post-hoc explainability methods take a trained model as input and extract the underlying relationships that the model has learned to construct a white-box surrogate model,that is a model that approximates the original model behavior;
- *intrinsic explainability* is based on models that can be considered transparent due to their simple structure. This allows to understand how they work by looking at their structure and therefore this type of model is considered explainable by itself. Example of this type of models are the Short Decision Trees and Sparse Linear Models [53].

2.3.2 Requirement of High Computing Power

ML and DL methods require high computational power and memory storage. In particular, the training of the DL models has a high computational complexity that can be reduced by iteratively refining the several parameters of the model to improve the performance. Likewise, the inference phase of the DL models is computationally expensive due to the potentially high dimensionality of the input data and due to the several computations that need to be performed [54]. With the latest advances in Graphics Processing Units (GPUs) and with the help of the parallel computing techniques, nowadays it is possible to improve the performance of the DL models training [55].

2.3.3 Bias in AI Algorithms

One important issue in AI is the risk of introducing bias. AI bias is a phenomenon that occurs when an AI-based algorithm produces results based on training data that are prejudiced due to erroneous assumptions and/or affected by human bias. This leads to biased outcomes or incorrect predictions. An example of AI-based system affected by bias is COMPAS. The imbalanced data can lead AI-based algorithms to a biased decision boundary [56]. The imbalanced data problem occurs when classes are not represented equally in the input dataset. The increasing recognition that AI algorithms can be affected by biases has highly motivated the development AI-based approaches that are free of bias [57].

2.3.4 Insufficient Data

Overfitting is one of most common obstacles that can occur in the development of learning algorithms. Overfitting means that an AI model has learned many patterns from training data and it has lost the dominant trend. This implies that the model is not generalizable to new data.

One of the most common cause of overfitting is the scarcity of the training data. Indeed, if the training data size is too small, it does not contain sufficient data samples to accurately represent all possible input data. For this reason, collecting more data could help prevent overfitting, but often the data that can be accessed are limited. Among the techniques used to address this type of issue are the cross-validation and the data augmentation. Cross-validation is a technique where the algorithm is trained on a training set, and its performance is measured on a validation set [58].

Data augmentation is one of the most common methods used to artificially enlarge the size of a training dataset by transforming or altering the data in the original dataset to create new data instances. Considering image analysis, image variants such as for instance rotated images or with changed features (e.g., brightness, noise, and contrast) are artificially generated [59, 60].

2.3.5 Limited Knowledge of the Potential of AI

Artificial intelligence can provide substantial improvements in all areas of healthcare but a low knowledge and awareness of its potential is also reflected in a low adoption of these tools in the clinical practice [45].

2.3.6 Legal and Ethical Issues in AI

The use of AI-based systems in the medical domain is increasing, consequently several ethical issues of fairness, transparency and privacy have raised [61]. Fairness, transparency and privacy are focused by the GDPR regulation that requires organizations to comply with strict rules regarding data collection and processing. AI decision-making algorithms might lead to fairer and more robust outcomes than human judgment but very often they are discriminating. Fairness can be defined such as the absence of prejudice or preference for an individual or group based on categories such as gender, race, and sexual orientation [62]. Transparency is an other fundamental challenge because the AI-based decision-making processes often directly affect people lifes and health.

Therefore, transparency can increase the trust in AI systems by the people and consequently their acceptance and effective adoption in the clinical practice [63]. Furthermore, as enormous amounts of personal data are collected and then used into AI algorithms, there are important concerns regarding the protection of patient privacy rights. Therefore, strict legal/ethical requirements must be met to preserve patient privacy [64]. Under the GDPR, an explicit consent from individuals before collecting their data must be obtained.

Furthermore, organizations must ensure that sensitive data are processed lawfully, fairly, and transparently. The doctors, blindly come to (non-explainable) diagnostic or therapeutic solution suggested by the machines, facing challenges regarding their moral and legal responsibility for the patient care.

2.4 Conclusion

Artificial intelligence is a branch of computer science concerned with building machines that are able to simulate the human intelligence. Machine learning is a subfield of AI which uses statistical techniques to enable machines to learn and improve from experience without being explicitly programmed. Thanks to the several advances in computer science, AI is rapidly becoming an integral part of modern healthcare. AI-based tools are being used to support medical professionals in clinical settings to improve the outcomes in healthcare. Although AI has already proven its potential and it has brought new opportunities, many challenges still need to be faced for its successful adoption in the medical domain.

Funding This work was funded by the Next Generation EU—Italian NRRP, Mission 4, Component 2, Investment 1.5, call for the creation and strengthening of" Innovation Ecosystems", building" Territorial R&D Leaders"(Directorial Decree n. 2021/3277)—project Tech4You—Technologies for climate change adaptation and quality of life improvement, n. ECS0000009. This work reflects only the authors' views and opinions, neither the Ministry for University and Research nor the European Commission can be considered responsible for them.

References

1. Arfi S, Srivastava N, Sharma N. Artificial intelligence: an emerging intellectual sword for battling carcinomas. Curr Pharmaceut Biotechnol. 2023.
2. Samuel AL. Some studies in machine learning using the game of checkers. IBM J Res Dev. 1959;3(3):210–29.
3. Lalehzarian S, Gowd A, Liu J. Machine learning in orthopaedic surgery. World J Orthoped. 2021;12:685–99.
4. Saravi B, Hassel F, Men S, Zink A, Shavlokhova V, Couillard-Despres S, Boeker M, Obid P, Lang GM. Artificial intelligence-driven prediction model-

ing and decision making in spine surgery using hybrid machine learning models. J Pers Med. 2022;12(4):509.
5. Mahbubur Rahman M, Kundu D, Suha SA, RaihanSiddiqi U, Dey SK. Hospital patients' length of stay prediction: a federated learning approach. J King Saud Univ – Comput Inf Sci. 2022;34(10, Part A):7874–84.
6. Colombo T, Mangone M, Agostini F, Bernetti A, Paoloni M, Santilli V, Palagi L. Supervised and unsupervised learning to classify scoliosis and healthy subjects based on non-invasive rasterstereography analysis. PLoS One. 2021;16(12):e0261511.
7. Galbusera F, Casaroli G, Bassani T. Artificial intelligence and machine learning in spine research. JOR Spine. 2019;2:e1044.
8. Orgueira AM, Rez MS, Arias JD, Ol L, Oriol A, Teruel AI, Lopez JM, Palomera L, Granell M, Blanchard MJ, de la Rubia J, de la Guia AP, Rios R, Sureda A, Hernandez MT, Bengoechea E, Calasanz MJ, Gutierrez N, Martin ML, Blade J, Lahuerta JJ, Miguel JS, Mateos MV, Orgueira AM, Rez MS, Arias JD, Ol L, Oriol A, Teruel AI, Lopez JM, Palomera L, Granell M, Blanchard MJ, de la Rubia J, de la Guia AP, Rios R, Sureda A, Hernandez MT, Bengoechea E, Calasanz MJ, Gutierrez N, Martin ML, Blade J, Lahuerta JJ, Miguel JS, Mateos MV. Unsupervised machine learning improves risk stratification in newly diagnosed multiple myeloma: an analysis of the Spanish Myeloma Group. Blood Cancer J. 2022;12(4):76.
9. Seoud L, Adankon M, Labelle H, Dansereau J, Cheriet F. Towards non invasive diagnosis of scoliosis using semi-supervised learning approach. 2010;6112:10–9.
10. Hammoudeh A. A concise introduction to reinforcement learning. 2018.
11. Hornung A, Chris Hornung G, Michael Mallow J, Barajas AJR, ArashSayari FG, Wilke H-J, Colman M, Phillips F, An H, Samartzis D. Artificial intelligence in spine care: current applications and future utility. Eur Spine J. 2022;31:2057–81.
12. Tajdari M, Pawar A, Li H, Tajdari F, Maqsood A, Cleary E, Saha S, Zhang YJ, Sarwark JF, Liu WK. Image-based modelling for adolescent idiopathic scoliosis: mechanistic machine learning analysis and prediction. Comput Methods Appl Mech Eng. 2021;374:113590.
13. Sze V, Chen Y-H, Yang T-J, Emer J. Efficient processingof deep neural networks: a tutorial and survey. Proc IEEE. 2017;105:2295–329.
14. Yamashita R, Nishio M, Do R, Togashi K. Convolutionalneural networks: an overview and application in radiology. Insights Imag. 2018;9:611–29.
15. Huang X, Luo M, Liu L, Wu D, You X, Deng Z, Xiu P, Yang X, Zhou C, Feng G, Wang L, Zhou Z, Fan J, He M, Gao Z, Pu L, Wu Z, Zhou Z, Song Y, Huang S. The comparison of convolutional neural networks and the manual measurement of Cobb angle in adolescent idiopathic scoliosis. Global Spine J. 2022:21925682221098672.
16. Chen H, Dou Q, Wang X, Qin J, Cheng JCY, Heng P-A. 3d fully convolutional networks for intervertebral disc localization and segmentation. In: Zheng G, Liao H, Jannin P, Cattin P, Lee S-L, editors. Medical imaging and augmented reality. Cham: Springer International Publishing; 2016. p. 375–82.
17. Cheng P, Yang Y, Yu H, He Y. Automatic vertebrae localization and segmentation in CT with a two-stage Dense-U-Net. Sci Rep. 2021;11(1):22156.
18. Kokabu T, Kanai S, Kawakami N, Uno K, Kotani T, Suzuki T, Tachi H, Abe Y, Iwasaki N, Sudo H. An algorithm for using deep learning convolutional neural networks with three dimensional depth sensor imaging in scoliosis detection. Spine J. 2021;21(6):980–7.
19. Ronneberger O, Fischer P, Brox T. U-net: convolutional networks for biomedical image segmentation. In: Navab N, Hornegger J, Wells WM, Frangi AF, editors. Medical image computing and computer-assisted intervention – MICCAI 2015. Cham: Springer International Publishing; 2015. p. 234–41.
20. Zongwei Zhou M, Siddiquee MR, Tajbakhsh N, JianmingLiang. Unet++: redesigning skip connections to exploit multiscale features in image segmentation. IEEE Trans Med Imaging. 2019;39(6):1856–67.
21. Yuxia Li Y, Si ZT, He L, Zhang J, Luo S, YushuGong. Mqanet: multi-task quadruple attention network of multi-object semantic segmentation from remote sensing images. Remote Sensing. 2022;14(24):6256.
22. Fan T, Wang G, Li Y, Wang H. Ma-net: a multi-scale attention network for liver and tumor segmentation. IEEE Access. 2020;8:179656–65.
23. Chi J, Han X, Chengdong W, Wang H, Ji P. X-net: multi-branch unet-like network for liver and tumor segmentation from 3d abdominal ct scans. Neurocomputing. 2021;459:81–96.
24. Murugan P. Learning the sequential temporal information with recurrentneural networks, 2018.
25. Feuerriegel S, Hartmann J, Janiesch C, Zschech P.Generative ai. 05 2023.
26. Ramdurai B. The impact, advancements and applications of generativeai. 06 2023.
27. Vaccari I, Orani V, Paglialonga A, Cambiaso E, MaurizioMongelli. A generative adversarial network (gan) technique for internet of medical things data. Sensors. 2021;21(11):3726.
28. Singh A, Ogunfunmi T. An overview of variational autoencoders for sourceseparation, finance, and biosignal applications. Entropy (Basel). 2021;24(1):55.
29. Kingma D, Welling M. An introduction to variational autoencoders. 01 2019.
30. Vaswani A, Shazeer N, Parmar N, Uszkoreit J, Jones L, Gomez AN, Kaiser L, Polosukhin I. Attention is all you need; 2023.
31. Vaswani A, Shazeer N, Parmar N, Uszkoreit J, Jones L,Gomez AN, Kaiser L, Polosukhin I. Attention is all you need. CoRR, abs/1706.03762, 2017.
32. Wolf T, Debut L, Sanh V, Chaumond J, Delangue C, Moi A, Cistac P, Rault T, Louf R, Funtowicz M, Davison J, Shleifer S, Platen P, Ma C, Jernite Y, Plu J,

Xu C, Scao T, Gugger S, Rush A. Transformers: state-of-theart natural language processing; 2020. p. 38–45.
33. Thakkar K, Jagdishbhai N. Exploring the capabilities and limitations of gpt and chat gpt in natural language processing. J Manage Res Anal. 2023;10:18–20.
34. Devlin J, Chang M-W, Lee K, Toutanova K. Bert: pretraining of deep bidirectional transformers for language understanding; 2019.
35. Koroteev M. Bert: a review of applications in natural language processingand understanding. 03 2021.
36. Thoppilan R, De Freitas D, Hall J, Shazeer N, Kulshreshtha A, Cheng H-T, Jin A, Bos T, Baker L, Du Y, Li YG, Lee H, Zheng HS, Ghafouri A, Menegali M, Huang Y, Krikun M, Lepikhin D, Qin J, Chen D, Xu Y, Chen Z, Roberts A, Bosma M, Zhou Y, Chang C-C, Krivokon I, Rusch W, Pickett M, Meier-Hellstern KS, Morris MR, Doshi T, Santos RD, Duke T, Soraker J, Zevenbergen B, Prabhakaran V, Diaz M, Hutchinson B, Olson K, Molina A, Hoffman-John E, Lee J, Aroyo L, Rajakumar R, Butryna A, Lamm M, Kuzmina V, Fenton J, Cohen A, Bernstein R, Kurzweil R, Arcas BA, Cui C, Croak M, Chi EH, Le Q. Lamda: language models for dialog applications. CoRR, abs/2201.08239, 2022.
37. Bi B, Li C, Chen W, Yan M, Wang W. PALM: pretraining anautoencoding&autoregressive language model for context-conditioned generation. CoRR, abs/2004.07159, 2020.
38. Scao T, Fan A, Akiki C, Pavlick E, Ili'c S, Hesslow D, Castagn'e R, Luccioni A, Yvon F, Gall'e M, Tow J, Rush A, Biderman S, Webson A, Ammanamanchi P, Wang T, Sagot B, Muennighoff N, Moral A, Wolf T. Bloom: a 176b-parameter open-access multilingual language model. 11 2022.
39. Touvron H, Martin L, Stone K, Albert P, Almahairi A, Babaei Y, Bashlykov N, Batra S, Bhargava P, Bhosale S, Bikel D, Blecher L, Ferrer C, Chen M, Cucurull G, Esiobu D, Fernandes J, Jeremy F, Wenyin F, Scialom T. Llama 2: Open foundation and fine-tuned chat models. 07 2023.
40. Raffel C, Shazeer N, Roberts A, Lee K, Narang S,Matena M, Zhou Y, Li W, Liu PJ. Exploring the limits of transfer learning with a unified text-to-text transformer. CoRR, abs/1910.10683, 2019.
41. Rahsepar AA, Tavakoli N, Grace HJ, Kim CH, Abtin F, Bedayat A. How ai responds to common lung cancer questions: Chatgpt versus google bard. Radiology. 2023;307(5):e230922.
42. Wang L, Xinyi Chen L, Zhang LL, Huang YB, Sun Y, Yuan X. Artificial intelligence in clinical decision support systems for oncology. Int J Med Sci. 2023;20:79–86.
43. Haug CJ, Drazen JM. Artificial intelligence and machine learningin clinical medicine, 2023. N Engl J Med. 2023;388(13):1201–8.
44. Rivera SC, Liu X, Chan A-W, Denniston AK, Calvert MJ, Ashrafian H, Beam AL, Collins GS, Darzi A, Deeks JJ, et al. Guidelines for clinical trial protocols for interventions involving artificial intelligence: the spirit-ai extension. Lancet Digital Health. 2020;2(10):e549–60.
45. Cannataro M, Guzzi PH, Agapito G, Zucco C, Milano M. Artificial intelligence in bioinformatics: from omics analysis to deep learning and network mining. Elsevier; 2022.
46. Rich Caruana, Yin Lou, Johannes Gehrke, Paul Koch, M. Sturm, Noemie Elhadad. Intelligible models for healthcare: predicting pneumonia risk and hospital 30-day readmission. In: Proceedings of the 21th ACM SIGKDD International Conference on Knowledge Discovery and Data Mining, 2015.
47. Tischbirek A. Artificial intelligence and discrimination: discriminating against discriminatory systems. Cham: Springer International Publishing; 2020. p. 103–21.
48. Flores AW, Bechtel K, Lowenkamp CT. False positives, false negatives, and false analyses: a rejoinder to "machine bias: There's software used across the country to predict future criminals. and it's biased against blacks". Federal Probation. 2016;80:38.
49. Aung YYM, Wong DCS, Ting DSW. The promise of artificialintelligence: a review of the opportunities and challenges of artificial intelligence in healthcare. Br Med Bull. 2021;139(1):4–15.
50. Mengnan D, Liu N, Xia H. Techniques for interpretable machinelearning. Commun ACM. 2019;63:68–77.
51. Hacker P, Passoth J-H. Varieties of ai explanations under thelaw. from the gdpr to the aia, and beyond. In: International workshop on extending explainable AI beyond deep models and classifiers. Springer; 2020. p. 343–73
52. Chuang Y-N, Wang G, Yang F, Liu Z, Cai X, Du M, Hu X. Efficient xai techniques: a taxonomic survey. arXiv preprint arXiv:2302.03225, 2023.
53. Molnar C, Casalicchio G, Bischl B. Interpretable machinelearning – a brief history, state-of-the-art and challenges, 10 2020.
54. Chen J, Ran X. Deep learning with edge computing: a review. Proc IEEE. 2019;107(8):1655–74.
55. Liyanage H, Liaw S-T, Jonnagaddala J, Schreiber R, Kuziemsky C, Terry AL, de Lusignan S. Artificial intelligence in primary health care: perceptions, issues, and challenges. Yearbook Med Inform. 2019;28(01):041–6.
56. Ashby SR, Zeithamova D. Category-biased neural representationsform spontaneously during learning that emphasizes memory for specific instances. J Neurosci. 2022;42(5):865–76.
57. DeCamp M, Lindvall C. Latent bias and the implementationof artificial intelligence in medicine. J Am Med Inform Assoc. 2020;27(12):2020–3.
58. Kaliappan J, Reddy A, Almal S, Mishra R, Hu Y-C, Srinivasan K. Impact of cross-validation on machine learning models for early detection of intrauterine fetal demise. Diagnostics. 2023;13:1692.
59. Mutasa S, Sun S, Ha R. Understanding artificial intelligence based radiology studies: what is overfitting? Clin Imaging. 2020;65:96–9.

60. Hung KF, Qi Yong H, Ai YY, Leung, and Andy Wai Kan Yeung. Potential and impact of artificial intelligence algorithms in dento-maxillofacial radiology. Clin Oral Investig. 2022;26(9):5535–55.
61. Cath C. Governing artificial intelligence: ethical, legal and technical opportunities and challenges. Philos Trans R Soc A. 2018;376(2133):20180080.
62. Asan O, Bayrak AE, Choudhury A. Artificial intelligence and human trust in healthcare: focus on clinicians. J Med Internet Res. 2020;22(6):e15154.
63. Kiseleva A, Kotzinos D, De Hert P. Transparency of ai inhealthcare as a multilayered system of accountabilities: between legal requirements and technical limitations. Front Artific Intell. 2022;5:879603.
64. Khalid N, Qayyum A, Bilal M, Al-Fuqaha A, JunaidQadir. Privacy-preserving artificial intelligence in healthcare: techniques and applications. Comput Biol Med. 2023:106848.

Machine Learning

3

Emin Suha Dedeogullari, Ataberk Beydemir, Zeynep Beyza Arik, Mahmut Nedim Doral, and Gazi Huri

3.1 Introduction

Orthopedic surgery has long been committed to improving the standard of patient care through cutting-edge biologic agents, implants, and surgical techniques. Orthopedic surgeons aim to assist patients in restoring mobility, manage pain, and increase functionality. However, orthopedics has challenges related to the demand for better clinical outcomes, the requirement for more individualized treatment plans, and the complexity of patient data that is accumulating.

The fusion of artificial intelligence (AI) and machine learning (ML) has emerged as an opportunity to address these issues in this era of data-driven healthcare [1]. The concept of AI, initially introduced in 1956, envisions machines capable of simulating human intelligence across a variety of tasks, from problem-solving to pattern recognition. Machine learning, first explicitly defined in 1959, represents a subset of algorithms designed to analyze incoming information, identify trends, predict outcomes, and continuously improve through the incorporation of past experiences. ML, a facet of artificial intelligence, holds the greatest potential for advancing the field of orthopedics [2, 3].

The fundamental idea behind ML is its capacity to identify complex correlations among enormous datasets. Selected AI subfields in orthopedic surgery demonstrate potential for improving clinical decision-making and enhancing patient care. ML has the potential to provide orthopedic experts with tools for more precise diagnoses and treatment suggestions, from the analysis of complicated medical images to the correlation of symptoms and biomarkers with disease characterization and prognosis [4].

The extraordinary potential of ML in orthopedics has not yet been fully explored. There are still issues to be resolved regarding data protection, model interpretability, and the requirement for easy incorporation into clinical processes. Despite this, orthopedic surgeons and researchers stand at the forefront of a transformative era that promises to raise patient care to new dimensions as research in this field keeps increasing.

This chapter explores the multifaceted relationship between ML and orthopedics, delving

E. S. Dedeogullari · A. Beydemir
Faculty of Medicine, Orthopaedics and Traumatology Department, Hacettepe University, Ankara, Turkey
e-mail: ededeogullari@ku.edu.tr

Z. B. Arik
Faculty of Medicine, Hacettepe University, Ankara, Turkey

M. N. Doral
Department of Orthopaedics, Magnet Hospital, Ankara, Turkey

G. Huri (✉)
Faculty of Medicine, Orthopaedics and Traumatology Department, Hacettepe University, Ankara, Turkey

Orthopaedcis and Sports Medicine Hospital, Aspetar FIFA Center of Excellence, Doha, Qatar

F. Familiari et al. (eds.), *Artificial Intelligence in Orthopaedic Surgery Made Easy*,
https://doi.org/10.1007/978-3-031-70310-2_3

into its applications, limitations, and the evolving landscape of data-driven decision-making in orthopedics.

3.2 What Is ML and What Are the Types of ML?

As a subfield of artificial intelligence, *machine learning* is a branch of science that includes an algorithm allowing software programs to predict outcomes more accurately without being explicitly programmed. In machine learning, input and output data are provided, and then the machine determines the process of generating labeled output data from the given inputs [5].

We can liken machine learning, in a simplified way, to a child learning certain information and patterns from their parents as they grow, distinguishing similarities and differences. As the child grows, it can be compared to the model learning a set of patterns, and with continuous input of new data, it may produce outputs that are different from what it learned in the past from the model's output sequence. Machine learning algorithms designed for extracting insights from more structured datasets encompass linear regression, random forest decision trees, nearest neighbors, k-means clustering, and support vector machines (SVM) [6].

Examining the data set and extracting useful information from it with these methods is called data mining. The more data given to the algorithm, the more likely it is that the resulting information will be more accurate. This is one advantage of machine learning over traditional statistics [7]. For this reason, the use of machine learning is increasing in a field with high data input, such as orthopedics.

Machine learning requires algorithms to identify patterns or connections in empirical datasets, whatever methodologies are utilized. Four different approaches—*supervised learning, unsupervised learning, semi-supervised learning, and reinforcement learning*—can be used to carry out this "learning" process (Fig. 3.1) [8].

In orthopedics, supervised learning is more commonly employed due to its ability to reach results in less time with less data. The specific organization of data obtained through interactive systems is referred to as *supervised learning* [5]. Input and output in this learning model are predetermined and often used for risk prediction. The primary goal of supervised learning is to predict a known output or target. In addition to choosing which subgroups to include in a new data sample, it also includes predicting an unknown parameter [9]. For example, when employing an ML algorithm to identify bone tumors in an ankle radiograph, a human must manually identify and label the characteristic features of a bone tumor, along with determining whether the radiograph is an example of a bone tumor [10]. *Unsupervised learning* is the process of analyzing data sets without explicit class labels. There is no predicted specified result in unsupervised learning. Instead, finding naturally occurring patterns or clusters within the data is its main goal. Because of this, evaluating unsupervised learning is intrinsically more difficult, and the value of such learned groups is typically assessed in terms of how well they perform in following supervised learning projects [11]. If we begin with the earlier example, the unsupervised learning process for identifying the distinctive attributes of a bone tumor does not involve explicit labeling, making the algorithm depend on self-organization. Additionally, *semi-supervised learning* is a machine learning technique that uses a small portion of labeled data and lots of unlabeled data to

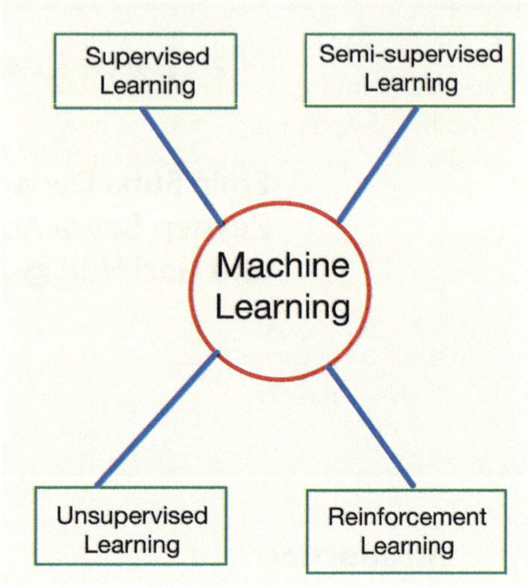

Fig. 3.1 Types of machine learning

train a predictive model. Lastly, *reinforcement learning* stands apart from both supervised and unsupervised learning, as it operates without the need for labeled data or a predefined training set. Instead, it relies on the capacity to observe and assess the consequences of the learning agent's actions [4].

3.3 Uses of Machine Learning in Orthopedic Surgery

Between 2010 and 2017, there was a tenfold increase in publications on the use of machine learning in orthopedics [6]. Especially in the field of musculoskeletal radiology, the substantial increase in imaging data has significantly boosted the use of machine learning in recent years in orthopedic research. The Food and Drug Administration (FDA) has approved six orthopedics-specific machine learning-based image analysis systems as of 2021. By evaluating radiography or computed tomography scans, these technologies help physicians diagnose primary and secondary osteoporosis, cervical spine fractures, vertebral compression fractures, rib fractures, and osteoarthritis (OA) [12].

Machine learning-based discriminative models can also be employed for the recognition of anatomical structures in magnetic resonance imaging. For example, to discriminate between the anterior and posterior cruciate ligaments, Zarychta used an unsupervised clustering process. With an accuracy rate of 89%, expert radiologists confirmed that the model correctly identified these ligaments in 66 of 74 T1-weighted magnetic resonance imaging (MRI) scans [13].

Bien et al. used a dataset of 1370 knee MRI scans to develop a model that can recognize meniscal and ACL tears and other abnormalities, among other diagnoses [14]. These studies highlight the potential for an automated image interpretation system to improve the diagnostic precision of orthopedic disorders, such as osteoarthritis of the hip and knee. In the case of OA-related research, Ashinsky et al. employed a machine learning algorithm that utilized T2-weighted maps of the central medial femoral condyle to forecast the progression to clinically symptomatic OA. The machine learning algorithm achieved a 75% accuracy rate in predicting the onset of OA [15]. Beyond the principles of image processing, ML is continuing to expand into other domains such as biomechanical and chemical sensors and video data [19]. Using these materials, Kotti et al. analyzed a group of subjects as they walked through a path of force plate sensors. The data concluded the degree of osteoarthritis with 73% accuracy during the evaluation [26]. Using a wide variety of data sets, ML can prosper personalized patient diagnosis and treatment by aiding in the analysis of patient-specific data in a brief amount of time with affordable costs.

In the field of orthopedic trauma, Olczak et al. utilized machine learning and achieved an 83% accuracy in fracture detection using a dataset comprising hand, wrist, and ankle radiographs [16]. Furthermore, Kruse et al. utilized a machine learning model to predict hip fracture risk with dual X-ray absorptiometry. Thanks to this advanced predictive modeling, they can predict hip fracture with a sensitivity of 100%, specificity of 69% for men, and a sensitivity of 88%, specificity of 81% for women [17].

In orthopedic oncology, machine learning is frequently used in the diagnosis of bone tumors and in the prediction and prevention of pathological fractures that may occur due to metastatic bone diseases. For instance, Oh et al. used machine learning (ML) methods to identify radiologic characteristics and predict pathological femoral fractures in patients with metastatic lung cancer using CT imaging data and clinical parameters. After that, they contrasted this ML model with one that solely utilized CT characteristics. Contrary to expectations, the ML model that included clinical features into account demonstrated higher predictive accuracy than the model that solely took CT features into account [18]. This study emphasized the increased accuracy in prediction with more data.

In the field of arthroplasty, when we look at the areas where machine learning is used, we can see that it is primarily employed in preoperative templating, implant detection, determining the position of the implant to be applied, and risk assessment. Machine learning can be used to minimize the difference between the implant size determined through preoperative templating and the implant size finally applied in surgery. In the literature, Polce and their colleagues successfully used machine learning to predict the fit of femoral and tibial components with high accuracy for 1801 patients in knee arthroplasty [19]. In total joint arthroplasty, proper implant positioning is crucial for achieving successful outcomes. With the assistance of machine learning, the implant position can be determined appropriately for each patient. Rouzrokh and others used machine learning to develop a model for the automatic radiographic measurement of acetabular inclination and version [20].

Additionally, in cases where revision arthroplasty is to be performed, the implant used in the patient's primary surgery needs to be pre-identified to obtain the appropriate surgical tools before the surgery. Machine learning approaches can also identify the manufacturer and model of orthopedic implants using radiographs [21]. Furthermore, machine learning models have been used to predict the risk of dislocation—a significant and undesirable complication in hip arthroplasty. Rouzrokh and colleagues developed a machine learning model to predict the risk of dislocation after primary hip arthroplasty, with a sensitivity of 88% and a negative predictive value of 99.5% [22].

In the field of spine surgery, advances in computer vision technology have grown alongside the use of computer-assisted navigation, robotic surgery, and augmented reality in the operating room. These technologies rely on creating detailed 3D spinal column reconstructions, usually from CT or MRI scans. Making these reconstructions involves using Artificial Neural Networks (ANNs) to automatically identify and outline vertebrae. Additionally, ML has facilitated significant advancements in the field of spine surgery, including automatic spine segmentation, detection of spinal stenosis and posterior element fractures, and lumbar stenosis grading [23]. In recent years, navigation systems commonly used in spinal surgery have also been developed through ML.

While machine learning has made great gains in the field of orthopedic surgery, it is crucial to consider both its benefits and drawbacks when deciding whether to use it in this field. By being aware of the potential advantages and challenges, orthopedic surgeons can use this technology safely while minimizing potential hazards.

3.4 The Advantages of Machine Learning in Orthopedic Surgery

The vast amount of investment made in this field of research has allowed physicians to use ML in the diagnosis of fractures, interpretation of radiographic imaging, implant detection, and measurements. Studies have been giving promising results of ML use in preoperative risk assessment and postoperative outcome predictions. This innovation can assist healthcare professionals as a support mechanism to provide high-quality patient care with minimal errors in a cost-effective manner [6].

Imaging studies in orthopedics are widely used to interpret musculoskeletal abnormalities. Therefore, Groot et al. have performed a review comparing imaging interpretation between ML and clinicians. The review concluded that ML models have surpassed in accurate radiographic imaging analysis to that of clinicians. Additionally, the ML model interpretations were comparably similar to those of radiologists and orthopedic surgeons when diagnosing fractures, osteoarthritis, and other abnormalities [24].

Ren et al. have evaluated 11 studies involving ML capacity to detect spine, shoulder, hip, or knee joint implants from radiographic images with the achievement of accuracy of 0.8–1.0 [21]. Moreover, one study exemplified that their prototype could decrease the amount of time necessary to detect the implant from 15 min to 0.06 s per image [7]. These results propose that ML can reduce the overall diagnosis and treatment period while also accurately predicting outcomes.

3.5 The Drawbacks of Machine Learning

The functionality of AI does bring along its limitations and is crucial to bring into consideration when using it as a side tool in medical practice. The more data provided to ML, the more training and learning will be processed, and the better the outcomes will be. However, the broad amount of data that must be provided can be expensive and inefficient. This training process can gain data sets from national or institutional databases, both of which have their limitations [7]. National databases have a larger population to study, but the data may not be accurate, may have missing data, and may not be readily available. Conversely, institutional databases have a smaller population, which may be useful when considering specific clinical questions but may not be useful when generalizing with a larger population [6].

When the ML model obtains input from a small amount of data with only specific examples during the training period, it will lack the ability to acknowledge the general concepts of the pathology. Hence, the machine will have accurate results with its own data but will work poorly with external data. This process called "overfitting" is one of the drawbacks that decrease the ability to implement ML in clinical settings [6]. For example, learning a new language from only one person with a unique accent and speaking style, you might become excellent at understanding and mimicking that person but struggle to understand others who speak with different accents. Groot et al. demonstrated that only 16% of the publicly accessible models that predict orthopedic surgical outcomes have been achieved with external databases [25]. The result of this review emphasizes the importance of external data and its relevance to gaining precise outputs using ML.

Current research offers ML models to detect and examine radiographic imaging on specific tasks. Even though these models may detect bone fractures, they still fail to analyze other abnormalities such as bone tumors and infections on computed tomography [11]. Therefore, it is vital that these models are supervised by medical professionals and that they are used to aid in the decision-making process rather than primarily providing the diagnosis. There are only a few products on the market that can detect multiple abnormalities, which in this case, increases the cost, time, and other risks of technical errors. The application field and the use of ML in a cost-effective manner is a crucial part of future research.

The evolution period to train an ML model takes an extensive amount of time to find, interpret, and apply the data to practical use. This prolonged period of training requires diligent work and decreases the efficiency of the model. Only a few of the models have been approved by the FDA, which only assesses the risk of harm and does not guarantee the algorithm's clinical effectiveness [7]. Hence, further research must be conducted to increase the ML model's success.

Another drawback is that there are ethical concerns that must be addressed from different aspects. It is crucial to collect input that can represent an entire population rather than a specific group to prevent unevaluated data, which may lead to faulty algorithms. These data sets must be carefully evaluated to prevent unconscious discrimination and keep track of the changing population, which is the foundation of the model's data set [26]. It is also important to prioritize patient consent and confidentiality, which may be difficult as AI technology can easily gain access to a specific patient population [27]. Therefore, informing patients about these types of procedures and their risks is important when obtaining consent. Furthermore, the increased use of analysis of radiographic imaging and automated surgical procedures may be a threat to the physician's knowledge and skill over time. This phenomenon called "deskilling" has been proposed when the clinician has a decline in experience when robotic procedures and technologies are overused [28]. This may especially pose an issue if ML models are not available during any inconvenience. For this reason, even if AI technologies can be used without the supervision of a physician, it is vital that conventional techniques are still used to keep surgical and clinical skills up to date.

3.6 Future Direction of ML in Orthopedic Surgery

The growing popularity of ML in the last decade is continuing to encourage researchers to use their curiosity to study in trials and apply models in clinical settings. The gradually increasing knowledge and experience in this field aim to find a more practical and cost-effective path to diagnose and treat patients. ML models can provide a second opinion to the medical practitioner and decrease the cost and time period of diagnosis and treatment by reducing the risk of errors. As these models are currently working in collaboration with physicians, future research must study to incorporate big data into ML models to lead to individualized precision medicine. In the meantime, the data used must be evaluated with increased accuracy with minimalized missing data. The passion for this novel finding continues to motivate researchers to find the most cost-effective and practical method to expand ML use in orthopedic surgery.

Nearly two decades ago, the concept of AI use in the operating room was applied to navigation-assisted arthroplasties [27]. The beginning goal was to arrange specific bony cuts and soft tissue balancing by using passive technology, which was entirely controlled by the surgeon. The next step is for ML to play a role in semi-active technology where the model provides feedback to the practitioner about its actions, such as in case of robotic arm-assisted total knee surgery. Active technology, on the other hand, allows the model to perform surgical tasks independently from the surgeon [29]. Batailler et al. portrayed that the current use of this novel technology in knee arthroplasty has a vital role in arranging surgeries, enhancing the validity of alignment of the lower extremity, positioning of implants, and calculating soft tissue balance [30]. Presently, AI can only be used under careful observation by the medical professional. Thereby, a mutual profit is generated by minimizing both machine-made and physician-made errors. However, future research may improve AI technology to create an environment where human presence is no longer necessary in the medical field.

Models that are currently approved by the FDA have several aforementioned drawbacks that must be taken into consideration. If prospective studies can overcome the setbacks of current ML models, medical professionals can enhance the ability to apply this technology in clinical settings.

3.7 Conclusion

Present applications of ML have made groundbreaking progress by using a vast amount of data in the analysis of imaging and aiding specific orthopedic procedures. As research continues to enhance ML technology, new dilemmas will come into question and may raise concerns about the applicability of these models. It is certain that advantages and disadvantages must be taken into consideration when using ML in the field of orthopedics. Despite the drawbacks that are faced during this journey, there is unlimited potential for future research to explore the world of ML and broaden its application into the field of orthopedics.

References

1. Makhni EC, Makhni S, Ramkumar PN. Artificial intelligence for the orthopaedic surgeon: an overview of potential benefits, limitations, and clinical applications. J Am Acad Orthop Surg. 2021;29(6):235–43.
2. McCarthy J, Minsky ML, Shannon CE. A proposal for the Dartmouth summer research project on artificial intelligence - August 31, 1955. AI Mag. 2006;27(4):12–4.
3. Samuel AL. Some studies in machine learning using the game of checkers. IBM J Res Dev. 1959;3(3):211.
4. Lalehzarian SP, Gowd AK, Liu JN. Machine learning in orthopaedic surgery. World J Orthop. 2021;12(9):685–99.
5. Sarker IH. Machine learning: algorithms, real-world applications and research directions. SN Comput Sci. 2021;2(3):160.
6. Cabitza F, Locoro A, Banfi G. Machine learning in orthopedics: a literature review. Front Bioeng Biotechnol. 2018;6:75.
7. Padash S, Mickley JP, Vera Garcia DV, Nugen F, Khosravi B, Erickson BJ, et al. An overview of machine learning in orthopedic surgery: an educational paper. J Arthroplast. 2023;38:1938.

8. Sidey-Gibbons JAM, Sidey-Gibbons CJ. Machine learning in medicine: a practical introduction. BMC Med Res Methodol. 2019;19(1):64.
9. Poduval M, Ghose A, Manchanda S, Bagaria V, Sinha A. Artificial intelligence and machine learning: a new disruptive force in orthopaedics. Indian J Orthop. 2020;54(2):109–22.
10. Myers TG, Ramkumar PN, Ricciardi BF, Urish KL, Kipper J, Ketonis C. Artificial intelligence and orthopaedics: an introduction for clinicians. J Bone Joint Surg Am. 2020;102(9):830–40.
11. Deo RC. Machine learning in medicine. Circulation. 2015;132(20):1920–30.
12. van Leeuwen KG, Schalekamp S, Rutten M, van Ginneken B, de Rooij M. Artificial intelligence in radiology: 100 commercially available products and their scientific evidence. Eur Radiol. 2021;31(6):3797–804.
13. Zarychta P. Features extraction in anterior and posterior cruciate ligaments analysis. Comput Med Imaging Graph. 2015;46(Pt 2):108–20.
14. Bien N, Rajpurkar P, Ball RL, Irvin J, Park A, Jones E, et al. Deep-learning-assisted diagnosis for knee magnetic resonance imaging: development and retrospective validation of MRNet. PLoS Med. 2018;15(11):e1002699.
15. Ashinsky BG, Bouhrara M, Coletta CE, Lehallier B, Urish KL, Lin PC, et al. Predicting early symptomatic osteoarthritis in the human knee using machine learning classification of magnetic resonance images from the osteoarthritis initiative. J Orthop Res. 2017;35(10):2243–50.
16. Olczak J, Fahlberg N, Maki A, Razavian AS, Jilert A, Stark A, et al. Artificial intelligence for analyzing orthopedic trauma radiographs. Acta Orthop. 2017;88(6):581–6.
17. Kruse C, Eiken P, Vestergaard P. Machine learning principles can improve hip fracture prediction. Calcif Tissue Int. 2017;100(4):348–60.
18. Oh E, Seo SW, Yoon YC, Kim DW, Kwon S, Yoon S. Prediction of pathologic femoral fractures in patients with lung cancer using machine learning algorithms: comparison of computed tomography-based radiological features with clinical features versus without clinical features. J Orthop Surg (Hong Kong). 2017;25(2):2309499017716243.
19. Polce EM, Kunze KN, Paul KM, Levine BR. Machine learning predicts femoral and tibial implant size mismatch for total knee arthroplasty. Arthroplast Today. 2021;8:268–77 e2.
20. Rouzrokh P, Wyles CC, Philbrick KA, Ramazanian T, Weston AD, Cai JC, et al. A deep learning tool for automated radiographic measurement of acetabular component inclination and version after Total hip arthroplasty. J Arthroplast. 2021;36(7):2510–7 e6.
21. Ren M, Yi PH. Artificial intelligence in orthopedic implant model classification: a systematic review. Skeletal Radiol. 2022;51(2):407–16.
22. Rouzrokh P, Ramazanian T, Wyles CC, Philbrick KA, Cai JC, Taunton MJ, et al. Deep learning artificial intelligence model for assessment of hip dislocation risk following primary total hip arthroplasty from postoperative radiographs. J Arthroplast. 2021;36(6):2197–203 e3.
23. Kim YJ, Ganbold B, Kim KG. Web-based spine segmentation using deep learning in computed tomography images. Healthc Inform Res. 2020;26(1):61–7.
24. Groot OQ, Bongers MER, Ogink PT, Senders JT, Karhade AV, Bramer JAM, et al. Does artificial intelligence outperform natural intelligence in interpreting musculoskeletal radiological studies? A systematic review. Clin Orthop Relat Res. 2020;478(12):2751–64.
25. Groot OQ, Bindels BJJ, Ogink PT, Kapoor ND, Twining PK, Collins AK, et al. Availability and reporting quality of external validations of machine-learning prediction models with orthopedic surgical outcomes: a systematic review. Acta Orthop. 2021;92(4):385–93.
26. Loftus TJ, Tighe PJ, Filiberto AC, Efron PA, Brakenridge SC, Mohr AM, et al. Artificial intelligence and surgical decision-making. JAMA Surg. 2020;155(2):148–58.
27. Kaya Bicer E, Fangerau H, Sur H. Artifical intelligence use in orthopedics: an ethical point of view. EFORT Open Rev. 2023;8(8):592–6.
28. Cabitza F, Rasoini R, Gensini GF. Unintended consequences of machine learning in medicine. JAMA. 2017;318(6):517–8.
29. Zhang J, Ndou WS, Ng N, Gaston P, Simpson PM, Macpherson GJ, et al. Robotic-arm assisted total knee arthroplasty is associated with improved accuracy and patient reported outcomes: a systematic review and meta-analysis. Knee Surg Sports Traumatol Arthrosc. 2022;30(8):2677–95.
30. Batailler C, Shatrov J, Sappey-Marinier E, Servien E, Parratte S, Lustig S. Artificial intelligence in knee arthroplasty: current concept of the available clinical applications. Arthroplasty. 2022;4(1):17.

Deep Learning

4

Ataberk Beydemir, Emin Suha Dedeogullari, Zeynep Beyza Arik, Erdi Özdemir, and Gazi Huri

4.1 Introduction

Deep learning (DL) is a subset of machine learning, in which multiple layers of artificial neural networks are utilized to process data in order to extract progressively higher-level features [1, 2]. Structurally, DL aims to process data by mimicking the neural network in the human brain [3]. After raw data is processed by neural networks in the initial layer, the results obtained are then transmitted to the neural networks in the next layer. This way, the results of the previous layer form the inputs for the subsequent layer. This process continues across multiple layers, ultimately yielding a final result (e.g., the presence or absence of a fracture, classification into a specific class, etc.).

A. Beydemir · E. S. Dedeogullari
Faculty of Medicine, Orthopaedics and Traumatology Department, Hacettepe University, Ankara, Turkey
e-mail: ededeogullari@ku.edu.tr

Z. B. Arik
Faculty of Medicine, Hacettepe University, Ankara, Turkey

E. Özdemir
Department of Orthopaedics and Traumatology, Güven Hospital, Ankara, Turkey

G. Huri (✉)
Faculty of Medicine, Orthopaedics and Traumatology Department, Hacettepe University, Ankara, Turkey

Orthopaedics and Sports Medicine Hospital, Aspetar FIFA Center of Excellence, Doha, Qatar

Even though DL is a subfield of machine learning, it differs in terms of how data is introduced to the algorithm [4]. In machine learning, when assigning a task to an algorithm, it is necessary to provide a training dataset that teaches the algorithm how to classify the data based on specific features (Fig. 4.1). For example, if we want the algorithm to classify distal radius fractures from X-rays, first we need to introduce the parameters used in fracture classification (such as displacement amount, intra-articular extension, fracture configuration, etc.) to the algorithm in a smaller dataset and teach it which fractures belong to which class. Through the analysis of this set, which encompasses diverse instances of distal radius fractures, the algorithm learns the correlations between specific features and distinct fracture types.

Note that in the example, it is crucial for the programmer to know which features are relevant to classify a distal radius fracture. If a distal radius fracture is consistently and incorrectly labeled, the algorithm's accuracy will be compromised initially. Moreover, in machine learning, the programmer must present the data to the computer in a comprehensible form [4]. Typically, this involves transforming the data into a comprehensive spreadsheet with numerous rows and columns, each containing distinct numerical values (referred to as "structured data"). This task can be challenging in healthcare, where a significant portion of the information is found in "unstruc-

F. Familiari et al. (eds.), *Artificial Intelligence in Orthopaedic Surgery Made Easy*,
https://doi.org/10.1007/978-3-031-70310-2_4

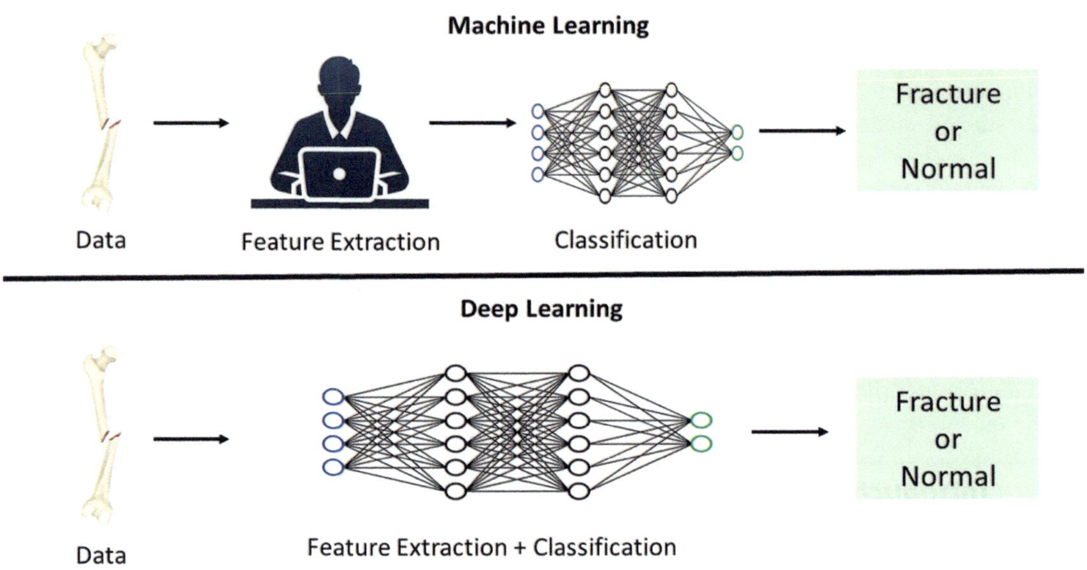

Fig. 4.1 Workflow difference between machine learning and deep learning

tured" datasets, mainly composed of clinical chart notes. Given the time-consuming nature of designing and selecting features, to handle vast datasets and unstructured data lacking well-defined features, scientists developed statistical models termed Artificial Neural Networks (ANNs) [4]. DL is an umbrella term that contains multiple layers of ANNs, hence the adjective "deep", that are capable of learning to extract features from a raw dataset without introduction [4]. For both DL and machine learning the efficacy of the learning process is amplified with a larger and more varied training set, underscoring the significance of "big data" in refining the algorithm's precision. Furthermore, through feedback loops that evaluate decisions as correct or incorrect, the algorithm possesses the capability to autonomously adjust itself, effectively "learning" and adapting its coding to enhance performance over time.

Artificial neuron concept was first proposed by Warren McCulloch and Walter Pitts in 1943 [5]. Although this concept has been revolutionized by other scientists through time; in 2012, the work of Geoffrey Hinton and his team in image recognition accelerated the wide use of DL [6]. These technological advancements spread to the field of medicine resulting in various applications of DL. In the medical literature, the main focus of DL is on the analysis of medical imaging, making orthopedics, closely related to musculoskeletal imaging, one of the pioneering fields in this area [7]. Fracture detection, localization and classification, tumor recognition, implant position, implant loosening, spinal deformity analysis, and sagittal vertebral profile calculations are examples of the use of DL in orthopedics [8–12]. Furthermore, the medical applications of DL are not limited to image analysis; examples are increasingly emerging in various areas such as suggesting treatment algorithms, organizing clinical and operating room workflows, and improving efficiency [13–15].

While DL holds promise for the development of numerous innovations in the medical field, it also has its drawbacks. Data dependency, interpretability, need for resources, bias and ethical considerations, and regulatory challenges are some of the main dilemmas that DL faces [16]. This chapter explores the logic behind DL, the integration of DL in orthopedics surgery reveals its applications and confronts its drawbacks while illustrating the continuous advancements of this model in the new era of medicine.

4.2 How Deep Learning Works?

Since image recognition is one of the most commonly studied areas of DL in orthopedics, the working principles of DL will be outlined using image recognition algorithms in this chapter. As an example how a DL method called Convolutional Neural Networks (CNNs) enables a computer to "read" radiographs will be explained (Fig. 4.2).

At its core, DL is fundamentally a mathematical computer algorithm [17]. Computers operate based on numerical data, so to interpret a radiograph, the image information needs to be converted into a format that computers can process, compute, and analyze. Consequently, computers perceive a digitized image as numerical data and interpret these numerical representations using mathematical functions. In essence, CNNs are specialized mathematical functions designed for image analysis. Like any mathematical function, CNNs take inputs (in this case, the numerical representation of the image) and produce a final output (a numerical prediction of the image content) [18].

The original inspiration behind the mathematical architecture of all DL systems, including CNNs, stemmed from the network of neurons found in the brain [5]. Instead of utilizing a network of biological neurons, DL systems employ a network of mathematical functions known as an Artificial Neural Network (ANN) [17]. While biological neurons transmit information via electrical signals, the artificial neurons within an ANN exchange the results of their mathematical computations. Conceptually, the ANN can be envisioned as a complex mathematical function comprised of numerous simpler mathematical functions. These functions "connect" and "transmit signals" between each other [17]. ANNs are structured into layers comprising interconnected neurons, where each layer functions collectively at a specific depth within the network [3]. Within each neuron, the mathematical operation involves processing weighted inputs, and these inputs are aggregated to generate an output. Subsequently, this output is transmitted to the neuron(s) in the following layer of the network, where it serves as a weighted input of the new layer [3].

The layers in an ANN serve distinct purposes and are typically classified as "input", "hidden", and "output" layers [18]. Each ANN begins with an input layer and concludes with an output layer (Fig. 4.3). As expected, the input layer receives the inputs (such as a radiograph) while the output layer provides the final answer (e.g., whether a radiograph depicts a fracture) [17]. Additionally, ANNs typically contain a variable number of hidden layers, positioned between the input and output layers. These hidden layers consist of stacks of mathematical functions and serve as intermediaries in the network.

The hidden layers are where most of the work is done. This is because the inclusion of hidden layers of mathematical functions adds depth to the neural network, hence the term "deep" [17]. A deep ANN may contain numerous hidden layers, each with its own characteristics [18]. Various types of hidden layers utilize different mathematical functions, with some layers being better suited for specific tasks than others. For instance; convolutional layers, pooling layers, and fully connected layers are the most commonly used types of layers in image recognition [18].

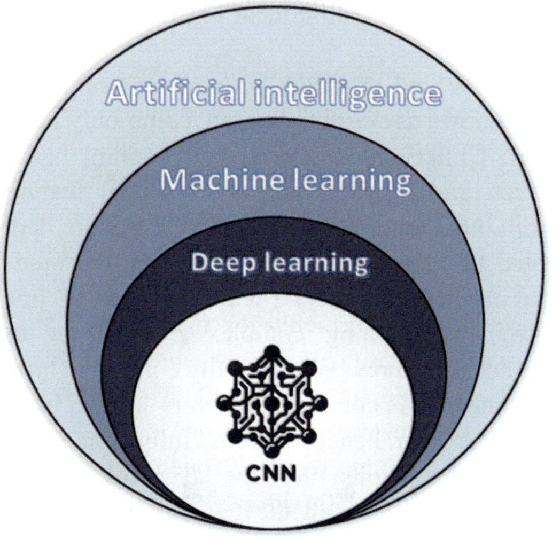

Fig. 4.2 Convolutional Neural Networks (CNN) as a subtype of deep learning

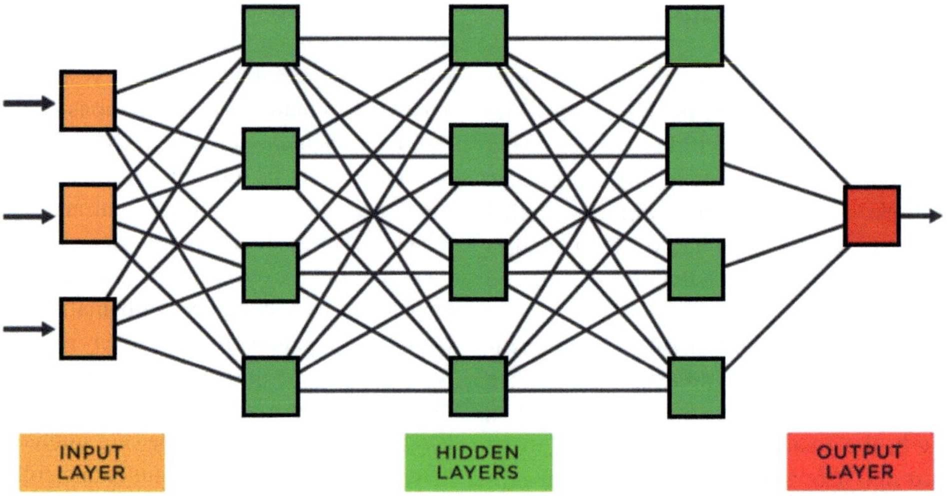

Fig. 4.3 Representation of Artificial Neural Networks (ANNs) in deep learning

CNNs, a subtype of ANN, employ interconnected layers of artificial neurons to detect various shapes or visual features within an image [19]. These layers of mathematical functions gradually define image details, starting with simple elements and progressively identifying complete objects [17]. CNNs do not perceive the shapes within the image, they rather function through pixels. Moreover, they do not identify pixels as colored dots but as numeric values according to their brightness [20]. For instance, in X-rays white pixels would get a value of 1, black pixels would get a value of 0, and any tone of gray is somewhere in between. Consequently, X-ray image is a matrix of numbers to DL [17].

In CNNs, a *feature map* refers to a two-dimensional representation of features detected within an input image by a specific filter [21]. Each filter is designed to detect particular patterns or features, such as edges, textures, or shapes. When the filter is *convolved* with the input image, the resulting output, known as a feature map, highlights areas of the image where the desired feature is present [22]. The intensity of each pixel in the feature map corresponds to the degree of similarity between the filter and the corresponding region of the input image. Feature maps from multiple filters are typically stacked together to form the output of a *convolutional* layer in the CNN [18]. These feature maps serve as inputs to subsequent layers in the network for further processing and feature extraction. *Pooling layers* can be used to reduce the spatial dimensions of feature maps. This leads to a more compact representation of the input while retaining essential information (i.e. focusing on cortical density and reducing input from X-ray's black background) for subsequent layers to learn from [17].

At the end of CNNs *fully connected layers*, also known as *dense layers*, are commonly found [23]. Unlike convolutional and pooling layers, which are designed to extract spatial features from input data, fully connected layers are dedicated to addressing the question that the model was trained to answer (i.e., what type of fracture?) by learning complex patterns in the extracted features [17]. In a fully connected layer, each neuron is connected to every neuron in the previous layer, hence the term "fully connected". These connections allow the layer to learn relationships between all the features extracted by the preceding layers [18].

4.3 Deep Learning Applications in Orthopedics

We have started to witness numerous examples of DL in the field of orthopedics, and the number of applications in this area is steadily increasing. Examples of applications include fracture diagnosis and classification in the trauma subspecialty, implant recognition and implant position analysis in arthroplasty, sagittal vertebral analysis in the spine, and evaluation of ligament reconstructions in sports surgery [8–12, 24–26].

In a retrospective study to evaluate the accuracy of eight different DL models for diagnosis of knee osteoarthritis grade as per the Kellgren-Lawrence scale, 2068 radiographs were used [27]. About 70% of the images were used as a training set, 10% as a testing set, and 20% as validation set. As a control group, three orthopedic surgeons graded the radiographs and reached agreement via consensus in case of disagreement. As a result, DL networks showed 54% to 93% accuracy in diagnozing knee osteoarthritis through X-rays. The DenseNet model showed the highest accuracy, at 93%.

Increased posterior tibial slope (PTS) is a known risk factor for graft failure after anterior cruciate ligament reconstruction [28]. Since there might be potential interobserver variability with manual measurements and performing measurements in large databases for research purposes can be laborious, a DL model was trained for PTS measurements [24]. 300 post-op lateral knee X-rays were used, in a manner of 80% to 20% train-validation scheme, to train U-Net model. For the control group, two researchers manually measured PTS via validated technique. The DL model reached a mean similarity coefficient of 0.885 on the validation cohort. The mean difference between manual measurements and DL model measurements was statistically insignificant. More than five disagreements were reported <5% of cases.

The assessment of sagittal balance is essential for characterizing, classifying, and subsequently planning treatment for adult spinal deformities [29]. Sacral slope (SS), pelvic tilt (PT), pelvic incidence (PI), lumbar lordosis (LL), and sagittal vertical axis (SVA) are among the most commonly used radiographic parameters [30]. Ensuring accurate and reliable measurement of these radiographic parameters is crucial. Typically, this assessment is conducted manually with software assistance, a process that is both time-consuming and examiner-dependent. In order to automatically perform such measurements a DL algorithm is trained [8]. Its accuracy on 118 preoperative and 125 postoperative lateral spinal X-rays was compared to manual measurements of two independent researchers. This study showed that the DL algorithm was able to measure all of the aforementioned parameters 91.5% and 84.8% in pre-op and post-op X-rays, respectively. The ICC between the manual measurements and the DL measurements was 0.71–0.99 for the preoperative and 0.72–0.96 for the postoperative analysis. Authors also reported that DL algorithm showed similar accuracy in implanted or cement-augmented post-op X-rays as well.

DL has several applications in musculoskeletal oncology such as tumor detection, grading, tumor volume calculation, classification, tumor necrosis rate, prognosis prediction, etc. [31–34]. X-rays, magnetic resonance images (MRI), computerized tomography (CT) images, positron emission tomography (PET) images even histopathological slides are widely used in training DL networks [9]. The introduction of patient demographic information and clinical notes has been shown to increase the accuracy of DL [34]. A CNN model was developed to classify viable and necrotic tumor regions in histopathological slides of osteosarcoma [25]. The model was trained on 536 non-tumor tiles, 263 necrotic tumor tiles, and 345 viable tumor tiles labeled by two pathologists. It achieved an accuracy of 91.2% in differentiating osteosarcoma slides into viable tumor, necrotic tumor, and non-tumor categories in H&E-stained images. Tumor-prediction maps generated by the model were used to visualize tumor regions and types, as well as to calculate the percentage of necrotic regions and display the tumor area across the slides.

Fracture detection and classification is one of the pioneering subfields for DL in orthopedics. There are many DL models trained for fracture recognition, localization, and classification in use [35–37]. In a retrospective study, ResNet DL model was trained to classify proximal humerus fractures based on Neer's classification system [38]. In total 1891 images consisting of 515 normal shoulders, 346 great tuberosity, 514 surgical neck, 269 3-part, and 247 4-part fractures were used in this study. To compare with human evaluation randomized radiographs were evaluated by 28 general physicians, 11 general orthopedists, and 19 shoulder specialists. As a result, DL algorithm showed 96% accuracy in differentiating normal shoulders from fractures. Also, it showed 65–86% accuracy for classifying fracture type, superior performance of the CNN being more marked in complex 3- and 4-part fractures. Moreover, DL outperformed general physicians and general orthopaedists, performed similarly to shoulder specialists.

In the arthroplasty literature, DL studies mostly focus on implant recognition along with subjects like hip dislocation risk, periprosthetic fracture detection, etc. [10, 26, 39]. Identifying the manufacturer of in-situ implants in revision cases is crucial. This process can be challenging, especially for young surgeons. In a recent study, DL algorithm was trained and validated with 1766 AP hip views of post-op total hip arthroplasty (THA) patients to identify 18 different implant models [26]. Consequently, DL model was able to classify radiographs according to implant type with an accuracy of 99.6%. Another study group trained ResNet18 DL model to assess the risk of hip dislocation based on postoperative AP pelvis radiographs [10]. In total, the analysis encompassed 1490 radiographs from dislocated THAs and 91,094 radiographs from non-dislocated THAs. As a result, DL algorithm succeeded in achieving high sensitivity (89%) and high negative predictive value (99%) in the external testing data set.

The examples of DL used in orthopedics can be extended. A common conclusion of many studies is that DL performs similarly to humans if not superiorly [17]. Moreover, it is worth noting that in many studies, thousands of data were used. While evaluating such a large amount of data manually requires significant time and effort, research in many fields may become more practical thanks to DL algorithms. The continued development of DL is predicted to lead to an increasing practical use. Nevertheless, it is important to emphasize that DL algorithms also have their drawbacks.

4.4 Drawbacks of Deep Learning

The increasing trend of DL use in the medical field is continuing to take part in diagnostic roles while questioning its accuracy and whether it can entirely replace physicians. These state-of-the-art models are designed to minimize missed diagnoses and physician-made errors while preventing unnecessary procedures [40]. Multiple studies based on DL-driven diagnoses of vertebral disease, bone fractures, and other orthopedic pathologies have shown the use of these AI models has assisted physicians in patient care and showed the potential for improved patient outcomes [41, 42]. However, most of the time interpretability of DL models is challenging. DL models are often considered *"black boxes"* because they provide predictions without clear explanations of how they arrived at those decisions [1]. This lack of interpretability can be problematic in medical contexts where understanding the reasoning behind diagnoses or treatment recommendations is crucial. Despite the intense ongoing research on DL use, for now, these models cannot be used alone but perhaps as an aid to physicians during the diagnostic and treatment period.

DL algorithms require large amounts of high-quality data for training, which may not always be readily available in the medical field due to issues like privacy concerns and data scarcity [2]. Also, training DL models require significant computational resources, including high-performance hardware and large amounts of memory. Implementing and maintaining such infrastructure can be costly and challenging for healthcare institutions.

Despite the increasing reliance on AI algorithms' diagnostic measures, it is important to take patient privacy, confidentiality, and consent into consideration [16]. This newly introduced model and its use is continuing to develop as it is being discovered. Meanwhile, both physicians and patients should be aware of its benefits and risks by receiving consent [43]. AI use often has the ability to gain access to stored data of a particular patient population. This may invade patient privacy and violate data protection regulations. Therefore, patients must be aware of these risks and must have the right to withdraw their consent [16]. Caution must be taken when relying on these models because Finlayson et al. emphasized that it is always easier to break systems than to protect them [44]. These problems may create regulatory challenges and slow down the translation of research findings into clinical practice.

AI relies on the big data applied to its input. The big data may unconsciously contain big biases as the data represented may not always apply to a specific subset of patient groups [16]. DL algorithms can inherit biases present in the training data, leading to unfair or discriminatory outcomes, especially if the data used for training is not representative of diverse patient populations. For this reason, the quality of data must be monitored, regulated, and updated at regular intervals [16]. When gathering input, it is vital to use accurate social factors, gender, and race information without discrimination [43]. *Overfitting* is another problem of big data dependency similar to machine learning [7]. DL models may become overly specialized to the training data, leading to poor generalization performance on unseen data. If DL models can overcome these drawbacks by identifying biased information, this novel machine can have higher accuracy and increase its use in diagnostic and therapeutic procedures.

4.5 Future Considerations of Deep Learning

The progress of AI continues to evolve traditional medical procedures into more practical applications used in disease diagnosis, treatment selection, and early forms of clinical reasoning [43]. These machine models in DL have gained popularity and are near to taking over the manual approaches which have been time-consuming and tiring for physicians. The DL algorithms that are currently being used as diagnostic tools in imaging are on the verge of achieving physician-level accuracy, leaving behind an era where diagnostic measures were dependent primarily on human expertise [43, 45].

DL has the potential to decrease the diagnosis period while increasing its accuracy. Liu et al. released a study led in the United Kingdom between 2013 and 2018, showing imaging tools such as CT and MRI use has increased by 54% and 48%, while human sources in this field grew only by 19% [40, 46]. The major advantage used by these machines is that they minimize errors made by physicians associated with fatigue, burnout, or carelessness while carrying a vast amount of tasks. Meanwhile, DL can enhance physicians' time spent on patient care, to maximize the efficacy of treatment and prognosis.

Another future goal for DL integration into medical practice would be increasing patient safety. These models may be a vital diagnostic modality when aiming to decrease radiation and contrast exposure during diagnostic procedures. There are several applications of DL-based image reconstruction to reduce radiation dose [47–49]. One study showed that DL-based reconstruction improved the subjective and objective image quality of multiphase hepatic CT compared with standard techniques, even at approximately half the radiation dose [48]. Another study concluded that utilizing a deep neural network for fully automated delimitation of the scan range leads to a considerable decrease in radiation exposure during CT coronary angiography when compared to manual examination planning [49]. A recent study showed that DL-based reconstructed chest

CT images showed comparable image quality and non-inferior nodule detectability relative to conventional low-dose CT images while exposing the patient to a quarter of the radiation dose [47]. It is undeniable that similar applications will be implemented in orthopedics, which is one of the medical specialties where radiation exposure is high for both patients and surgeons.

4.6 Conclusion

In conclusion, DL represents a groundbreaking advancement in machine learning, leveraging multiple layers of artificial neural networks to process data and extract progressively higher-level features. Its structural mimicry of the human brain's neural network allows for complex data processing and analysis, leading to remarkable applications across various fields, including orthopedics. By autonomously extracting features from raw data without explicit introduction, DL eliminates the need for manual feature selection, making it particularly suitable for processing vast datasets and unstructured information commonly found in healthcare. In orthopedics, DL has shown remarkable potential, revolutionizing tasks such as fracture detection, tumor recognition, implant recognition, and sagittal vertebral analysis. However, despite its promise, DL also presents challenges, including interpretability issues, resource requirements, biases, and ethical considerations. It is essential to address these limitations while harnessing the full potential of DL in orthopedics. Nevertheless, with ongoing advancements and increasing practical applications, DL is poised to play a transformative role in the future of orthopedic surgery, enhancing diagnostic accuracy, treatment selection, and patient safety.

References

1. Tg M, Pn R, Bf R, Kl U, Kipper J, Ketonis C. Artificial intelligence and orthopaedics: an introduction for clinicians. J Bone Joint Surg Am. 2020;102(9):830–40. https://doi.org/10.2106/Jbjs.19.01128.
2. Olczak J, Pavlopoulos J, Prijs J, Ffa I, Jn D, Lundstrom C, et al. Presenting artificial intelligence, deep learning, and machine learning studies to clinicians and healthcare stakeholders: an introductory reference with a guideline and a clinical Ai research (Cair) checklist proposal. Acta Orthop. 2021;92(5):513–25. https://doi.org/10.1080/17453674.2021.1918389.
3. Phs K, Sanduleanu S, Primakov S, Wu G, Jochems A, Refaee T, et al. Deep learning in fracture detection: a narrative review. Acta Orthop. 2020;91(2):215–20. https://doi.org/10.1080/17453674.2019.1711323.
4. Sa B. Artificial intelligence, machine learning, deep learning, and cognitive computing: what do these terms mean and How will they impact health care? J Arthroplast. 2018;33(8):2358–61. https://doi.org/10.1016/J.Arth.2018.02.067.
5. Mcculloch Ws, Pitts W. A logical calculus of the ideas immanent in nervous activity. 1943. Bull Math Biol. 1990;52(1–2):99–115; Discussion 73-97.
6. Krizhevsky A, Sutskever I, Hinton G. Imagenet classification with deep convolutional neural networks. Neural Inf Process Syst. 2012;60:25. https://doi.org/10.1145/3065386.
7. Borjali A, Chen A, Muratoglu O, Morid M, Varadarajan K. Deep learning in orthopedics: how do we build trust in the machine? Healthcare Transformation. 2020; https://doi.org/10.1089/Heat.2019.0006.
8. Lochel J, Putzier M, Dreischarf M, Grover P, Urinbayev K, Abbas F, et al. Deep learning algorithm for fully automated measurement of sagittal balance in adult spinal deformity. Eur Spine J. 2024; https://doi.org/10.1007/S00586-023-08109-1.
9. Zhou X, Wang H, Feng C, Xu R, He Y, Li L, et al. Emerging applications of deep learning in bone tumors: current advances and challenges. Front Oncol. 2022;12:908873. https://doi.org/10.3389/Fonc.2022.908873.
10. Rouzrokh P, Ramazanian T, Cc W, Ka P, Jc C, Mj T, et al. Deep learning artificial intelligence model for assessment of hip dislocation risk following primary total hip arthroplasty from postoperative radiographs. J Arthroplast. 2021;36(6):2197–203 E3. https://doi.org/10.1016/J.Arth.2021.02.028.
11. Krogue J, Kv C, Km H, Toogood P, Eg M, Ej G, et al. Automatic hip fracture identification and functional subclassification with deep learning. Radiol Artif Intell. 2020;2(2):E190023. https://doi.org/10.1148/Ryai.2020190023.
12. Rf S, Sa B, Am M, Pedoia V, Tp V. Incremental inputs improve the automated detection of implant loosening using machine-learning algorithms. Bone Joint J. 2020;102-B(6_Supple_A):101–6. https://doi.org/10.1302/0301-620x.102b6.Bjj-2019-1577.R1.
13. Ka T, Kondrashova O, Bradley A, Ed W, Pearson JV, Waddell N. Deep learning in cancer diagnosis, prognosis and treatment selection. Genome Med. 2021;13(1):152. https://doi.org/10.1186/S13073-021-00968-X.

14. Tanzi L, Piazzolla P, Vezzetti E. Intraoperative surgery room management: a deep learning perspective. Int J Med Robot. 2020;16(5):1–12. https://doi.org/10.1002/Rcs.2136.
15. Lee S, Lee Y. Improving emergency department efficiency by patient scheduling using deep reinforcement learning. Healthcare (Basel). 2020;8(2) https://doi.org/10.3390/Healthcare8020077.
16. Kaya Bicer E, Fangerau H, Sur H. Artifical intelligence use in orthopedics: an ethical point of view. Efort Open Rev. 2023;8(8):592–6. https://doi.org/10.1530/Eor-23-0083.
17. Bg H, Krogue J, Ds J, Pl S. Deep learning and imaging for the orthopaedic surgeon: how machines "read" radiographs. J Bone Joint Surg Am. 2022;104(18):1675–86. https://doi.org/10.2106/Jbjs.21.01387.
18. Goodfellow I, Bengio Y, Courville A. Deep learning. Mit Press; 2016.
19. Hubel D, Tn W. Receptive fields of single neurones in the cat's striate cortex. J Physiol. 1959;148(3):574.
20. Da F, Ponce J. Computer vision: a modern approach. Prentice Hall Professional Technical Reference; 2002.
21. Szeliski R. Computer vision: algorithms and applications. Springer Nature; 2022.
22. Bb T, Kamsu-Foguem B, Tangara F. Deep convolution neural network for image recognition. Eco Inform. 2018;48:257–68.
23. Alzubaidi L, Zhang J, Aj H, Al-Dujaili A, Duan Y, Al-Shamma O, et al. Review of deep learning: concepts, Cnn architectures, challenges, applications, future directions. J Big Data. 2021;8:1–74.
24. Lu Y, Pareek A, Yang L, Rouzrokh P, Khosravi B, Kr O, et al. Deep learning artificial intelligence tool for automated radiographic determination of posterior tibial slope in patients with Acl injury. Orthop J Sports Med. 2023;11 https://doi.org/10.1177/23259671231215820.
25. Hb A, Mishra R, Daescu O, Cederberg K, Rakheja D, Sengupta A, et al. Viable and necrotic tumor assessment from whole slide images of osteosarcoma using machine-learning and deep-learning models. PLoS One. 2019;14:e0210706. https://doi.org/10.1371/Journal.Pone.0210706.
26. Jm K, Hs H, Bc L, Al R, Rm M, Lm N, et al. Artificial intelligence to identify arthroplasty implants from radiographs of the hip. J Arthroplast. 2021;36(7s):S290–S4 E1. https://doi.org/10.1016/J.Arth.2020.11.015.
27. Tiwari A, Poduval M, Bagaria V. Evaluation of artificial intelligence models for osteoarthritis of the knee using deep learning algorithms for orthopedic radiographs. World J Orthop. 2022;13(6):603–14. https://doi.org/10.5312/Wjo.V13.I6.603.
28. Lj L, Akpinar B, Rj M. Tibial slope and anterior cruciate ligament reconstruction outcomes. Jbjs Rev. 2020;8(4):E0184. https://doi.org/10.2106/Jbjs.Rvw.19.00184.
29. Jc LH, Roussouly P. Sagittal Spino-pelvic balance is a crucial analysis for normal and degenerative spine. Eur Spine J. 2011;20(Suppl 5):556–7. https://doi.org/10.1007/S00586-011-1943-Y.
30. Jc LH, Thompson W, Mohsinaly Y, Barrey C, Faundez A. Sagittal balance of the spine. Eur Spine J. 2019;28(9):1889–905. https://doi.org/10.1007/S00586-019-06083-1.
31. He Y, Pan I, Bao B, Halsey K, Chang M, Liu H, et al. Deep learning-based classification of primary bone tumors on radiographs: a preliminary study. EBioMedicine. 2020;62:103121. https://doi.org/10.1016/J.Ebiom.2020.103121.
32. Fr E, Bao B, Wu J, Dalal D, Liao W, He Y, et al. Deep learning for classification of bone lesions on routine Mri. EBioMedicine. 2021;68:103402. https://doi.org/10.1016/J.Ebiom.2021.103402.
33. Navarro F, Dapper H, Asadpour R, Knebel C, Mb S, Schwarze V, et al. Development and external validation of deep-learning-based tumor grading models in soft-tissue sarcoma patients using Mr imaging. Cancers (Basel). 2021;13(12) https://doi.org/10.3390/Cancers13122866.
34. He Y, Guo J, Ding X, Pma VO, Zhang Y, Chen A, et al. Convolutional neural network to predict the local recurrence of giant cell tumor of bone after curettage based on pre-surgery magnetic resonance images. Eur Radiol. 2019;29(10):5441–51. https://doi.org/10.1007/S00330-019-06082-2.
35. Hy C, Bw H, Yk Y, Lin F, Yang T, Rs Y, et al. Application of deep learning algorithm to detect and visualize vertebral fractures on plain frontal radiographs. PLoS One. 2021;16(1):E0245992. https://doi.org/10.1371/Journal.Pone.0245992.
36. Ct C, Ty H, Ty L, Cc C, Cc C, Cc C, et al. Application of a deep learning algorithm for detection and visualization of hip fractures on plain pelvic radiographs. Eur Radiol. 2019;29(10):5469–77. https://doi.org/10.1007/S00330-019-06167-Y.
37. Kitamura G, Cy C, Be M. Ankle fracture detection utilizing a convolutional neural network ensemble implemented with a small sample, De novo training, and multiview incorporation. J Digit Imaging. 2019;32(4):672–7. https://doi.org/10.1007/S10278-018-0167-7.
38. Sw C, Ss H, Lee Jw O, Ks KN, Jp Y, et al. Automated detection and classification of the proximal humerus fracture by using deep learning algorithm. Acta Orthop. 2018;89(4):468–73. https://doi.org/10.1080/17453674.2018.1453714.
39. Sj J, Alpaugh K, Kn K, Ty L, Dj M, Jm V, et al. Deep-learning automation of preoperative radiographic parameters associated with early periprosthetic femur fracture after Total hip arthroplasty. J Arthroplast. 2023;39:1191. https://doi.org/10.1016/J.Arth.2023.11.021.
40. Kg VL, De Rooij M, Schalekamp S, Van Ginneken B, How RM. Does artificial intelligence in radi-

ology improve efficiency and health outcomes? Pediatr Radiol. 2022;52(11):2087–93. https://doi.org/10.1007/S00247-021-05114-8.

41. Lx W, Zhu Z, Qc C, Wb J, Yz W, Nk S, et al. Development and validation of a deep-learning model for the detection of non-displaced femoral neck fractures with anteroposterior and lateral hip radiographs. Quant Imaging Med Surg. 2024;14(1):527–39. https://doi.org/10.21037/Qims-23-814.
42. Wang Y, Su F, Lu Q, Zhang W, Liu T, Tao Y, et al. Deep learning-driven diagnosis of multi-type vertebra diseases based on computed tomography images. Quant Imaging Med Surg. 2024;14(1):800–13. https://doi.org/10.21037/Qims-23-685.
43. Mp M, Nm B. Corr synthesis: when should the orthopaedic surgeon use artificial intelligence, machine learning, and deep learning? Clin Orthop Relat Res. 2021;479(7):1497–505. https://doi.org/10.1097/Corr.0000000000001679.
44. Sg F, Bowers J, Ito J, Jl Z, Al B, Is K. Adversarial attacks on medical machine learning. Science. 2019;363(6433):1287–9. https://doi.org/10.1126/Science.Aaw4399.
45. Su Z, Adam A, Mf N, Ayob M, Punganan G. Skeletal fracture detection with deep learning: a comprehensive review. Diagnostics (Basel). 2023;13(20) https://doi.org/10.3390/Diagnostics13203245.
46. Kalidindi S, Gandhi S. Workforce crisis in radiology in the UK and the strategies to deal with it: Is artificial intelligence the saviour? Cureus. 2023;15(8):E43866. https://doi.org/10.7759/Cureus.43866.
47. Jo G, Ahn C, Hong J, Ds K, Park J, Kim H, et al. 75% radiation dose reduction using deep learning reconstruction on low-dose chest Ct. BMC Med Imaging. 2023;23(1):121. https://doi.org/10.1186/S12880-023-01081-8.
48. Nagayama Y, Goto M, Sakabe D, Emoto T, Shigematsu S, Taguchi N, et al. Radiation dose optimization potential of deep learning-based reconstruction for multiphase hepatic Ct: a clinical and phantom study. Eur J Radiol. 2022;151:110280. https://doi.org/10.1016/J.Ejrad.2022.110280.
49. Demircioglu A, Bos D, Demircioglu E, Qaadan S, Glasmachers T, Bruder O, et al. Deep learning-based scan range optimization can reduce radiation exposure in coronary Ct angiography. Eur Radiol. 2024;34(1):411–21. https://doi.org/10.1007/S00330-023-09971-9.

5 Artificial Intelligence in Hip Arthroplasty

Biagio Zampogna, Francesco Rosario Parisi, Andrea Zampoli, and Rocco Papalia

5.1 Introduction

Osteoarthritis (OA) is the most common degenerative joint disease, affecting women and men an estimated 18% and 10%, respectively, over 60 years old [1]. The importance of OA is due to its high socio-economic impact in developed countries. In this last case, pain and loss of function are debilitating and cost between 1.0% and 2.5% of gross domestic product (GDP) [2]. Hip OA is commonly associated with other diseases, and many studies show an association with frailty [3], an increased risk of all causes of mortality [4], mental health problems [5], and increased cardiovascular mortality [4]. THA represents one of the most effective orthopedic elective surgical procedures, and it improves the quality of life better than in the past. Each year, more than one million THA are worldwide [6–8]. Around 115,000 primary procedures were performed in Italy in 2021 [9]. The number of primary THA and its revision surgeries is increasing annually, demonstrating insensibility to macroeconomic downturns of the last two decades [10, 11]. Hip osteoarthritis is the main indication for total hip arthroplasty (90%), followed by femoral neck fracture (5%), femoral head avascular necrosis (AVN) (2%), developmental dysplasia of the hip (DDH) (2%), and inflammatory arthritis (1%) [12]. Even if we have improved our understanding of disease pathogenesis and increased the ability to identify patients at the most significant risk of disease, early diagnosis, and measure treatment efficacy, we have a limited solution. The average age of the primary THA in the UK is 69 years [12]. However, the number of younger patients undergoing surgery has increased in the USA, and younger than 65 could represent 52% of all patients by 2030 [13]. Another important data is the ratio between men and women; THA is more common in women than men by 1.5:1 [9, 14]. This data represents how hip disease and surgery treatment are relevant in the healthcare system and how much it is a problem for the patient and society. THA has demonstrated satisfactory

B. Zampogna
Operative Research Unit of Orthopaedic and Trauma Surgery, Fondazione Policlinico Universitario Campus Bio-Medico, Rome, Italy

Research Unit of Orthopaedic and Trauma Surgery, Department of Medicine and Surgery, Università Campus Bio-Medico di Roma, Rome, Italy

BIOMORF Department of Biomedical, Dental, Morphological and Functional Images, University of Messina, A.O.U. Policlinico "G.Martino", Messina, Italy
e-mail: f.parisi@unicampus.it

F. R. Parisi (✉) · A. Zampoli · R. Papalia
Operative Research Unit of Orthopaedic and Trauma Surgery, Fondazione Policlinico Universitario Campus Bio-Medico, Rome, Italy

Research Unit of Orthopaedic and Trauma Surgery, Department of Medicine and Surgery, Università Campus Bio-Medico di Roma, Rome, Italy
e-mail: f.parisi@unicampus.it

F. Familiari et al. (eds.), *Artificial Intelligence in Orthopaedic Surgery Made Easy*,
https://doi.org/10.1007/978-3-031-70310-2_5

survival rates [15–17], with over 90% survivorship over 10 years, thanks to continuous technological advancements [15]. However, as total joint arthroplasty surgeries and life expectancy increase, the revision THA proportion will likely rise further [16, 18]. Several perioperative complications have been described [16], including leg length discrepancy [17], implant dislocation [19], periprosthetic fracture [20], septic (PJI) or aseptic loosening [21, 22], and stress-shielding [23, 24], and all of which can lead to a THA failure. In orthopedics, technological advancements are discovering new pathways to enhance surgical procedures' performance, accuracy, and outcomes. Considering the projected unsustainable spending, identifying patients at risk for bad outcomes and implant failure is crucial for healthcare providers. The evolving applications of AI highlight how it can improve epidemiological studies, surgical planning, and patient outcomes in THA.

5.2 Background

Although we have heard about AI for over 50 years, AI health applications like machine learning (ML) and deep learning (DL) have only been developing for a few years, thanks to higher computational power and lesser costs than in the past. Besides, the more significant effect is increased knowledge about healthcare data collection and analysis. AI has been extensively employed in evaluating primary and revision hip surgery. Machine learning (ML), a type of artificial intelligence that uses computational algorithms to learn and improve with experience, and deep knowledge (DL), a subset of ML, has significantly enhanced clinical practice. Artificial intelligence (AI), particularly ML with deep understanding, has found widespread applications in orthopedics, especially in primary surgery. These new technologies were recently applied in image analysis, diagnosis, and care progress, and they have increased in the last two decades. AI and ML have been employed at various stages, including estimating risk factors, selecting and implanting prosthetic implants, detecting primary hip replacement failure early, and choosing future hip replacements [24]. These innovative tools in hip arthroplasty offer several advantages. With increasing awareness of healthcare costs, a predictive model for the need for surgery remains an essential tool for surgeons. AI and ML models can aid in predicting postoperative complications and developing personalized treatment protocols to minimize or manage complications and maximize outcomes. They have also shown promise in predicting postoperative pain, including identifying individuals at high risk of prolonged postoperative opioid prescriptions [25–28]. They may also allow surgeons to tailor treatment for their patients better, potentially offering nonoperative management, particularly when revision surgery or significant postoperative problems are anticipated. AI is emerging as a revolutionary frontier in the THA sphere [28]; for these reasons, it is evident that in the future, this innovative predictive tool will concretely support surgeons in every step of hip surgery and clinical decision-making. The AI world might be helpful in extensive studies for assessing hip OA features and outcomes and primary and revision THA surgery, identifying intricate patterns. This chapter aims to examine the applications of AI in THA and how it can offer solutions in preoperative planning, surgical assistance, and postoperative monitoring to guarantee the precision management of challenges associated with this complex surgical procedure.

5.3 Imaging

Imaging techniques are essential in THA, from preoperative planning to postoperative follow-up. Therefore, image analysis is an important part of the surgery decision-making. In current practice, hip OA is diagnosed by X-ray imaging, which is cost-efficient, easy, and rapid [29]. The main scoring systems for hip OA grading are Kellgren and Lawrence [30] and the Osteoarthritis Research Society International [31]. Preoperatively, X-rays assess joint disease, bone quality, and the location of the hip joint's anatomical landmarks [32]. Computed tomography

(CT scan) and magnetic resonance imaging (MRI) are other imaging methods. CT scans offer more comprehensive information than traditional X-rays [30] because of the detailed cross-sectional images of the hip joint and surrounding structures. CT scans are essential for evaluating complex anatomic variations, deformities, or fractures that may not be visible on X-rays [31]. Soft tissues, like muscles, tendons, ligaments, and the joint capsule, can be helpfully evaluated by MRI [33]. Three-dimensional (3D) Imaging techniques, such as 3D CT, MRI reconstructions, and 3D modeling, provide a detailed view of the hip joint in three dimensions [34]. 3D images allow more accurate planning and visualization of patient-specific anatomy, resulting in personalized implant selection and surgical approach. In this scenario, the use of AI is recent, as Cabitza et al. [28] showed applications in image analysis for detecting and predicting OA in bone and cartilage segmentation. AI can help preoperative planning to recognize acetabulum and femur morphology, instantly matching the optimal implant and size. AI is increasingly used in 3D preoperative planning, with authors demonstrating its superiority over 2D planning for stem and acetabular cup size. Interestingly, as the volume of data entered increases, the accuracy of the acetabular cup and femoral stem measurements gradually improves. The uses of AI in image analysis are uncountable, and they are growing fast and well over primary hip surgery [35].

5.3.1 Preoperative Assessment

ML has been used to recognize OA by analyzing pixels in an image to identify relevant structures, extracting specific features, and applying preprogrammed mathematical methods and measurements to cluster all relevant information in a model. Once the model is created, the algorithm can be applied to an unknown image using a known model for OA [36]. Through thousands of iterations of results, the machine efficiently refines its ability to analyze images without human intervention. This algorithm can be utilized in both research and clinical settings to diagnose the presence of OA on radiographs and determine whether a patient requires surgery or can be treated conservatively [37]. The AI is transforming THA's preoperative imaging assessment process, allowing orthopedic surgeons to increase understanding and support during the planning [38]. Preoperative imaging assessment of the THA focuses on correct OA severity staging, hip landmarks identification, hip anatomy measurements identification, and confirming surgical indication. Several DL models were developed for the diagnosis and the severity grading analysis of hip OA by radiograph. Hip OA is traditionally diagnosed with specific features, including the Kellgren-Lawrence score, narrowing of the joint space, formation of the osteophytes on the femoral head and acetabulum, and the development of subchondral sclerosis and cysts. In literature, several papers showed how AI and its subset (machine learning and deep learning) achieved high sensitivity and specificity compared to the chief physicians [39]. Yanping Xue et al. [40] showed that hip OA diagnosis has an accuracy of 92.8% compared to the expert physicians, a significant result for the growth of image diagnosis practice. Von Schacky et al. [41] analyzed 15,364 hip joints using 7738 weight-bearing anterior-posterior pelvic radiographs, and they developed a DL model to extract the features we discussed earlier to radiographic automatically. They showed how the DL model has higher reliabilities for grading femoral head osteophytes and narrowing joint space. It is evident how these specific AI, ML, and DL models may be helpful in large-scale studies for assessing hip OA features. An important study was conducted by Schwarz et al. [42] for the use of AI (HIPPO—Hip Positioning Assistant 1.03, Image Biopsy Lab, Vienna) in the evaluation of pelvic radiographs about specific measures: lateral center-edge angle (LCE angle), neck-diaphyseal angle, sharp angle, femoral head coverage, extrusion index, and pelvic obliquity. They showed that it is possible to have a reliable alternative to manual evaluation on pelvic X-rays. Their study demonstrated how AI software is accurate in 94.3% of all cases, with the results for each measurement in line with the literature. These steps are essential in developing new parameters and improving the knowledge around OA, dysplasia, and femoral-acetabular hip impingement.

5.3.2 Digital Planning

AI is making considerable progress in several areas of THA, and planning is one of them. Traditionally, THA planning involves manual measurements, assessments, and decision-making by orthopedic surgeons based on their experience and knowledge. 2D X-ray is the most used planning method, but its accuracy is limited, ranging from 40.7 to 99.2% [42, 43]. Preoperative digital templating resulted in 30% to 90% accuracy for femoral stem measurements and 50% to 90% for acetabular cup measurements [44–46]. X-ray-based planning precision can be limited by several factors, including surgeon experience, magnification error, the patient's position, and the bi-dimensionality of X-ray images [47]. Furthermore, the process can be time-consuming and subject to some variability [47]. Another method is computed tomography (CT) based on 3D preoperative planning, which provides critical and detailed parameters on a 3-dimensional scale. It is an evident improvement concerning 2D planning, and it has relatively stable intergroup and intragroup consistency [48], as well as strong repeatability and accuracy [49]. The accuracy of femoral stem measurements by 3D computerization was between 84% to 100% and between 80% to 100% in acetabular cup measurements [49, 50]. The difficulty with this method is the long training time and the process, which includes image segmentation, pelvic correction, deformity recognition, and postoperative simulation. As a result, the application of CT-based planning systems is restricted because they are especially time-consuming and require multidisciplinary expertise [51]. With AI technology evolution, different planning systems have been developed. AI-HIP software (Beijing Changmugu Medical Technology Co., Ltd., Beijing, China) is a planning software based on AI technology that can quickly and automatically identify the hip joint shape and match the optimal implant size. AI has still shown promising results in processing medical images with high accuracy and significantly reduced time requirements [52, 53]. For these reasons, AI achieved a significant role in an essential phase of the surgery as the planning, with potential benefits in improving efficacy and accuracy. AI can contribute to hip arthroplasty planning in different phases:

1. Image Analysis and Segmentation: The AI algorithms can analyze preoperative imaging data, X-rays, CT scans, and MRI to precisely identify and segment relevant anatomical structures like the hip joint, femur, and surrounding tissues. Different ways of solving these problems have been proposed [54, 55], with intelligent convolutional neural network CNN-based methods (deep learning model), and their application in hip segmentation has been successful [51, 56]. Despite better segmentation quality, these networks of deep neurons take time and require a lot of pixel labeling. Besides, these networks need help to handle gaps in segment results. In this development, a revolutionary study about this process was conducted by Dong Wu et al. [57], who showed a greater accuracy of the segmentation and the execution time of their DL than in the past and how this model is a reliable method. This finding makes it important for clinicians to observe the anatomical structures of hip joints, even in cases of severe disease.
2. Implant Selection: Each patient's hip anatomy can change significantly, and AI can help the surgical plan to the individual's specific needs. AI can assist in selecting the most appropriate hip implant for a particular patient. By analyzing a vast amount of patient data, AI algorithms can recommend the best implant size, type, and design, which may improve implant fit and reduce the risk of complications. In recent years, several studies in this field were conducted; an important workflow was shown

by Xi Chen et al. [58]; they demonstrated the efficacy and reliability of the AI-HIP planning software achieved from 1.2 million CT scans. AI-HIP reduced the time and workforce activity to realize detailed preoperative plans while being more accurate than the traditional method. Another critical study was produced by Xuzhuang Ding et al. [58], and it showed how AI-HIP software could help during implant selection with excellent reliability in component size prediction and implant position. The results in this analysis between AI-HIP and conventional planning were about stem agreement of 87.7% and 58.9%, respectively, and the cup agreement of 94.0% and 65.2%, respectively.

3. Surgical Simulation: AI-powered surgical simulation tools enable surgeons to practice and refine their approach before the actual operation; it could help develop confidence, improve skills, and anticipate potential challenges [59].
4. Workflow Optimization: AI can streamline the preoperative planning process, reducing the time and effort required by the surgical team. Automated tools can assist in generating comprehensive reports, surgical checklists, and other necessary documentation [60].

5.3.3 Intraoperative Assessment

The image intraoperative assessment represents an essential step during THA, and fluoroscopy is commonly used to guide the surgical procedure. As previously mentioned, AI has become a transformative tool in various orthopedic hip surgery fields, and integrating AI with fluoroscopy is a remarkable application. The problem and the need around this approach is the human-assisted observation of the intraoperative image. The combination of AI and fluoroscopy allows surgeons to receive real-time guidance and make informed decisions and adjustments, leading to more accurate implant placements, reduced risks, and improved postoperative recovery for patients undergoing THA. Recent research about this application was conducted by Robert B. Grupp et al. [61]. They showed how it is possible to apply the CNN model for automatic anatomical fluoroscopy observation to create the first accurate dataset of hip fluoroscopy. This study demonstrated that performance in fluoroscopic segmentation and landmark localization could be achieved using these datasets as training for neural networks. Utilizing AI algorithms to analyze fluoroscopic images can provide surgeons with valuable insights into the patient's anatomy, joint alignment, and potential complications during the surgery. However, a study by Yasuhiro Homma et al. [62] discussed an application of AI during THA, analyzing the intraoperative assessment of the sound produced by the hammer while placing non-cemented stems. This recent research has introduced a prediction model employing an ML algorithm to identify the last scraping sound recorded after surgery. The study's findings pave the way for a novel approach to differentiate between accurate and incorrect pounding sounds during surgery, thus preventing potential problems in total hip arthroplasty, especially intraoperative fractures. The application of AI allowed for an objective examination of the collected data, resulting in higher precision in detecting the appropriate hammering noises.

5.3.4 Postoperative Assessment

AI is increasingly important in image postoperative assessments of THA. After the surgery, monitoring the patient's imaging is critical to guarantee success and identify potential complications. The AI shows his contribution in image postoperative assessments of the hip arthroplasty and could help in the early detection of postoperative complications, such as infections or implant-related problems. By analyzing imaging scans, AI algorithms can alert to potential issues requiring immediate attention. Among the several studies in the literature that have shown interesting results, a recent paper by Albano et al.

[63] shows how an MRI-based ML model can help recognize and identify signs of periprosthetic joint infection (PJI). The AI was employed to discriminate septic from non-septic THA failure based on preoperative MRI features. The study utilized an ML and support vector machine (SVM) to examine specific MRI characteristics that could predict THA infection. The results revealed that bone edema, synovitis, synovial stratification, and extracapsular edema were the most significant predictors of disease, with an accuracy range of 75.1% to 81.5%. The AI-based SVM identified bone edema as the most reliable predictor, achieving an 80% accuracy rate. These findings demonstrate the potential benefits of AI-based machine learning classifiers as adjunct diagnostic tools, especially in challenging scenarios like distinguishing between septic and aseptic THA failure. This model may be a valuable aid for radiologists in detecting THA infections. The study of Murphy et al. [64] demonstrated that a model of AI could accurately calculate the correct version of the cups on radiographs of patients with THA. It is essential because dislocation is a rare complication following THA associated with discomfort, reduced function, the possibility of future revision surgery, and significant healthcare expenses. On the same topic, Rozurokh et al. [65, 66] demonstrated how to evaluate the risk of THA dislocation using a deep learning model based on postoperative pelvis X-ray. Their model showed a better sensibility and negative prediction value than the competitors, making it a valuable tool to be used in conjunction with clinical risk factor information, providing a rapid assessment of dislocation risk following THA. In this context, the help of AI that analyses data could be decisive in the assessment. About the implant failure analysis, several studies have been published: Shah et al. [67] have shown an innovative algorithm of machine learning to diagnose hip and knee prosthesis loosening by using radiographs and patient features with accuracy, sensitivity, and specificity of 88.3%, 70.2%, and 95.6% respectively, a result higher than a model based on radiographs alone. Another study by M Loppini et al. [68] showed the use of the convolutional neural network (CNN) in detecting implant failure on 630 patients, demonstrating a greater sensitivity, specificity, and accuracy of 96.7% for each one. At the least, a critical study was conducted by Man-Soo Kim et al. [69], who wrote a systematic review and Meta-Analysis about the influence of machine learning on prosthetic loosening detection in hip and knee arthroplasty. They analyzed around ten studies, 3236 images, and 2442 cases of total hip arthroplasty. They showed that the most used machine learning system is DenseNet, and the pooled sensitivity and specificity across studies were 93% and 96%, respectively. Machine learning results on plain radiographs were promising, with reasonable accuracy, sensitivity, and specificity in detecting loosening around total hip arthroplasty. Prosthetic loosening screening programs can be incorporated with the use of machine learning. To accurately judge the machine learning model's ability to detect loosening around joint arthroplasty, more research results will be necessary. An interesting application of AI is recognizing prosthetic implants in the postoperative phase. DL approaches based on CNN can effectively recognize and identify unique THA patterns using anteroposterior radiographic images. The significant benefit of this technique lies in its ability to create a comprehensive database, which allows surgeons to identify patients easily and quickly. Moreover, DL systems can continuously incorporate new knowledge as it becomes available, enabling long-term development of the method and iterative improvements to its categorization capacity. Adopting this DL system can rapidly decrease the risks of delayed reoperation, increased perioperative morbidity and mortality, and excessive resource utilization resulting from failing to identify hip arthroplasty implants preoperatively.

5.4 Outcomes Analysis

5.4.1 Satisfaction

Patient satisfaction is a crucial outcome measure in total hip arthroplasty (THA) [70] due to its ability to reflect subjective improvements in quality of life and the fulfillment of preoperative expectations [71, 72]. Adopting machine learning (ML) algorithms to predict patient satisfaction following THA has been widely embraced. Over the years, numerous pre- and postoperative scores have been developed to assess a range of motion (ROM), discomfort, and patient satisfaction before and after the procedure. Zhang et al. used a machine learning algorithm to predict patient satisfaction after total hip arthroplasty [70]. Comorbidities and preoperative patient-reported outcome measures (PROMs) such as Short Form-36 (SF-36), physical component summary (PCS), mental component summary (MCS), Western Ontario and McMaster's Universities Osteoarthritis Index (WOMAC), Oxford Hip Score (OHS), and Harris Hip Score have been utilized to evaluate function and satisfaction. Particularly significant predictors of unhappiness were found to be preoperative WOMAC [73] and SF-36 MCS [74], aligning with earlier research that suggested a link between post-THA discontent and poorer preoperative physical and mental health [66, 69]. Notably, patients' perceptions of their disabilities and pain sensitivity can be influenced by their mental health, potentially diminishing their level of satisfaction [25]. Younger patients tend to express higher levels of dissatisfaction, possibly due to their elevated expectations and more demanding functional needs [65, 70]. The most significant indicators of dissatisfaction included patient age, preoperative WOMAC score, number of comorbidities, preoperative MCS, prior lumbar spine surgery, low body mass index (18.5), and comorbidities. Regarding predicting patient satisfaction following THA, machine learning systems have demonstrated a strong capacity for discrimination. Our findings indicate that preoperative counseling and health optimization before THA are determinants of postoperative satisfaction, both of which can be modifiable and non-modifiable factors that may enhance overall patient satisfaction.

5.4.2 Fall Risk

In the initial post-THA recovery period, two intriguing clinical applications of AI involve forecasting the probability of falling and recognizing patients at low and high risk [75]. The associated risk variables are complex and multifaceted and can vary from patient to patient [72, 73]. Moreover, most clinically utilized fall risk assessment instruments still rely on subjective measures, making it challenging to forecast a patient's fall risk accurately. In a study conducted by Polus et al. [75], wearable sensors were utilized to collect objective data defining the functional ability of patients, enabling the classification of fall risk. Patients were equipped with sensors and asked to complete timed walk tests during preoperative, 2-week, and 6-week follow-up sessions. The study revealed that gait impairments and patient age are sensitive predictors of falls following THA. Notably, a significant difference in physician Harris's Hip Score total scores among patient groups supported this finding. Combining wearable sensors and machine learning has facilitated valuable data acquisition for stratifying fall risk using objective prediction models. Before surgery, it is advantageous to identify and alert patients at a high risk of falling. Low-risk patients can be directed toward more effective recovery aid programs, such as outpatient THA, which has been demonstrated to reduce costs, shorten hospital stays, and improve patient satisfaction [74, 76]. For high-risk patients, doctors can offer supplemental treatment and refer them to fall prevention education, which can reduce the likelihood and impact of falls [77, 78]. Overall, using this fall risk assessment tool, which stratifies patients to optimize their postoperative pathways, promotes improved patient management and contributes to a more efficient healthcare system.

5.5 Conclusion

This chapter examined how integrating AI technology and its subsets can significantly improve orthopedics, especially in the hip adult reconstruction sector. AI is revolutionizing epidemiological studies, etiological knowledge, preoperative assessment, planning process, intraoperative assistance, and postoperative monitoring, enabling a more precise, personalized, and efficient surgery to address the challenges related to hip prostheses. With the help of AI, orthopedic surgeons can achieve more data from various sources than in the past, including radiological data, patient records, and past procedure outcomes. These data are analyzed by machine learning algorithms, which give a detailed evaluation of the patient's anatomy and can optimize implant selection and accurate planning. AI gets involved in the surgical phase and offers advantages in postoperative monitoring. By analyzing data collected and applying predictive algorithms, AI can control the patient's progress, identifying any warning signs and allowing timely intervention in case of complications. However, it is essential to understand that AI should not replace the experience and expertise of orthopedic surgeons. AI should be considered an important support tool for orthopedic surgeons, increasing their knowledge of the competencies of AI to achieve the best possible patient outcomes. In conclusion, artificial intelligence represents a frontier in orthopedic surgery, exploring new possibilities to improve success and safety, especially hip arthroplasty.

References

1. Woolf AD, Pfleger B. Burden of major musculoskeletal conditions. Bull World Health Organ. 2003;81(9):646–56.
2. Hiligsmann M, Cooper C, Arden N, Boers M, Branco JC, Luisa Brandi M, et al. Health economics in osteoarthritis: an Expert's consensus paper from the European Society for Clinical and Economic Aspects of osteoporosis and osteoarthritis (ESCEO). Semin Arthritis Rheum. 2013;43(3):303–13.
3. Wise BL, Parimi N, Zhang Y, Cawthon PM, Barrett-Connor E, Ensrud KE, et al. Frailty and hip osteoarthritis in men in the MrOS cohort. J Gerontol A Biol Sci Med Sci 1 maggio 2014;69(5):602–608.
4. Barbour KE, Lui LY, Nevitt MC, Murphy LB, Helmick CG, Theis KA, et al. Hip osteoarthritis and the risk of all-cause and disease-specific mortality in older women: a population-based cohort study. Arthritis Rheumatol Hoboken NJ. 2015;67(7):1798–805.
5. Cook C, Pietrobon R, Hegedus E. Osteoarthritis and the impact on quality of life health indicators. Rheumatol Int. 2007;27(4):315–21.
6. OECD Health statistics. OECD.
7. Gollings J. The AOANJRR is funded by the Australian Government Department of Health.
8. Ben-Shlomo Y, Blom A, Boulton C, Brittain R, Clark E, Dawson-Bowling S, et al. The National Joint Registry 18th annual report 2021 [internet]. London: National Joint Registry; 2021 [citato 8 agosto 2023]. (National Joint Registry Annual Reports). Disponibile su: http://www.ncbi.nlm.nih.gov/books/NBK576858/
9. GQr4Pb-Report_PNE_2022.pdf.
10. Kurtz SM, Ong KL, Lau E, Bozic KJ. Impact of the economic downturn on total joint replacement demand in the United States: Updated Projections to 2021. J Bone Jt Surg. 2014;96(8):624–30.
11. Singh JA, Yu S, Chen L, Cleveland JD. Rates of total joint replacement in the United States: future projections to 2020–2040 using the national inpatient sample. J Rheumatol. 2019;46(9):1134–40.
12. RRCjA2-NJR-15th-Annual-Report-2018.pdf.
13. Kurtz SM, Lau E, Ong K, Zhao K, Kelly M, Bozic KJ. Future Young patient demand for primary and revision joint replacement: National Projections from 2010 to 2030. Clin Orthop. 2009;467(10):2606–12.
14. Glyn-Jones S, Palmer AJR, Agricola R, Price AJ, Vincent TL, Weinans H, et al. Osteoarthritis. The Lancet. 2015;386(9991):376–87.
15. Galley J, Sutter R, Stern C, Filli L, Rahm S, Pfirrmann CWA. Diagnosis of periprosthetic hip joint infection using MRI with metal artifact reduction at 1.5 T. Radiology. 2020;296(1):98–108.
16. Huo J, Huang G, Han D, Wang X, Bu Y, Chen Y, et al. Value of 3D preoperative planning for primary total hip arthroplasty based on artificial intelligence technology. J Orthop Surg. 2021;16(1):156.
17. Maloney WJ, Keeney JA. Leg length discrepancy after total hip arthroplasty. J Arthroplasty. 2004;19(4 Suppl 1):108–10.
18. Schwaiger BJ, Gassert FT, Suren C, Gersing AS, Haller B, Pfeiffer D, et al. Diagnostic accuracy of MRI with metal artifact reduction for the detection of periprosthetic joint infection and aseptic loosening of total hip arthroplasty. Eur J Radiol. 2020;131:109253.
19. Seagrave KG, Troelsen A, Malchau H, Husted H, Gromov K. Acetabular cup position and risk of dislocation in primary total hip arthroplasty. Acta Orthop. 2017;88(1):10–7.
20. Lindberg-Larsen M, Jørgensen CC, Solgaard S, Kjersgaard AG, Kehlet H. Lunbeck foundation centre for fast-track hip and knee replacement. Increased risk of intraoperative and early postoperative periprosthetic femoral fracture with uncemented stems. Acta Orthop. 2017;88(4):390–4.
21. Streit MR, Innmann MM, Merle C, Bruckner T, Aldinger PR, Gotterbarm T. Long-term (20- to

25-year) results of an uncemented tapered titanium femoral component and factors affecting survivorship. Clin Orthop. 2013;471(10):3262–9.
22. Pitto RP, Bhargava A, Pandit S, Munro JT. Retroacetabular stress-shielding in THA. Clin Orthop. 2008;466(2):353–8.
23. Sanki T, Endo H, Tetsunaga T, Furumatsu T, Yamada K, Ozaki T. Ten-year outcomes of total hip arthroplasty using fit-and-fill type cementless collared straight stem implants: relationship between the initial contact status and stress shielding. Acta Med Okayama. 2020;74(1):7–15.
24. Lopez CD, Gazgalis A, Boddapati V, Shah RP, Cooper HJ, Geller JA. Artificial learning and machine learning decision guidance applications in Total hip and knee arthroplasty: a systematic review. Arthroplasty Today. 2021;11:103–12.
25. Gandhi R, Davey JR, Mahomed NN. Predicting patient dissatisfaction following joint replacement surgery. J Rheumatol. 2008;35(12):2415–8.
26. Katakam A, Karhade AV, Schwab JH, Chen AF, Bedair HS. Development and validation of machine learning algorithms for postoperative opioid prescriptions after TKA. J Orthop. 2020;22:95–9.
27. Karhade AV, Schwab JH, Bedair HS. Development of machine learning algorithms for prediction of sustained postoperative opioid prescriptions after total hip arthroplasty. J Arthroplasty. 2019;34(10):2272–2277.e1.
28. Cabitza F, Locoro A, Banfi G. Machine learning in orthopedics: a literature review. Front Bioeng Biotechnol. 2018;6:75.
29. Guermazi A, Hayashi D, Roemer FW, Felson DT. Osteoarthritis: a review of strengths and weaknesses of different imaging options. Rheum Dis Clin North Am. 2013;39(3):567–91.
30. Weber MA, Merle C, Rehnitz C, Gotterbarm T. Modern radiological imaging of osteoarthritis of the hip joint with consideration of predisposing conditions. RöFo - Fortschritte Auf Dem Geb Röntgenstrahlen Bildgeb Verfahr. 2016;188(07):635–51.
31. Bishi H, Smith JBV, Asopa V, Field RE, Wang C, Sochart DH. Comparison of the accuracy of 2D and 3D templating methods for planning primary total hip replacement: a systematic review and meta-analysis. EFORT Open Rev. 2022;7(1):70–83.
32. Roux CH, Mazieres B, Verrouil E, Rat AC, Fardellone P, Fautrel B, et al. Femoro-tibial knee osteoarthritis: one or two X-rays? Results from a population-based study. Joint Bone Spine. 2016;83(1):37–42.
33. Mamisch TC, Zilkens C, Siebenrock KA, Bittersohl B, Kim YJ, Werlen S. Hip MRI and its implications for surgery in osteoarthritis patients. Rheum Dis Clin N Am. 2009;35(3):591–604.
34. Kohli A, Xia S, Wells JE, Chhabra A. Three-dimensional CT and 3D MRI of hip- important aids to hip preservation surgery. Semin Ultrasound CT MR. 2023;44(4):252–70.
35. Loftus TJ, Tighe PJ, Filiberto AC, Efron PA, Brakenridge SC, Mohr AM, et al. Artificial intelligence and surgical decision-making. JAMA Surg. 2020;155(2):148–58.
36. Gurung B, Liu P, Harris PDR, Sagi A, Field RE, Sochart DH, et al. Artificial intelligence for image analysis in total hip and total knee arthroplasty: a scoping review. Bone Jt J. 2022;104-B(8):929–37.
37. McBride TJ, Prakash D. How to read a postoperative total hip replacement radiograph. Postgrad Med J. 2011;87(1024):101–9.
38. Borjali A, Chen AF, Muratoglu OK, Morid MA, Varadarajan KM. Detecting total hip replacement prosthesis design on plain radiographs using deep convolutional neural network. J Orthop Res. 2020;38(7):1465–71.
39. Ramkumar PN, Karnuta JM, Navarro SM, Haeberle HS, Iorio R, Mont MA, et al. Preoperative prediction of value metrics and a patient-specific payment model for primary total hip arthroplasty: development and validation of a deep learning model. J Arthroplasty. 2019;34(10):2228–2234.e1.
40. Xue Y, Zhang R, Deng Y, Chen K, Jiang T. A preliminary examination of the diagnostic value of deep learning in hip osteoarthritis. PLoS One. 2017;12(6):e0178992.
41. von Schacky CE, Sohn JH, Liu F, Ozhinsky E, Jungmann PM, Nardo L, et al. Development and validation of a multitask deep learning model for severity grading of hip osteoarthritis features on radiographs. Radiology. 2020;295(1):136–45.
42. Schwarz GM, Simon S, Mitterer JA, Huber S, Frank BJ, Aichmair A, et al. Can an artificial intelligence powered software reliably assess pelvic radiographs? Int Orthop. 2023;47(4):945–53.
43. Della Valle AG, Padgett DE, Salvati EA. Preoperative planning for primary total hip arthroplasty. J Am Acad Orthop Surg. 2005;13(7):455–62.
44. Efe T, El Zayat BF, Heyse TJ, Timmesfeld N, Fuchs-Winkelmann S, Schmitt J. Precision of preoperative digital templating in total hip arthroplasty. Acta Orthop Belg. 2011;77(5):616–21.
45. Gamble P, de Beer J, Petruccelli D, Winemaker M. The accuracy of digital templating in uncemented total hip arthroplasty. J Arthroplasty. 2010;25(4):529–32.
46. Carter LW, Stovall DO, Young TR. Determination of accuracy of preoperative templating of noncemented femoral prostheses. J Arthroplasty. 1995;10(4):507–13.
47. Asnis SE, Heller YY. Total hip arthroplasty templating: a simple method to correct for radiograph magnification. Orthopedics [Internet]. 2019 [citato 8 agosto 2023];42(3). Disponibile su: https://doi.org/10.3928/01477447-20190307-01
48. Unnanuntana A, Wagner D, Goodman SB. The accuracy of preoperative templating in cementless total hip arthroplasty. J Arthroplasty. 2009;24(2):180–6.
49. Wako Y, Nakamura J, Miura M, Kawarai Y, Sugano M, Nawata K. Interobserver and Intraobserver reliability of three-dimensional preoperative planning software in total hip arthroplasty. J Arthroplasty. 2018;33(2):601–7.

50. Mainard D, Barbier O, Knafo Y, Belleville R, Mainard-Simard L, Gross JB. Accuracy and reproducibility of preoperative three-dimensional planning for total hip arthroplasty using biplanar low-dose radiographs : a pilot study. Orthop Traumatol Surg Res OTSR. 2017;103(4):531–6.
51. Chu C, Chen C, Liu L, Zheng G. FACTS: fully automatic CT segmentation of a hip joint. Ann Biomed Eng. 2015;43(5):1247–59.
52. Zhou XY, Guo Y, Shen M, Yang GZ. Application of artificial intelligence in surgery. Front Med. 2020;14(4):417–30.
53. Wang Z, Meng Y, Weng F, Chen Y, Lu F, Liu X, et al. An effective CNN method for fully automated segmenting subcutaneous and visceral adipose tissue on CT scans. Ann Biomed Eng. 2020;48(1):312–28.
54. Chang Y, Yuan Y, Guo C, Wang Y, Cheng Y, Tamura S. Accurate pelvis and femur segmentation in hip CT with a novel patch-based refinement. IEEE J Biomed Health Inform. 2019;23(3):1192–204.
55. Kim JJ, Nam J, Jang IG. Fully automated segmentation of a hip joint using the patient-specific optimal thresholding and watershed algorithm. Comput Methods Programs Biomed. 2018;154:161–71.
56. Wang C, Connolly B, De Oliveira Lopes PF, Frangi AF, Smedby Ö. Pelvis segmentation using multi-pass U-net and iterative shape estimation. In: Vrtovec T, Yao J, Zheng G, Pozo JM, editors. Computational methods and clinical applications in musculoskeletal imaging [internet], Lecture Notes in Computer Science, vol. 11404. Cham: Springer International Publishing; 2019. p. 49–57. https://doi.org/10.1007/978-3-030-11166-3_5.
57. Wu D, Zhi X, Liu X, Zhang Y, Chai W. Utility of a novel integrated deep convolutional neural network for the segmentation of hip joint from computed tomography images in the preoperative planning of total hip arthroplasty. J Orthop Surg. 2022;17(1):164.
58. Chen X, Liu X, Wang Y, Ma R, Zhu S, Li S, et al. Development and validation of an artificial intelligence preoperative planning system for total hip arthroplasty. Front Med. 2022;9:841202.
59. Alastruey-López D, Ezquerra L, Seral B, Pérez MA. Using artificial neural networks to predict impingement and dislocation in total hip arthroplasty. Comput Methods Biomech Biomed Engin. 2020;23(10):649–57.
60. Birkhoff DC, van Dalen ASHM, Schijven MP. A review on the current applications of artificial intelligence in the operating room. Surg Innov. 2021;28(5):611–9.
61. Grupp RB, Unberath M, Gao C, Hegeman RA, Murphy RJ, Alexander CP, et al. Automatic annotation of hip anatomy in fluoroscopy for robust and efficient 2D/3D registration. Int J Comput Assist Radiol Surg. 2020;15(5):759–69.
62. Homma Y, Ito S, Zhuang X, Baba T, Fujibayashi K, Kaneko K, et al. Artificial intelligence for distinguishment of hammering sound in total hip arthroplasty. Sci Rep. 2022;12(1):9826.
63. Albano D, Gitto S, Messina C, Serpi F, Salvatore C, Castiglioni I, et al. MRI-based artificial intelligence to predict infection following total hip arthroplasty failure. Radiol Med (Torino). 2023;128(3):340–6.
64. Murphy MP, Killen CJ, Winfrey SR, Schmitt DR, Hopkinson WJ, Wu K, et al. Artificial intelligence autonomously measures cup orientation, corrects for pelvis orientation, and identifies retroversion from antero-posterior pelvis radiographs. J Arthroplasty. 2023;38(7 Suppl 2):S319–23.
65. Rouzrokh P, Ramazanian T, Wyles CC, Philbrick KA, Cai JC, Taunton MJ, et al. Deep learning artificial intelligence model for assessment of hip dislocation risk following primary total hip arthroplasty from postoperative radiographs. J Arthroplasty. 2021;36(6):2197–2203.e3.
66. Vail TP. Deep learning dramatically reduces the work associated with image cataloguing and analysis: commentary on an article by Pouria Rouzrokh, MD, MPH, MHPE, et al.: Applying deep learning to establish a total hip arthroplasty radiography registry. A stepwise approach. J Bone Joint Surg Am. 2022;104(18):e82.
67. Shah RF, Bini SA, Martinez AM, Pedoia V, Vail TP. Incremental inputs improve the automated detection of implant loosening using machine-learning algorithms. Bone Jt J. 2020;102-B(6_Supple_A):101–6.
68. Loppini M, Gambaro FM, Chiappetta K, Grappiolo G, Bianchi AM, Corino VDA. Automatic identification of failure in hip replacement: an artificial intelligence approach. Bioeng Basel Switz. 2022;9(7):288.
69. Kim MS, Kim JJ, Kang KH, Lee JH, In Y. Detection of prosthetic loosening in hip and knee arthroplasty using machine learning: a systematic review and meta-analysis. Med Kaunas Lith. 2023;59(4):782.
70. Zhang S, Chen JY, Pang HN, Lo NN, Yeo SJ, Liow MHL. Development and internal validation of machine learning algorithms to predict patient satisfaction after total hip arthroplasty. Arthroplasty. 2021;3(1):33.
71. Palazzo C, Jourdan C, Descamps S, Nizard R, Hamadouche M, Anract P, et al. Determinants of satisfaction 1 year after total hip arthroplasty: the role of expectations fulfilment. BMC Musculoskelet Disord. 2014;15(1):53.
72. Hamilton DF, Lane JV, Gaston P, Patton JT, MacDonald D, Simpson AHRW, et al. What determines patient satisfaction with surgery? A prospective cohort study of 4709 patients following total joint replacement. BMJ Open. 2013;3(4):e002525.
73. Siljander MP, McQuivey KS, Fahs AM, Galasso LA, Serdahely KJ, Karadsheh MS. Current trends in patient-reported outcome measures in total joint arthroplasty: a study of 4 major orthopaedic journals. J Arthroplasty. 2018;33(11):3416–21.
74. Mancuso CA, Salvati EA, Johanson NA, Peterson MGE, Charlson ME. Patients' expectations and satisfaction with total hip arthroplasty. J Arthroplasty. 1997;12(4):387–96.
75. Polus JS, Bloomfield RA, Vasarhelyi EM, Lanting BA, Teeter MG. Machine learning predicts the fall risk of

total hip arthroplasty patients based on wearable sensor instrumented performance tests. J Arthroplasty. 2021;36(2):573–8.
76. Anakwe RE, Jenkins PJ, Moran M. Predicting dissatisfaction after total hip arthroplasty: a study of 850 patients. J Arthroplasty. 2011;26(2):209–13.
77. Lo CWT, Tsang WWN, Yan CH, Lord SR, Hill KD, Wong AYL. Risk factors for falls in patients with total hip arthroplasty and total knee arthroplasty: a systematic review and meta-analysis. Osteoarthritis Cartilage. 2019;27(7):979–93.
78. Elliott S, Leland NE. Occupational therapy fall prevention interventions for community-dwelling older adults: a systematic review. Am J Occup Ther. 2018;72(4):7204190040p1–11.

6 Artificial Intelligence in Knee Arthroplasty

Enrico Bertugli, Sébastien Lustig, Sébastien Parratte, Fabio Catani, and Cécile Batailler

6.1 Introduction

This chapter aims to present the current concepts regarding artificial intelligence (AI) and explain its potential applications in knee arthroplasty. Many studies reporting the interest in AI-based tools in the orthopedic field have been published during the last few years, with the growing interest in AI-based tools in knee arthroplasty.

A literature review was conducted about the use of AI in knee arthroplasty up until May 2023. This research was done to identify available articles on the comprehensive clinical relevance of AI-based tools used before, during, and after knee arthroplasty. AI could become of paramount importance before knee arthroplasty (diagnosing, planning, and surgical training), during knee arthroplasty (surgical guidance, real-time assistance in intraoperative navigation), and postoperatively (analyzing clinical and radiological data from previous patients, predicting postoperative outcomes and monitoring patients remotely examining data such as gait, knee flexion angle, and recovery progress).

6.2 AI Before Knee Arthroplasty

AI has numerous preoperative applications that mainly concern the selection of the most appropriate diagnostic and therapeutic decision-making process for the patient. Moreover, AI can aid in the surgeon's training. From a clinical perspective, AI could allow greater diagnostic accuracy in conditions such as osteoarthritis and loosening, leading to more precise surgical indications. Furthermore, through specific algorithms, it enhances accuracy in preoperative planning, including determining the needed implant size, positioning, and identifying the implant in cases requiring revision surgery.

In terms of surgical education and training, it enables the use of augmented reality tools that allow surgeons to study anatomy and surgical techniques in an advanced manner. Surgeons can practice surgical steps and study complex cases without the surgical complications that may arise

E. Bertugli · F. Catani
Department of Orthopaedic Surgery, Azienda Ospedaliero-Universitaria Policlinico di Modena, University of Modena and Reggio-Emilia, Modena, Italy
e-mail: fabio.catani@unimore.it

S. Lustig · C. Batailler (✉)
Orthopaedic Surgery and Sports Medicine Department, Croix-Rousse Hospital, Lyon University Hospital, Lyon, France

Univ Lyon, Claude Bernard Lyon 1 University, IFSTTAR, LBMC UMR_T9406, Lyon, France

S. Parratte
International Knee and Joint Centre, Abu Dhabi, United Arab Emirates

Institute for Locomotion, Aix-Marseille University, Marseille, France

F. Familiari et al. (eds.), *Artificial Intelligence in Orthopaedic Surgery Made Easy*,
https://doi.org/10.1007/978-3-031-70310-2_6

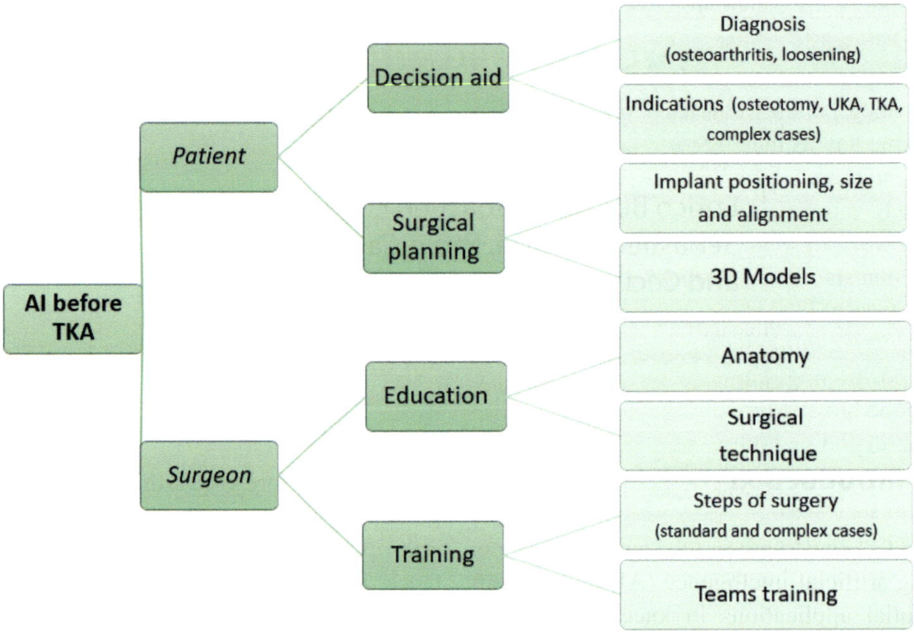

Fig. 6.1 Chart of the preoperative AI applications

during actual procedures on human beings (Fig. 6.1).

Ensuring appropriate *patient selection (diagnosis and indications)* is paramount for the success of knee arthroplasty. However, studies suggest that approximately 33% of patients may be inaccurately selected, leading to unsatisfactory outcomes [1]. The American Academy of Orthopedic Surgeons has developed practice guidelines and machine learning-based algorithms to address this issue. These algorithms aim to standardize the patient selection process by considering factors such as medical history, symptom severity, osteoarthritis severity, previous treatment failures, and more. The predictive algorithm models require effective communication between the patients and surgeons. Patient demographics, preoperative patient-reported outcome measurements (PROMs), preferences, values, and needs, as well as their knowledge about treatments, risks, benefits, and alternatives, are all relevant and validated predictive factors [1–3].

AI-based algorithms can assist in defining preoperative parameters, grading the *severity of knee osteoarthritis*, and reducing inter-observer variability. In revision knee arthroplasty, it can be used to diagnose *prosthetic loosening* on X-ray (with a precision of >95%) and *identify implant models* [4, 5]. Lau LCM et al. found that an image-based machine learning model can detect knee arthroplasty loosening with high accuracy and predictability, and the class activation heatmap can potentially assist surgeons in identifying the sites of loosening [6].

Navarro et al. demonstrated excellent validity in predicting *length of stay (LOS)* and cost before primary TKA [7, 8]. A recent study by Liu et al. focused on the development of a *hospital stay extension model*, which demonstrated a good performance in both the training and validation groups [9].

Kunze et al. described another efficient model with good discriminative capacity for identifying patients at greatest risk for *dissatisfaction* after TKA, and the most important predictors of dissatisfaction were age, number of medical comorbidities, presence of one or more drug allergies, preoperative patient-reported health state score, and preoperative KSS [10].

In 2021 Wei et al. used studied a model to determine the preoperative and perioperative variables that could predict *same-day discharge for TKA patients*. Using both ANN modeling and logistic regression analysis, the study identified clinically significant factors that could accurately predict which patients can safely be discharged on the same day as their TKA procedure (preoperative sodium, preoperative international normalized ratio, BMI, age, anesthesia type, operating time, dyspnea status, functional status, race, anemia status, and chronic obstructive pulmonary disease) [7, 11].

Surgical planning includes limb alignment, implant positioning, gap balancing, and implant size. Preoperatively, proper *TKA component size* can be predicted using formulas based on demographic data such as sex, height, weight, age, ethnicity, and shoe size.

Wallace et al. demonstrated that demographic-based multivariate linear regression models can be used to predict more accurate implant size than digitally-templated sizes for femoral ($P = 0.04$) and tibial ($P < 0.01$) components [12].

Also, Kunze et al. verified that ML algorithms can accurately predict the size of TKA components in real time [13]. An application to predict component size is freely accessible at the following link: https://orthopedics.shinyapps.io/TKASizing_Calculator/ [1].

A study by Klag et al. analyzed the difference in templating between 2D to 3D imaging technology and the 2D digital templating done by surgeons. The first one accurately predicted tibial and femoral component sizes compared to the latter. The improved accuracy of implant size predictions through the use of 3D templating technology has the potential to enhance intraoperative efficiency, reduce costs, and decrease surgical time [14].

In 2021, Farooq et al. conducted a study to determine the *optimal sagittal component position* in TKA. Using machine learning algorithms, the researchers predicted the likelihood of achieving higher levels of patient satisfaction, along with the knee "feeling normal", based on specific parameters. They found higher satisfaction levels with a tibial slope change closer to native (−2 to +2°) and a femoral component flexion of 0 to +7°. Poorer outcomes were predicted with any femoral component extension, femoral component flexion beyond +10°, and the addition or removal of >5° of the native tibial slope. The authors conducted a level III evidence study utilizing machine learning algorithms to identify the optimal sagittal position of the implant that could predict the most favorable outcomes [7, 15].

Surgeons' education and training are traditionally performed on real patients in the operating room and supervised by senior surgeons. This is undergoing substantial change with AI development. Extended reality technologies allow surgeons to visualize patient-specific anatomy in real time, improving preoperative planning and providing valuable guidance during surgery [16]. Surgeons can benefit from extended reality technologies by assessing implant choices and placement, monitoring procedural errors and efficiency, and reducing overall completion time. By incorporating technical and cognitive practices, surgeons can minimize implant malalignment and surgical complications in primary and revision knee arthroplasty procedures [1]. Using the assistive mode, the surgeon can obtain feedback on key steps (planning bone resection, implant positioning, sizing, assessing the virtual range of motion, and gap balancing) to anticipate difficulties or achieve a surgical target.

Augmented reality and Virtual reality offer a way for medical professionals to enhance their skills in doing TKA and revising TKA by simulating various clinical settings, which shifts the learning curve [17]. The surgeons can obtain learning experience without direct supervision and collect data all along the training process. Replicating real-life procedures through virtual simulations eliminates the risks associated with injuries and the need for costly resources like cadavers. However, there are certain drawbacks to consider, such as limited image quality, the potential for cyber-sickness, device-related challenges (e.g., battery capacity and wireless technology), and considerations regarding the cost-benefit ratio [1].

6.3 AI During Knee Arthroplasty

AI provides a range of important possibilities during TKA. In particular, it allows for proper positioning and alignment of the implant through the analysis of numerous factors, including anatomical data, balancing of soft tissues, bone preservation, and especially intraoperative feedback (image-based, augmented reality, or robotic-assisted) (Fig. 6.2).

Robotic-assisted knee arthroplasty is defined as a machine capable of automatically carrying out complex actions. This system integrates information from preoperative imaging or intraoperative surface mapping, specific bone landmarks (bone shape, tibial and femoral alignment), and the ligament balancing intraoperatively.

There are three categories of robotic systems: passive, semi-autonomous, and autonomous.

A *passive system* provides a 3D virtual model allowing accurate preoperative planning but does not prepare the bone.

The *autonomous* and semi-autonomous systems incorporate safeguards against bone removal beyond the 3D plane.

The *semi-autonomous* robotic-assisted system combines the benefits of a navigation system and an autonomous robotic system and is a typical example of an AI-based tool. The collected data include bone and implant alignment algorithms and soft-tissue balance to propose surgical planning, secondarily adjusted according to the surgeon's requests and targets. A robotic arm allows performing bone resections or positioning a cutting guide with a real-time automatic feedback system following knee movements or cut progression.

A widespread example of a semi-autonomous robotic-assisted system is the Mako System, robotic-assisted THA, and TKA (Mako Surgical Corp. [Stryker], Fort Lauderdale, Florida). The system utilizes three elements: pre-op 3D CT-based planning and image-based intra-op navigation, pre-resection implant modifications with integrated alignment, implant position and gap data, and a semi-constrained robotic arm-assisted execution of bone resection with "haptic" boundaries. The Mako System allows for improved implant placement utilizing CT guidance, bone resection accuracy, and flex-

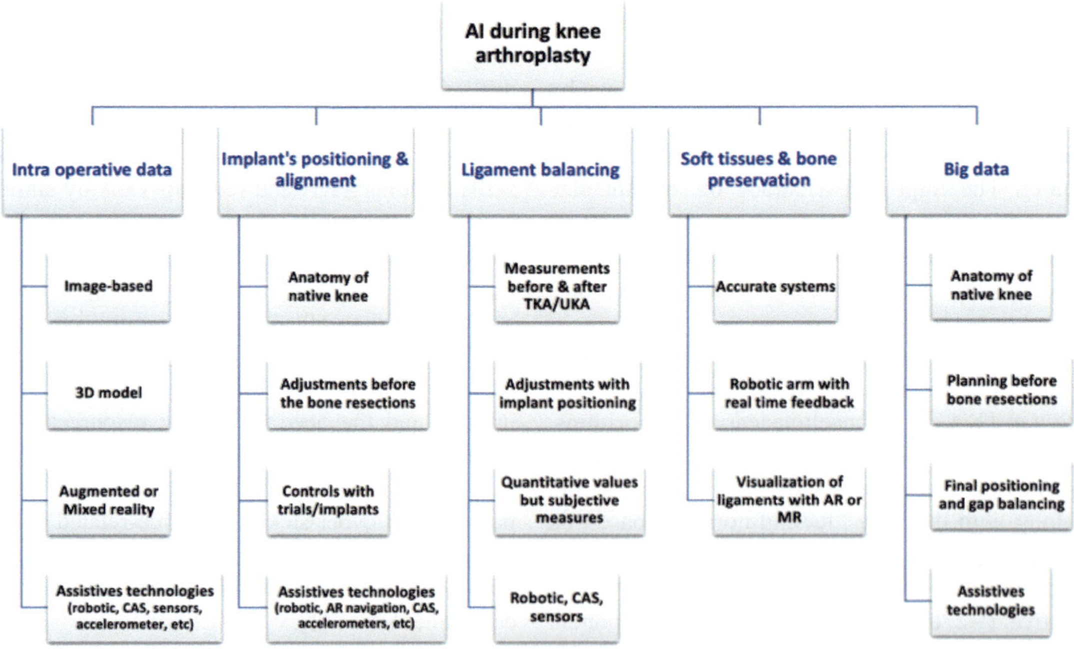

Fig. 6.2 Structure chart presenting the intraoperative features of AI tools

ibility for functional implant placement with gap balancing [18].

Progressively, the algorithms of robotic systems integrate machine learning models to improve surgical planning according to the previous surgery. During surgery, a *feedback loop* is created when bone cutting is controlled, or the cutting guide is positioned (Fig. 6.3). This control improves the surgeon's accuracy and decreases the risk of errors. The robotic systems aim not to replace surgeons but to be an accurate and consistent delivery tool. The major benefit of robotic systems is accurate and reproducible bone preparation thanks to the robotic interface, regardless of the system used [1, 19]. Most currently available robotic platforms assess ligament balancing according to intraoperative bone cutting and implant positioning. Therefore, implementing robotics in TKA ensures a patient-specific alignment path by enhancing the understanding of intraoperative gap geometry [20].

There are several limitations associated with robotic-assisted TKA. These include the need for significant capital investment and ongoing expenses for operating room consumables. Additionally, surgeons and staff require extensive education to ensure robotics's safe and efficient utilization. Using specific hardware with bony trackers and a bulky robotic unit may prove impractical in certain cases. Furthermore, robotic-assisted TKA often requires longer operative times and necessitates a learning curve for the surgical team. Moreover, a robotic system is usually compatible only with one type of implant. The laxity assessment at the beginning of surgery is manual and thus lacks accuracy [1].

Augmented reality-based navigation systems superimpose clinical information into the surgeon's sight and have been developed to guide TKA implantation. Augmented reality platforms require three processes: tracking, computing, and visualization.

Tracking of object position is achieved by contact, semi-contact, and contactless methods. The semi-contact system involves attachment to the anatomy and marker and a contactless link between the features and cameras. The marker's 3D positions are used to triangulate the marker's 2D position in each camera of the optical system. Contactless systems are still to be developed. Tracking is done without the need for attachment to the object or patient and has been made possible with the apparition of depth cameras. Depth cameras are active sensors that project a structured light pattern onto a scene, creating a pattern used to reconstruct the 3D surface of the object.

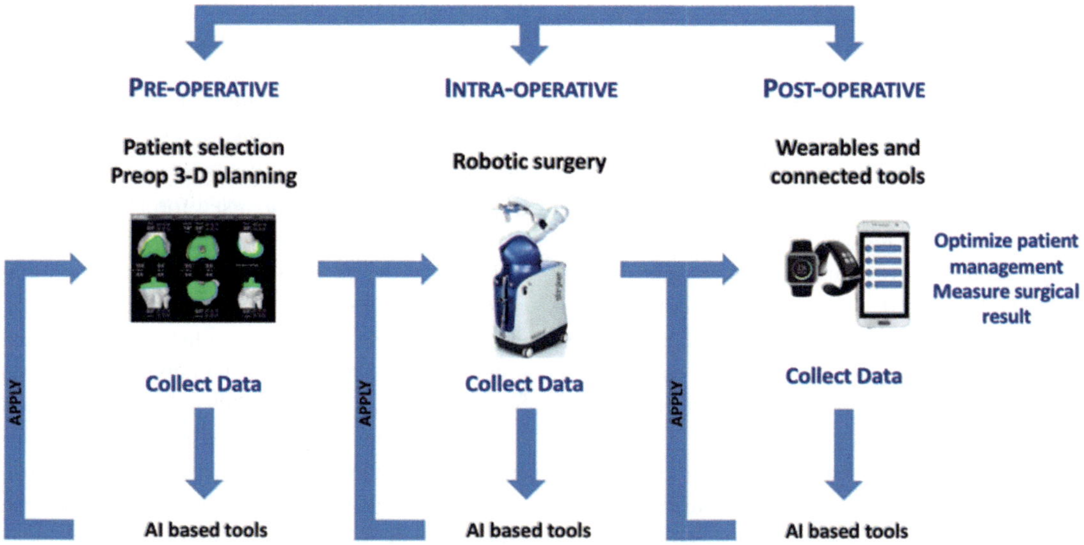

Fig. 6.3 Graphic explanation of the Feedback Loop: data collection (before, during, and after surgery) via the connected tools to create mega data information for adjusting the surgical plan

Computing requires two operations: the first is to register the anatomical features tracked with the preoperative images. The second is to compute the clinical index from raw information, which compares the actual situation with the preoperative plan. By assessing the actual situation against the initial plan, surgeons can identify any deviations or variations that may have occurred during the procedure.

The final step is *visualization* which produces an image for the user. In augmented reality, the digital image must align with the surgeons' reality. Augmented reality technology helps the surgeon focus on the patient by directly overlaying feedback information into the surgical field. Compared to the robotic-assisted systems, the advantages of augmented reality platforms are a smaller physical footprint, a lower cost (no capital investment), the ability to have the intraoperative data in the same field of view, the absence of intraosseous trackers, and an easier workflow [1].

The Pixee Medical system is a computer-assisted orthopedic surgery solution using AR to support TKA (Pixee Medical, Besancon, France). The software installed in smart glasses is combined with minimally invasive surgical instrumentation. The connected glasses precisely calculate the 3D coordinates of the instruments thanks to the analysis of their specific markers (QR-Code), filmed by the integrated camera. The navigation information is displayed in the surgeon's field of view, which interacts with the application thanks to the glasses' accelerometers.

The NextAR™ system (Medacta, Castel San Pietro, Switzerland), another AR-based navigation system for TKA, requires sensors anchored to the femur and tibia using pins inserted within the surgical wound. A preoperative plan is generated based on CT imaging and a dedicated algorithm to identify ligament origin and insertion to monitor balance during intraoperative navigation.

Fucentese et al. presented a novel augmented reality-based surgical guidance system for TKA (GMK Efficiency, Medacta International SA, Castel San Pietro, Switzerland) in which, before any bone resection, the resting length of the collateral ligaments was acquired with the knee in full extension, to be used as a reference for the rest of the procedure. Compensating for cartilage wear while acquiring the resting length can indicate the native length of the collateral ligaments. This novel approach allows for a 3-dimensional assessment of the effect of each planning parameter on ligament contracture and elongation. In particular, the impact of tibia rotation can be adequately evaluated. A qualitative assessment of the measurements obtained with the system on cadaveric specimens has confirmed that the results are in line with the pattern of collateral ligament elongation measured in vivo for the same implant in another published study [21].

Tsukada et al. reviewed 11 consecutive unicompartmental knee arthroplasties performed using an AR-based portable navigation system for proximal tibial resection. The extramedullary tibial cutting guide of the AR-based navigation system carries two markers with Quick Response (QR) codes. The extramedullary tibial cutting guide of the AR-based navigation system was set on the patient's lower leg, similar to the standard cutting guide. The absolute differences between the preoperative target resection angles and postoperative measured angles were 1.9° ± 1.5° in coronal alignment and 2.6° ± 1.2° in sagittal alignment. This study could not conclusively demonstrate the clinical effectiveness of the AR-based navigation system [22].

To the best of our knowledge, the majority of studies involve cadaveric research, with only a few isolated cases of augmented reality (AR) or mixed reality (MR) being used for TKA [23].

Despite the increasing media attention surrounding these devices, their impact on patient outcomes and cost-effectiveness still lacks clear evidence. It is crucial to conduct well-designed clinical studies to evaluate the benefits and drawbacks of these technologies to make informed decisions about their implementation in healthcare settings. Continued research and publication of clinical studies are necessary to understand the effectiveness and value of these novel devices comprehensively.

6.4 AI After Knee Arthroplasty

Remote patient monitoring (RPM) through smartphones enables the collection of continuous subjective and objective data during the postoperative period. RPM is a system that relies on network-enabled connectivity and includes interconnected computing devices, mechanical devices, digital machines, and objects. Each entity is assigned unique identifiers (UIDs) and can transfer data over a network autonomously, eliminating the need for direct human-to-human or human-to-computer interaction [24]. A machine learning-based remote patient monitoring system has been developed using an open-source software development kit designed for smartphones [1]. These devices enable real-time tracking of patient engagement in physical therapy and home exercise programs through their smartphones. This allows the surgical team to monitor and assess their rehabilitation progress. If patients are not meeting the expected postoperative milestones, the surgical team can intervene by scheduling additional clinic visits or making phone calls to provide necessary support and guidance. These devices have advanced machine learning capabilities, allowing the software to automate processes through AI principles, probability theory, statistical physics, data mining, and pattern recognition from empirical data. Kurtz et al. found that TKA patients were highly receptive to using wearable technology in their treatments, whereas nonoperative OA knee patients were generally unreceptive [25].

A study by Li L. focused on postoperative rehabilitation of knee joint injuries. The results showed that, compared with traditional methods, the rehabilitation training method based on AR showed strong advantages in alleviating postoperative pain and helping structural and functional recovery [26].

Predictive models and machine learning can be used to estimate *postoperative improvement and patient satisfaction* and to learn for future patient and surgeon decision-making. The increasing availability of extensive digital healthcare datasets has enabled the advancement of PM in postoperative outcomes following TKA. These PMs analyze a wide range of variables, including patient-specific characteristics, functional scores, preoperative pain, comorbidities, psychological features, socioeconomic indicators, and the location of perioperative recovery. They aim to understand how these factors influence clinical outcomes and improve the prediction of postoperative results after TKA.

The main preoperative predictive factors described in the literature for the postoperative outcomes after TKA are pain scores (VAS and back pain), knee-specific PROMs (such as KOOS and WOMAC), range of motion, quality of life PROMs (EQ-5D) and mental health (assessed by anxiety and depression scales and SF-12) [1]. Other factors that have also been evaluated are comorbidities (ASA score), demographic data (such as BMI, sex age), previous knee surgery, the severity of osteoarthritis, and preoperative knee alignment [1].

Constructing a reliable data set is a significant challenge when using PM in healthcare. The accuracy of PM in evaluating postoperative outcomes based on preoperative parameters heavily relies on the quality of the initial data set. It is crucial for the initial data set to represent the patient population for which the PM will be employed.

To enhance the reliability of PM, utilizing data from large populations and incorporating objective preoperative 3D anatomy assessment is recommended. The PM can yield more accurate predictions and insights by leveraging extensive data sets and comprehensive anatomical evaluations. In contrast, relying on limited data sets may introduce biases and limitations, potentially compromising the reliability and effectiveness of the PM system. Therefore, utilizing data from larger populations and incorporating objective preoperative assessments enhances the strength and reliability of PM applications [1].

To the best of our knowledge, none of the currently available PM systems have successfully replicated the clinical understanding of surgeons or become practical tools for clinical use. While PM holds great potential in healthcare, it is important to acknowledge that it has not yet reached a stage where it can fully replace or replicate the expertise and judgment of skilled clinicians.

Significant apprehensions arise regarding AI bias. If the data used to train AI systems contain any form of bias, it can lead to pervasive and systematic analytical errors.

Finally, the next challenge will be to *"close the loop"* using accurate interconnected data sets and predictive monitoring during the above-mentioned phases (before, during, and after knee arthroplasty) to help surgeons and healthcare providers in their decision-making (Fig. 6.3).

The ultimate goal is to promote collaborative decision-making between healthcare professionals and AI-based tools, combining the expertise of doctors with the capabilities of artificial intelligence. This approach, known as *collaborative intelligence*, aims to optimize patient management by leveraging predictive models and clinical experience to enhance surgical outcomes for every individual.

6.5 Conclusions

Knee arthroplasty benefits from the integration of AI-based tools, which enhance the decision-making process, surgical planning, and the precision and consistency of surgical procedures. Collaborative intelligence aims to optimize patient management by leveraging predictive models and clinical experience to enhance surgical outcomes. It is important to note that the implementation of collaborative intelligence requires ongoing research, validation, and refinement of AI algorithms, as well as appropriate regulations and ethical considerations to maintain patient safety, privacy, and trust in the healthcare system.

The final goal is to exploit data and connected devices so that surgeons can make more informed decisions, adjust surgical plans, and improve patient outcomes based on a deeper understanding of the complexities involved in individual cases.

References

1. Batailler C, Shatrov J, Sappey-Marinier E, Servien E, Parratte S, Lustig S. Artificial intelligence in knee arthroplasty: current concept of the available clinical applications. Arthroplasty. 2022;4:17.
2. Hawker GA, Bohm E, Dunbar MJ, Faris P, Jones CA, Noseworthy T, Ravi B, Woodhouse LJ, Marshall DA. Patient appropriateness for total knee arthroplasty and predicted probability of a good outcome. RMD Open. 2023;9:e002808.
3. Noonan VK, Lyddiatt A, Ware P, et al. Montreal accord on patient-reported outcomes (PROs) use series - paper 3: patient-reported outcomes can facilitate shared decision-making and guide self-management. J Clin Epidemiol. 2017;89:125–35.
4. Yi PH, Wei J, Kim TK, Sair HI, Hui FK, Hager GD, Fritz J, Oni JK. Automated detection & classification of knee arthroplasty using deep learning. Knee. 2020;27:535–42.
5. Klemt C, Uzosike AC, Cohen-Levy WB, Harvey MJ, Subih MA, Kwon Y-M. The ability of deep learning models to identify total hip and knee arthroplasty implant design from plain radiographs. J Am Acad Orthop Surg. 2022;30:409–15.
6. Lau LCM, Chui ECS, Man GCW, Xin Y, Ho KKW, Mak KKK, Ong MTY, Law SW, Cheung WH, Yung PSH. A novel image-based machine learning model with superior accuracy and predictability for knee arthroplasty loosening detection and clinical decision making. J Orthop Translat. 2022;36:177–83.
7. Rodríguez-Merchán EC. The current role of the virtual elements of artificial intelligence in total knee arthroplasty. EFORT Open Rev. 2022;7:491–7.
8. Navarro SM, Wang EY, Haeberle HS, Mont MA, Krebs VE, Patterson BM, Ramkumar PN. Machine learning and primary total knee arthroplasty: patient forecasting for a patient-specific payment model. J Arthroplast. 2018;33:3617–23.
9. Liu B, Ma Y, Zhou C, Wang Z, Zhang Q. A novel predictive model of hospital stay for total knee arthroplasty patients. Front Surg. 2022;9:807467.
10. Kunze KN, Polce EM, Sadauskas AJ, Levine BR. Development of machine learning algorithms to predict patient dissatisfaction after primary total knee arthroplasty. J Arthroplast. 2020;35:3117–22.
11. Wei C, Quan T, Wang KY, et al. Artificial neural network prediction of same-day discharge following primary total knee arthroplasty based on preoperative and intraoperative variables. Bone Joint J. 2021;103-B:1358–66.
12. Wallace SJ, Murphy MP, Schiffman CJ, Hopkinson WJ, Brown NM. Demographic data is more predictive of component size than digital radiographic templating in total knee arthroplasty. Knee Surg Relat Res. 2020;32:63.
13. Kunze KN, Polce EM, Patel A, Courtney PM, Levine BR. Validation and performance of a machine-

learning derived prediction guide for total knee arthroplasty component sizing. Arch Orthop Trauma Surg. 2021;141:2235–44.
14. Klag EA, Lizzio VA, Charters MA, Ayoola AS, Wesemann L, Banka TR, North WT. Increased accuracy in templating for total knee arthroplasty using 3D models generated from radiographs. J Knee Surg. 2022;36:837. https://doi.org/10.1055/s-0042-1743496.
15. Farooq H, Deckard ER, Arnold NR, Meneghini RM. Machine learning algorithms identify optimal sagittal component position in total knee arthroplasty. J Arthroplast. 2021;36:S242–9.
16. Goh GS, Lohre R, Parvizi J, Goel DP. Virtual and augmented reality for surgical training and simulation in knee arthroplasty. Arch Orthop Trauma Surg. 2021;141:2303–12.
17. Mandal P, Ambade R. Surgery training and simulation using virtual and augmented reality for knee arthroplasty. Cureus. 14:e28823.
18. M R. The MAKO robotic-arm knee arthroplasty system. Arch Orthop Trauma Surg. 2021;141:2043. https://doi.org/10.1007/s00402-021-04208-0.
19. Batailler C, Fernandez A, Swan J, Servien E, Haddad FS, Catani F, Lustig S. MAKO CT-based robotic arm-assisted system is a reliable procedure for total knee arthroplasty: a systematic review. Knee Surg Sports Traumatol Arthrosc. 2021;29:3585–98.
20. von Eisenhart-Rothe R, Hinterwimmer F, Graichen H, Hirschmann MT. Artificial intelligence and robotics in TKA surgery: promising options for improved outcomes? Knee Surg Sports Traumatol Arthrosc. 2022;30:2535–7.
21. Fucentese SF, Koch PP. A novel augmented reality-based surgical guidance system for total knee arthroplasty. Arch Orthop Trauma Surg. 2021;141:2227–33.
22. Tsukada S, Ogawa H, Kurosaka K, Saito M, Nishino M, Hirasawa N. Augmented reality-aided unicompartmental knee arthroplasty. J Exp Orthop. 2022;9:88.
23. Su S, Lei P, Wang C, Gao F, Zhong D, Hu Y. Mixed reality technology in total knee arthroplasty: an updated review with a preliminary case report. Front Surg. 2022;9:804029.
24. Myers TG, Ramkumar PN, Ricciardi BF, Urish KL, Kipper J, Ketonis C. Artificial intelligence and orthopaedics. J Bone Joint Surg Am. 2020;102:830–40.
25. Kurtz SM, Higgs GB, Chen Z, Koshut WJ, Tarazi JM, Sherman AE, McLean SG, Mont MA. Patient perceptions of wearable and smartphone technologies for remote outcome monitoring in total knee arthroplasties. J Knee Surg. 2022;36:1253. https://doi.org/10.1055/s-0042-1755378.
26. Li L. Effect of remote control augmented reality multimedia technology for postoperative rehabilitation of knee joint injury. Comput Math Methods Med. 2022;2022:9320063.

7 Artificial Intelligence in Shoulder Arthroplasty

Edward G. McFarland, Piotr Łukasiewicz, and Sarah I. Goldfarb

7.1 Introduction

The rapid growth of artificial intelligence (AI) has been extended to applications that include a variety of issues regarding total shoulder arthroplasty (TSA). ChatGPT itself, when queried by Michael King, MD, at Vanderbilt [1] concluded that "The potential of AI in surgery is truly exciting. We can expect to see AI being used in increasingly sophisticated ways to assist with surgical procedures and improve patient outcomes. The excitement over what AI can potentially accomplish in medicine in general and also in shoulder arthroplasty is certainly on the rise."

AI has already had an impact on several areas of clinical practice, but the applications clinically for shoulder arthroplasty are only in their infancy. Areas of study of AI include risk prediction and patient outcomes of shoulder arthroplasty [2]; prediction of healthcare costs associated with shoulder arthroplasty [3]; the technology of image recognition [4] to identify the type and manufacturer of shoulder implants that have been implanted in the patient's shoulder [1]; and how AI can interface with robotic assistance, virtual reality and "force-space navigation" [5] (device navigation using force feedback). On the academic side, there is also hope that AI will be instrumental in translational research, but ChatGPT's response to an editorial by Douglas Mann, MD, was that "while AI has the potential to be a useful tool in the field of translational medicine, it is unlikely to be the future of this field" [6].

7.2 Clinical Applications

For clinicians, the bottom line is how AI can assist in procuring better clinical results for patients. Ideally, AI could assist in the clinic, where the history and results of the examination would become part of deep knowledge. Interpretations of radiographic studies (including radiographs, computed tomography, magnetic resonance imaging, and bone scans) and laboratory studies (sedimentation rates, C-reactive protein, blood cell types and counts, joint fluid aspirates, and histological studies) could also be processed.

However, the use of AI with the needed degree of accuracy clinically for all of these purposes is far from a reality at this point, as all of these tasks depend upon the data available at the time of the analysis. Few issues in shoulder arthroplasty exhibit homogeneity of the disease process and data good enough to make concrete conclusions about the pathophysiology, clinical evaluation,

E. G. McFarland (✉) · P. Łukasiewicz
S. I. Goldfarb
Division of Shoulder and Elbow Surgery, Department of Orthopedic Surgery, The Johns Hopkins University School of Medicine, Baltimore, MD, USA
e-mail: emcfarl1@jhmi.edu

F. Familiari et al. (eds.), *Artificial Intelligence in Orthopaedic Surgery Made Easy*,
https://doi.org/10.1007/978-3-031-70310-2_7

diagnosis, surgical interventions, and subsequent results of shoulder arthroplasty. As other authors have noted, this is the conundrum of AI: its ability to collate large amounts of information and look for patterns not discernable by researchers but yield results that are only as accurate as the available scientific evidence. While AI may use models to collate the data, the consensus is that the aphorism "garbage in, garbage out" applies to reliance on current literature regarding shoulder arthroplasty.

Another challenge to the clinical application of AI-derived information is the current variation in how the data are processed. A study by Kumar et al. [7] evaluated the accuracy of three different machine-learning techniques for their ability to predict clinical outcomes of patients who underwent either primary anatomic TSA (aTSA) (N = 1895) or primary reverse TSA (rTSA) (N = 2887). Each of these models was asked to predict clinical outcomes using 291 data points for each patient. The implants were from one manufacturer, and all patients had preoperative and postoperative clinical evaluations from one of 30 different surgeons [8]. The three different models were machine-learning techniques linear regression, XGBoost [9], and Wide and Deep [10].

There was little difference in prediction accuracy for each machine-learning technique. The lower absolute error for every measure demonstrated that the Wide and Deep model had the highest accuracy, followed by XGBoost. The most predictive feature of clinical results in all three models was the length of time from surgery. Of the patient-reported outcome measures, the Shoulder and Pain Disability Index (SPADI) and American Shoulder and Elbow Surgeons (ASES) scores, along with four preoperative measures of range of motion, were highly predictive, as were whether it was the dominant arm, whether the sex was female, and whether the patient had had previous surgery [7].

In the study by Kumar et al., the authors delineate a number of issues with the use of AI when considering clinical studies, warning that "the generalizability of any predictive model is limited by the quality of the underlying data" [7]. The authors point out that the usual demographic information, clinical features of the cohort, and any other data points should be delineated in any clinical study. This study by Kumar et al. also analyzed patients from a large database, from which 1428 were excluded for a variety of reasons, creating a bias similar to that seen in some published clinical studies. Not all data points were present for all patients, which also plagues clinical studies, and the study did not include patients with other diagnoses, such as revision, short stem, fracture, and humeral resurfacing implant. Predictive models also should account for whether the implants studied include aTSA, rTSA, or both. Finally, the modeling process and strategy in any study using AI should be reported so that there is complete transparency and so that it can be determined if the modeling is appropriate. Forsberg suggests that in the future any coding or test data be available to readers and that the models and algorithms used in publications be open and transparent [8].

AI has also been used to predict patient satisfaction and clinical improvement after aTSA and rTSA [11, 12]. Polce et al. used supervised machine learning (SML) in a retrospective study of 413 patients, of whom 331 (83%) were satisfied at 2 years [11]. The authors used Guidelines for Developing and Reporting Machine Learning Predictive Models in Biomedical Research [13] in their analysis and found that the five best predictor variables for postoperative satisfaction that were used in the machine-learning models were baseline Single Assessment Numeric Evaluation (SANE) score, preoperative exercise and activity, insurance status, diagnosis, and preoperative duration of symptoms. The study also revealed that patients with higher preoperative SANE scores actually scored lower in the likelihood of satisfaction, probably because they had a higher physical function at baseline, and that patients who had had symptoms for over 2 years prior to surgery were more likely to report that they were satisfied after surgery. However, the authors acknowledged that only 30% of patients responded to the satisfaction question and the postoperative patient-reported outcome measures. Consequently, they commented that the study should be considered an indication of the possible utility of SML in clinical studies in the future.

7.3 Length of Stay and Economic Studies

Other uses of AI in shoulder arthroplasty have been in studies of factors related to patient length of stay [2, 3, 14], discharge readmission rates to the hospital [15], and inpatient costs of shoulder arthroplasty [3]. Machine learning was used by Gowd et al. to predict the total healthcare cost of primary aTSA and rTSA in the Nationwide Readmissions Database [16]. The authors found that readmissions were the major contributor to perioperative costs, others being hospital characteristics such as volume of shoulder arthroplasty cases and the geographic area of the hospital. Arvind et al. studied five different machine-learning techniques to determine which variables were best at predicting readmission within 30 days [15]. They found that using a Random Forest algorithm [17], readmission could be predicted with five variables: high bilirubin (>1.9 mg/dL), age > 65 years, race, presence of chronic obstructive pulmonary disease, and American Society of Anesthesiologists score of ≥3 [15]. Also using the National Readmissions Database, Karnuta et al. [3] studied which artificial neural networks could accurately predict total cost, length of stay, and disposition for both chronic/degenerative lesions and acute/traumatic conditions. They found that the machine learning using a "neural network development" (Fig. 7.1) predicted accuracy and area under the curve (AUC) of 76.5% and 70.3, respectively, for total cost; accuracy of 91.8% and AUC of 0.89 for length of stay; and accuracy of 72% and AUC of 0.79 for discharge disposition [3]. They concluded that AI has the potential to predict for patients and providers the inpatient and outpatient costs of TSA and "expectation management between health care providers, patients, and payers" [3].

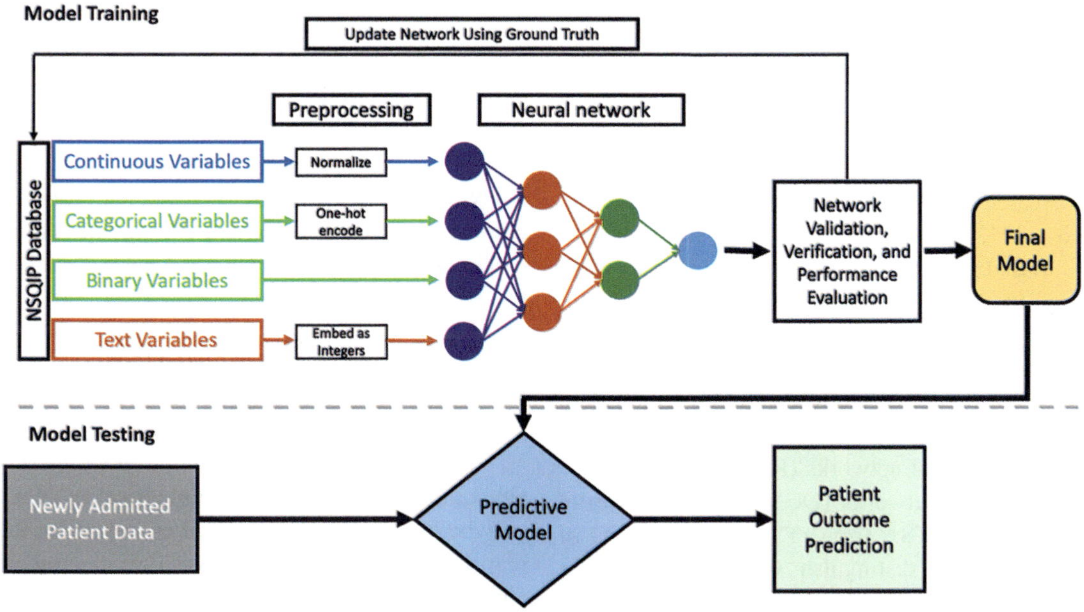

Fig. 7.1 Diagram depicting the pathway of data processing and outcome prediction using machine learning modeling. This study has used this process for final model development, although external testing and outcome prediction remains as a future step. Reproduced with permission from Karnuta et al. 2020, p. 2388 [3]

7.4 Implant Recognition

An area that has received attention has been the use of AI for recognizing the types of shoulder implants when the prosthesis has failed, which requires identification of the implant when it is to be removed. This is important, as shoulder arthroplasties performed in the past 30 years are now failing due to implant loosening. For aTSA, the estimated survival rates (95% confidence interval [CI]) were 97% (92%–100%) at 5 years, 97% (91%–100%) at 10 years, and 84% (71%–98%) at 15 years, and 83.2% (70.5%–97.8%) at 20 years [18, 19]. For rTSA, implant survival without reoperation (95% confidence interval [CI]) was 97.3% (96%–98%) at 5 years, 95.3% (93%–97%) at 10 years, and 94.1% (91%–96%) at 15 years [20]. As a result, the necessity for revision of shoulder arthroplasties has become increasingly acute. Along with this is the need to be able to identify the type of device and the manufacturer in order to have the proper instrumentation and equipment for implant removal. A survey of knee arthroplasty surgeons found that it took a median time of 20 min per case to identify the implant components and that 10% of the implants could not be identified at all [21]. This inability to identify components was speculated to result in increased operating room time due to lack of proper instrumentation; increased morbidity, including increased blood and bone loss; increased surgical complexity; and increased costs [21, 22].

Based on these findings, several studies were performed with the intent of using deep learning or AI to facilitate the identification of shoulder arthroplasty using plain radiographs [22–25]. Many of these studies were highly technical in nature. For example, the study by Yi et al. [24] utilized residual networks (ResNet) deep convoluted neural networks (DCNN) to successfully differentiate aTSA from rTSA with an AUC of 0.97 but could distinguish, with class activation map (CAM) analysis, a Stryker Solar shoulder arthroplasty (AUC of 0.86). As part of the analysis, "heat maps" through class activation mapping (CAM) were employed to determine if the DCNN was actually learning to discern the arthroplasty from other "confounding objects in the image."

Yi et al. [24] evaluated only five shoulder arthroplasty models; other studies of the ability of AI to distinguish the different types and manufacturers of shoulder arthroplasty share a similar concern. An "IMFC-Net model" of only four different prostheses was investigated by Sultan et al. [24], who reported an accuracy of 89% and a precision rate of 90%. X-rays of four different manufacturers and 16 different models were analyzed by Urban et al. [22], who found that deep learning was able to identify the correct manufacturer of the different implants approximately 80% of the time. Finally, Kunze et al. [21] studied 22 different aTSAs and rTSAs from 8 implant manufacturers. They reported an accuracy of 97%, but in a subset of implants used at their institution the accuracy was 99.4% and the sensitivity was over 0.97. While these results are encouraging, their clinical application has not been studied, so it is not known whether they produce any measurable benefit; from a clinical point of view, anything short of 100% accuracy would be a disappointment. Finally, because the studies are limited to the number and variety of implants included, generalizability may not be as broad. Another issue is the ability of AI to recognize both anatomic and reverse TSAs, as there are at least over 45 types of each on the market in past or current use. The ability to identify this many prostheses will be a challenge for AI, although the rapidity of change in this field may make this possible much sooner than expected.

7.5 AI and Robotics and Virtual, Augmented, and Mixed Reality

One of the more clinically important values of AI may be its use in the area of robotics and virtual reality. Robotic systems have the theoretical advantages of accurate and precise osteotomies and preparation of the glenoid for the glenoid component of aTSA and the baseplate of rTSA. While not yet as developed in shoulder arthroplasty as in total knee arthroplasty, AI has the potential also to aid in the modeling of soft tissue balance around the joint. There has been significant interest in patient-specific instrumentation (PSI), which can be used to place the components more accurately. Iannotti et al. demonstrated that when using PSI, the risks of malpositioning of the glenoid version and inclination were reduced by 90% and 96%, respectively [26]. Custom glenoid components that closely match the anatomy of the glenoid can now be manufactured [27].

AI also has the potential to assist in the use of virtual, augmented, and mixed-reality applications when performing shoulder arthroplasty [5]. Virtual reality is the technology that involves a computer-generated environment within which the surgeon performs the procedure. In augmented reality, the superimposition of an image onto the real-world anatomy by the surgeon is used to guide the procedure on the screen [28]. Augmented reality has the potential to be used for training but also intraoperatively. Mixed-reality systems have the same images as augmented reality but also use a hologram to provide better depth perception and navigation [5].

The growth and use of these technologies will increase once it is proven that they are accurate and warrant the time and expense necessary for their implementation. Smith et al. [29] compared the accuracy of a robotic system to that of an experienced shoulder surgeon. The study was performed on saw bones, so there were no soft tissue constraints. They found that the errors for the robot were 2.16 mm for implant position and 2.89 mm for orientation for both the standard shoulder model and the B2 glenoid implant. For the surgeon, errors for the standard shoulder were 1.6 mm and 5.04 mm for implant position and orientation, respectively; for the B2 glenoid, errors were 3.01 mm and 4.54 mm for position and orientation, respectively.

The study of the use of these novel technologies clinically is hindered by several limitations. Similar to studies in the hip and knee literature, although more accurate, replacement of the components has not been proven to be of any clinical significance when used for shoulder replacement surgery. While accurate positioning of the glenoid component, the humeral component, and baseplates are important from an engineering point of view, complex biological systems with bony, ligamentous, and muscular contributions to motion are difficult to include in any modeling of joint kinematics and kinetics. The error of several millimeters when positioning a component may make no difference in the clinical result. Finally, the time and the cost of these devices will need to be considered.

7.6 The Future of AI in Shoulder Arthroplasty

While there currently is enthusiasm for the application of AI to shoulder surgery, there are several cautions regarding its use and implementation. First, it has been noted by many observers that the shoulder presents challenges to understanding the anatomy, biomechanics, and examination findings; distinguishing normal from symptomatic lesions; and interpreting radiologic studies. The pathophysiology of rotator cuff disease remains unknown so that predicting who warrants arthroplasty surgery and who does not has yet to be determined. The variables that indicate who should have nonoperative vs surgical treatment involve a combination of facts and patient preferences, and it is unlikely that AI will be able to determine all the emotive and experiential feelings involved in the decision-making for arthroplasty surgery. There is a long way to go before knowledge of the pathophysiology and subsequent clinical course will be thorough enough to trust that AI will be capable of giving adequate answers for each pathology.

D'Amico et al. [30] asked ChatGPT about the potential of chatbot technology in the field of neurosurgery. The response included the comment "One concern is the potential for chatbots to misdiagnose or provide incorrect information, which could have serious consequences for patients." This observation relates to the evaluation and treatment of shoulders, including shoulder arthroplasty. The editorial also lists several concerns regarding chatbot technology. These include privacy concerns, as patient data could be vulnerable to discovery or manipulation by outside forces. There is also an ethical concern, as chatbot recommendations might be used as standards that do not fit every patient, and it is conceivable that clinicians could be penalized for not following guidelines. Currently, the guidelines from ChatGPT do not produce AUCs above 0.9 [3], which can create ethical concerns when discussing treatment. In addition, the available literature will be the source for chatbot technology, and this may only amplify the biases of those data in the algorithms. There also could be legal issues with the publication of guidelines based upon AI that may be mistaken for or interpreted as the standard of care for shoulder arthroplasty and other treatments. The validity of AI technology should also be open for evaluation, including what the data sources were, and the mechanics of the algorithms should be available when interpreting the conclusions and recommendations made as a result of AI [8]. Last, it is possible that AI technologies will be used as adjuncts to clinical decision-making and not interpreted as rigid guidelines, which could impede clinicians from making decisions with the patient. Every clinician should be allowed the liberty to grow and learn and not be fettered by AI algorithms in their care of patients.

7.7 Conclusion

AI for shoulder arthroplasty is in its infancy but the applications will continue to expand. However, there are major concerns about the ability of AI to deal with the deficiencies in our understanding of how the shoulder works and the inherent variability of patient physiology, anatomy, pathophysiology, and expectations.

References

1. King MR. The future of AI in medicine: a perspective from a chatbot. Ann Biomed Eng. 2023;51:291–5. https://doi.org/10.1007/s10439-022-03121-w.
2. Biron DR, Sinha I, Kleiner JE, Aluthge DP, Goodman AD, Sarkar IN, Cohen E, Daniels AH. A novel machine learning model developed to assist in patient selection for outpatient total shoulder arthroplasty. J Am Acad Orthop Surg. 2020;28:e580–5. https://doi.org/10.5435/JAAOS-D-19-00395.
3. Karnuta JM, Churchill JL, Haeberle HS, Nwachukwu BU, Taylor SA, Ricchetti ET, Ramkumar PN. The value of artificial neural networks for predicting length of stay, discharge disposition, and inpatient costs after anatomic and reverse shoulder arthroplasty. J Shoulder Elb Surg. 2020;29:2385–94. https://doi.org/10.1016/j.jse.2020.04.009.
4. Kurmis AP, Ianunzio JR. Artificial intelligence in orthopedic surgery: evolution, current state and future directions. Arthroplasty. 2022;4:9. https://doi.org/10.1186/s42836-022-00112-z.
5. Twomey-Kozak J, Hurley E, Levin J, Anakwenze O, Klifto C. Technological innovations in shoulder replacement: current concepts and the future of robotics in total shoulder arthroplasty. J Shoulder Elb Surg. 2023;S1058-2746(23)00417–2. https://doi.org/10.1016/j.jse.2023.04.022
6. Mann DL. Artificial intelligence discusses the role of artificial intelligence in translational medicine: a JACC: basic to translational science interview with ChatGPT. JACC Basic Transl Sci. 2023;8:221–3. https://doi.org/10.1016/j.jacbts.2023.01.001.
7. Kumar V, Roche C, Overman S, Simovitch R, Flurin P-H, Wright T, Zuckerman J, Routman H, Teredesai A. What is the accuracy of three different machine learning techniques to predict clinical outcomes after shoulder arthroplasty? Clin Orthop Relat Res. 2020;478:2351–63. https://doi.org/10.1097/CORR.0000000000001263.
8. Forsberg JA. CORR Insights®: what is the accuracy of three different machine learning techniques to predict clinical outcomes after shoulder arthroplasty? Clin Orthop Relat Res. 2020;478:2364. https://doi.org/10.1097/CORR.0000000000001344.
9. Chen T, Guestrin C. XGBoost: a scalable tree boosting system. In: Proceedings of the 22nd ACM SIGKDD international conference on knowledge discovery and data mining. New York: Association for Computing Machinery; 2016. p. 785–94.
10. Cheng H-T, Koc L, Harmsen J, Shaked T, Chandra T, Aradhye H, Anderson G, Corrado G, Chai W, Ispir M, Anil R, Haque Z, Hong L, Jain V, Liu X, Shah H. Wide & deep learning for recommender systems. 2016.
11. Polce EM, Kunze KN, Fu MC, Garrigues GE, Forsythe B, Nicholson GP, Cole BJ, Verma NN. Development of supervised machine learning algorithms for prediction of satisfaction at 2 years following total shoulder arthroplasty. J Shoulder Elb Surg. 2021;30:e290–9. https://doi.org/10.1016/j.jse.2020.09.007.
12. Marigi EM, Hao KA, Friedman RJ, Greene AT, Roche CP, Wright TW, King JJ, Schoch BS. Exactech Equinoxe anatomic versus reverse total shoulder arthroplasty for primary osteoarthritis: case controlled comparisons using the machine learning–derived shoulder arthroplasty smart score. J Shoulder Elb Surg. 2023;32:793–802. https://doi.org/10.1016/j.jse.2022.09.029.

13. Luo W, Phung D, Tran T, Gupta S, Rana S, Karmakar C, Shilton A, Yearwood J, Dimitrova N, Ho TB, Venkatesh S, Berk M. Guidelines for developing and reporting machine learning predictive models in biomedical research: a multidisciplinary view. J Med Internet Res. 2016;18:e5870. https://doi.org/10.2196/jmir.5870.
14. Lopez CD, Constant M, Anderson MJJ, Confino JE, Heffernan JT, Jobin CM. Using machine learning methods to predict nonhome discharge after elective total shoulder arthroplasty. JSES Int. 2021;5:692–8. https://doi.org/10.1016/j.jseint.2021.02.011.
15. Arvind V, London DA, Cirino C, Keswani A, Cagle PJ. Comparison of machine learning techniques to predict unplanned readmission following total shoulder arthroplasty. J Shoulder Elb Surg. 2021;30:e50–9. https://doi.org/10.1016/j.jse.2020.05.013.
16. Gowd AK, Agarwalla A, Beck EC, Rosas S, Waterman BR, Romeo AA, Liu JN. Prediction of total healthcare cost following total shoulder arthroplasty utilizing machine learning. J Shoulder Elb Surg. 2022;31:2449–56. https://doi.org/10.1016/j.jse.2022.07.013.
17. Cutler A, Cutler DR, Stevens JR. Random forests. In: Zhang C, Ma Y, editors. Ensemble machine learning: methods and applications. New York, NY: Springer; 2012. p. 157–75.
18. Schoch B, Schleck C, Cofield RH, Sperling JW. Shoulder arthroplasty in patients younger than 50 years: minimum 20-year follow-up. J Shoulder Elb Surg. 2015;24:705–10. https://doi.org/10.1016/j.jse.2014.07.016.
19. Sperling JW, Cofield RH, Rowland CM. Minimum fifteen-year follow-up of Neer hemiarthroplasty and total shoulder arthroplasty in patients aged fifty years or younger. J Shoulder Elb Surg. 2004;13:604–13. https://doi.org/10.1016/S1058274604001296.
20. Chelli M, Boileau P, Domos P, Clavert P, Berhouet J, Collin P, Walch G, Favard L. Survivorship of reverse shoulder arthroplasty according to indication, age and gender. J Clin Med. 2022;11:2677. https://doi.org/10.3390/jcm11102677.
21. Wilson NA, Jehn M, York S, Davis CM. Revision total hip and knee arthroplasty implant identification: implications for use of unique device identification 2012 AAHKS member survey results. J Arthroplast. 2014;29:251–5. https://doi.org/10.1016/j.arth.2013.06.027.
22. Kunze KN, Jang SJ, Fullerton MA, Vigdorchik JM, Haddad FS. What's all the chatter about? Bone Joint J. 2023;105-B:587–9. https://doi.org/10.1302/0301-620X.105B6.BJJ-2023-0156.
23. Urban G, Porhemmat S, Stark M, Feeley B, Okada K, Baldi P. Classifying shoulder implants in X-ray images using deep learning. Comput Struct Biotechnol J. 2020;18:967–72. https://doi.org/10.1016/j.csbj.2020.04.005.
24. Yi PH, Kim TK, Wei J, Li X, Hager GD, Sair HI, Fritz J. Automated detection and classification of shoulder arthroplasty models using deep learning. Skeletal Radiol. 2020;49:1623–32. https://doi.org/10.1007/s00256-020-03463-3.
25. Sultan H, Owais M, Park C, Mahmood T, Haider A, Park KR. Artificial intelligence-based recognition of different types of shoulder implants in x-ray scans based on dense residual ensemble-network for personalized medicine. J Pers Med. 2021;11:482. https://doi.org/10.3390/jpm11060482.
26. Iannotti J, Baker J, Rodriguez E, Brems J, Ricchetti E, Mesiha M, Bryan J. Three-dimensional preoperative planning software and a novel information transfer technology improve glenoid component positioning. J Bone Joint Surg Am. 2014;96:e71. https://doi.org/10.2106/JBJS.L.01346.
27. Rangarajan R, Blout CK, Patel VV, Bastian SA, Lee BK, Itamura JM. Early results of reverse total shoulder arthroplasty using a patient-matched glenoid implant for severe glenoid bone deficiency. J Shoulder Elb Surg. 2020;29:S139–48. https://doi.org/10.1016/j.jse.2020.04.024.
28. Daher M, Ghanimeh J, Otayek J, Ghoul A, Bizdikian A-J, Abiad RE. Augmented reality and shoulder replacement: a state-of-the-art review article. JSES Rev Rep Techniq. 2023. https://doi.org/10.1016/j.xrrt.2023.01.008
29. Smith CD, Athwal GS, Ferreira LM. Early experience with force-space navigated robotics for glenoid implantation during total shoulder arthroplasty. Ann Robotics Autom. 2021;5:1–10. https://doi.org/10.17352/ara.000007
30. D'Amico RS, White TG, Shah HA, Langer DJ. I asked a ChatGPT to write an editorial about how we can incorporate chatbots into neurosurgical research and patient care. Neurosurgery. 2023;92:663. https://doi.org/10.1227/neu.0000000000002414

8 Artificial Intelligence in Surgical Robotics

Filippo Calanna, Joil Ramazzotti, Pierrenzo Pozzi, Riccardo Compagnoni, Paolo Ferrua, and Pietro Simone Randelli

8.1 Introduction

The integration of artificial intelligence (AI) in the field of orthopedics has emerged as a transformative pathway to enhance patient care, optimize surgical interventions, and advance research initiatives.

Utilizing machine learning algorithms and deep learning networks, AI applications have been implemented for diagnostic augmentation, preoperative planning, intraoperative navigation, and postoperative monitoring. This chapter aims to highlight the various dimensions of AI applications within orthopedics and its integration with robotics, emphasizing the potential benefits and challenges accompanying this technological infusion.

8.2 History

A decade ago, healthcare robots were primarily designed to enhance surgical precision and minimize invasiveness. The integration of robotics in surgical procedures represents a significant advancement in modern medicine. These robotic systems are operated via specialized consoles equipped with haptic interfaces, allowing surgeons to receive tactile feedback as they navigate surgical instruments, thereby enhancing the intuitive control and precision of surgical interventions. These systems display high-resolution, magnified images, providing the surgical team with augmented visual information.

The CASPAR® (U.R.S.-ortho GmbH&Co. KG, Rastatt, Germany) is one of the earliest orthopedic robotic systems that showed promising and excellent clinical results and no major adverse events in a prospective study at 2 years of follow-up [1] (Fig. 8.1).

The Da Vinci® Surgical System (Intuitive Surgical, Sunnyvale, CA, USA) is one of the most recognized robotic systems designed for

F. Calanna · J. Ramazzotti (✉) · P. Pozzi
Clinica Ortopedica, ASST Centro Specialistico Ortopedico Traumatologico Gaetano Pini-CTO, Milan, Italy

R. Compagnoni · P. Ferrua
Clinica Ortopedica, ASST Centro Specialistico Ortopedico Traumatologico Gaetano Pini-CTO, Milan, Italy

Department of Biomedical, Surgical and Dental Sciences, Università degli Studi di Milano, Milan, Italy

P. S. Randelli
Clinica Ortopedica, ASST Centro Specialistico Ortopedico Traumatologico Gaetano Pini-CTO, Milan, Italy

Laboratory of Applied Biomechanics, Department of Biomedical Sciences for Health, Università degli Studi di Milano, Milan, Italy

Research Center for Adult and Pediatric Rheumatic Diseases (RECAP-RD), Department of Biomedical Sciences for Health, Università degli Studi di Milano, Milan, Italy

F. Familiari et al. (eds.), *Artificial Intelligence in Orthopaedic Surgery Made Easy*,
https://doi.org/10.1007/978-3-031-70310-2_8

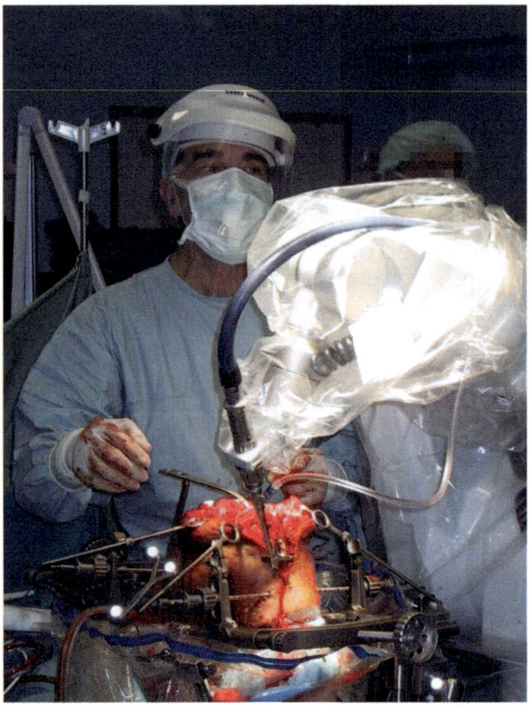

Fig. 8.1 View of the working CASPAR® robot guided by Prof. Giovanni Peretti in 2000 at Gaetano Pini Hospital, Milan, Italy. (Courtesy of Prof. Pietro S. Randelli)

laparoscopic surgery. Its high-fidelity 3D visualization and ergonomic interface, associated with haptic feedback, provide an immersive operative setting, resulting in precise surgical maneuvers with high fidelity.

Numerous clinical studies and trials have analyzed the safety and efficacy of this system across a variety of surgical disciplines including urology, gynecology, thoracic surgery, and general surgery among others [2]. The strong evidence generated over the years underscores the system's ability to facilitate precise surgical maneuvers and to minimize invasiveness: the result is less postoperative pain, faster recovery, and lower rates of complications when compared to traditional surgical approach. Unluckily, up to now, the Da Vinci® surgical systems do not have applications in orthopedic surgery.

In the domain of orthopedic surgeries, particularly those involving the knee and hip, the ROSA® (Robotic Surgical Assistant) Knee system (Zimmer Biomet, Warsaw, Indiana, USA) and the Mako Robotic Arm™ (Stryker, Warsaw, Indiana USA) are prominent examples [3]. The ROSA® enhances the precision of bone resections and implant placements in knee arthroplasty, while the MAKO™ system facilitates pre-surgical planning and real-time monitoring in hip and knee surgeries, ensuring accurate placement of implants.

The SpineAssist® (Mazor Robotics Ltd., Caesarea, Israel), a pioneering venture in robotic-assisted spine surgery, represents a significant stride toward enhancing the precision and safety of spinal interventions. The SpineAssist® system was the first of its kind to receive FDA approval in 2004, marking the inception of robotic-assisted spine surgery [4].

The operational mechanism of SpineAssist involves a patient-mounted track attached to an anatomical landmark on the spine, utilizing preoperative and/or intraoperative CT imaging for planning screw trajectories [5].

Together, these robotic systems represent innovative robotic technology and surgical expertise, potentially contributing to enhanced precision, improved patient safety, and favorable postoperative outcomes in different surgical settings.

The introduction of these robotic systems in the clinical setting could introduce new challenges for surgeons.

One of the foremost challenges associated with the utilization of robotic systems in orthopedic surgery is the introduction of substantial economic costs, including the acquisition, maintenance, and service contracts of the robotic equipment, as the introduction of dedicated instruments and accessories [6]. Another important factor is the longer operative time, especially during the learning curve. It is documented that the use of robotics may result in longer operative durations due to various factors including system setup, intraoperative adjustments, and potential technical difficulties during the surgical procedure [7]. Moreover, the physical footprint of these robotic systems was substantial, occupying a significant amount of space within the operating room [8].

Secondly, the different systems rely on the placement of percutaneous pins in order to ensure successful surgical outcomes in orthopedic procedures. New complications arise from pin-hole mobilization or fractures and also pin-related infections are documented in the literature [9].

Thus, while these robotic systems offered advantages in terms of precision and control, they also introduced complexities related to surgeon workload and operating room logistics.

The cost-benefit balance should be accurately evaluated [10]. It is still necessary a meticulous evaluation of the cost-effectiveness and the tangible benefits offered by robotic systems in orthopedic surgical settings.

8.3 AI Contribution to Robotics

Today, the landscape of surgical robotics has undergone a dramatic transformation. The focus has shifted from mere precision to enhanced autonomy, flexibility, and self-learning capabilities. Surgeons now expect these robots to be more than just extensions of their own skills. They want robots that can actively monitor changes in the operating room, detect errors, and even react autonomously to emergencies [11]. This shift has been made possible through the integration of advanced artificial intelligence technologies into robotic systems.

In this new paradigm, AI technologies employed in surgical robots can be broadly categorized into pattern recognition solutions, deep learning solutions, and computer vision solutions that will be discussed in the book [12]. Robots trained on a dataset of surgical procedures can learn and replicate patterns with advanced precision. For instance, a robot trained in tissue removal can adapt its surgical plan in real time if it detects tissue deformations during the procedure [13].

Deep learning algorithms may further enhance the robot's autonomy by incorporating scenarios from both pre- and postoperative stages. For example, a robot programmed for surgery on a patient with chronic kidney disease can analyze preoperative CT scans to predict the risks of kidney failure and adjust its actions during the surgery if it detects complications like bleeding. Computer vision technology specializes in pattern recognition within images, such as 3D scans, and videos captured during surgery: this capability enables the robot to replicate suturing gestures with greater accuracy, for instance.

8.4 Real Application in the OR

The integration of artificial intelligence (AI) and robotics in surgical practices is a transformative development that promises to revolutionize patient outcomes and surgical procedures. While orthopedics has been a significant beneficiary of these advancements, it is worth noting that other surgical domains, such as neurosurgery, are also undergoing a similar transformation.

A study by Sauson Soldozy et al. [14] highlights the challenges and opportunities in integrating robotic surgery into neurosurgical procedures, particularly pituitary surgery. The confined working space and the need for precise maneuvers in endoscopic endonasal surgery make the development of an effective and safe robotic system a complex endeavor. Despite these challenges, preclinical studies have demonstrated the feasibility of using the Da Vinci Surgical System in both transnasal and transoral approaches. This system integrates computational methods to create a pre-surgical reconstructive model, automating the line of dissection and enhancing the approach to the sphenoid sinus. Although surgical robotics for transsphenoidal surgery is still in its early stages, the preliminary findings are promising and suggest a significant role also for pituitary surgery in the future.

These advancements in neurosurgery offer valuable insights into the field of orthopedics. The challenges of working in confined spaces and the need for precise maneuvers are common in both fields.

The integration of artificial intelligence (AI) with robotics in orthopedic surgery is revolutionizing the way surgical procedures are planned, executed, and monitored. This transformation is driven by a confluence of factors, including an aging population, increasing healthcare demands, and the need for more efficient surgical procedures. AI in robotic surgery is making these machines an integral part of the operating room (OR) and hospital ecosystem, allowing them to interact seamlessly with other systems and access patient records.

One of the most compelling examples of this integration in the orthopedic world is the ROSA® [15] (Robotic Surgical Assistant) system by Zimmer Biomet, which received FDA clearance in 2019. ROSA® serves as a multi-purpose platform that integrates preoperative, intraoperative, and postoperative stages of knee surgery. It not only assists with knee replacement procedures but also functions as a digital healthcare platform. The system uses AI algorithms to refine surgical decisions and even has a mobile version that collects patient data post-surgery to select the best care plan. This level of integration makes the surgical process more efficient for both surgeons and patients.

Another noteworthy example is Maestro® by Moon Surgical (Paris, France) [16], a Franco–American team that recently raised significant funding for their project. Unlike traditional bulky robots that require extensive modifications to the OR suite, Maestro® is designed to fit effortlessly into any OR. It serves as an extra set of arms to assist the surgeon, ensuring full control over the instruments. Developed in cooperation with King's College London, the solution employs AI and machine learning algorithms to fit seamlessly into any surgical procedure without disrupting the workflow.

Financial constraints and supply chain disruptions have made it difficult for healthcare systems to adopt these advanced technologies. Moreover, the lengthy and costly FDA or other certification systems like CE in Europe, approval process remains a significant hurdle for new products. Despite these challenges, the positive trends in the market are encouraging both large holdings and innovative startups to invest in this niche, which is undergoing radical transformation.

The demand for fully autonomous solutions is also on the rise, as evidenced by the Smart Tissue Autonomous Robot (STAR) [13]. This system uses machine learning-based tracking algorithms, a 3D imaging system, and advanced control techniques to adapt in real time during surgery. It has been trained on thousands of motion profiles to predict tissue motion and guide the surgeon's plans. Although still in the experimental stage, STAR has shown promising results, outperforming human surgeons in animal surgeries.

Dynamic Adaptation and Real-time decision support are made possible by the nature of machine learning models: they are designed to evolve, unlike traditional static algorithms.

They can be continually updated and refined as new data streams become available, creating a system that is not just reactive but also proactive in its approach to surgical planning and execution.

This dynamic adaptability comes into play in particularly impactful ways during the surgical procedures themselves. For instance, real-time data obtained from intraoperative imaging, sensor feedback, or even patient vitals can be instantaneously incorporated into the machine learning model guiding the surgical robot or providing decision support to the surgeon. This enables the surgical plan to be modified on-the-fly, accommodating unforeseen complications or variations in tissue anatomy. The result is an additional layer of safety and surgical precision that was previously unattainable with more traditional surgical approaches.

By allowing for real-time adjustments based on live data, this dynamic adaptation mechanism serves as a robust real-time decision support system. It further fortifies the feedback loop initiated by postoperative data collection, thereby creating a comprehensive, cyclical system that aims for continuous improvement in surgical outcomes and patient safety.

In summary, the integration of AI with robotics in orthopedic surgery is ushering in a new era of precision, efficiency, and patient-centric care. These technologies are not only making surgical procedures more accurate but are also streamlining the entire surgical process, from preoperative planning to postoperative care. As AI algorithms continue to evolve and robotic systems become more sophisticated, we can expect even more groundbreaking innovations in the near future, setting the stage for a new paradigm in orthopedic surgery.

8.5 Personalization and Time-Preserving Robotic Surgeries

AI's capability to adapt to a surgeon's unique workflow has a direct impact on the efficiency of the operating room. The AI system's collection of the surgeon's preferences and techniques allows for a seamless transition from preoperative planning to intraoperative execution [17]. By having all the preparatory work translated efficiently into the OR, the surgical team can commence the procedure with all necessary parameters and instruments readily available in a setting of highly complicated surgeries adapted to robotic usage. This not only shortens the time spent in the OR but also minimizes the likelihood of complications arising from delays or miscommunications.

The synergy between AI and robotic systems in surgical settings is forging a new frontier in operational efficiency and adaptability. By harnessing AI's ability to learn and adapt to a surgeon's unique workflow, a bespoke surgical environment is curated, one that seamlessly transitions from preoperative strategizing to intraoperative execution [17].

Furthermore, the intuitive nature of AI-enhanced robotic systems alleviates the learning curve traditionally associated with robotic surgery. By automating and optimizing various procedural steps, AI diminishes the operational complexity, making robotic systems more user-friendly and accessible to the surgical team. This user-centric design, underpinned by AI's ability to assimilate the surgeon's preferences and techniques, emboldens a broader spectrum of healthcare providers to embrace robotic surgery.

Moreover, the time efficiency accrued through AI-driven workflow optimizations translates to a reduction in operational costs. Additionally, the enhanced precision and real-time decision support furnished by AI minimize the likelihood of costly postoperative complications and revisions.

Equally important is the facet of preventive care. The real-time monitoring and feedback provided by AI-empowered robotic systems can preemptively identify and correct potential issues before they escalate into serious complications.

In retrospect, the integration of AI with robotic systems in surgical settings is more than a mere augmentation of technological capacity. It represents a paradigm shift toward a more intuitive, efficient, and cost-effective surgical practice. By bridging the gap between preoperative planning and intraoperative execution, and simplifying the utilization of robotic systems, AI is not only elevating the standard of surgical care but is also making robotic surgery a more viable and affordable option across the healthcare spectrum.

Research centers and investors have recognized the immense potential of this integration, leading to increased funding and research in this domain. As a result, the medical robot market itself is poised for exponential growth in the coming years [18] more than ever.

8.6 IA and Robotic Integration in a Loop for the Future

The feedback mechanisms enabled by meticulous collection and analysis of postoperative data inject an additional layer of sophistication and adaptability into the integrated system of AI and robotics within orthopedic surgery. This database of postoperative data, whether analyzed in real-time during ongoing surgical procedures or evaluated retrospectively for future surgical planning, serves multiple pivotal functions. Firstly, it offers a robust metric for assessing the immediate and long-term effectiveness of surgical interventions, facilitating an evidence-based approach to clinical decision-making. Secondly, it provides invaluable insights into potential areas for surgical and procedural improvement, thereby serving as a guide for iterative refinements that may reconduct to the intraoperatory phase with high precision thanks to the robot application. All this integration creates a dynamic, adaptive system [19].

Post-surgery, the comprehensive data stored by the robots during the intraoperative phase becomes a linchpin for correlating with postoperative outcomes such as healing rate, infection occurrence, or implant functionality. This correlation unveils invaluable insights into how intraoperative actions and decisions reverberate through to postoperative recovery and overall surgical success.

Moreover, the closed-loop data system facilitates a retrospective analysis, linking postoperative results back to both preoperative planning and intraoperative data.

Unlike traditional surgical methods, where data collection was largely subjective and reliant on human observation, robotic systems generate highly specific, objective data points during each procedure. These data include variables such as instrument trajectory, force applied, and tissue response [20].

When these granular, objective data are subjected to machine learning algorithms, they can be rigorously analyzed to identify patterns, correlations, and optimal techniques that were previously inaccessible or not readily apparent to human observers. This marks a significant difference from earlier practices, where the lack of objective data hindered the development of evidence-based protocols [21].

The continuous aggregation and analysis of this objective data enable AI to pinpoint the most effective surgical approaches for various orthopedic pathologies. This dynamic data stream serves as an invaluable resource for healthcare providers, equipping them with empirical evidence to refine their surgical protocols. In this way, AI significantly may contribute to evidence-based medicine.

As a specific example, the objective data collected by robotic systems can be used to evaluate the relative efficacy of different surgical techniques in knee arthroplasty, such as mechanical alignment versus kinematic alignment. These techniques can then be correlated with long-term patient outcomes, including metrics like pain levels, range of motion, and quality of life. Thus, AI and robotics function synergistically as a robust platform for both the validation of clinical studies and the real-time optimization of surgical protocols.

8.7 Limitations and Ethical Considerations

While the fusion of artificial intelligence (AI) and robotics promises to revolutionize orthopedic practice, it is not without limitations and ethical issues. One of the most pressing concerns in the deployment of AI is its "black box" nature [22], a term that refers to the opacity in the algorithmic decision-making process. Although these algorithms can analyze vast datasets and make intricate calculations, the lack of transparency in how they arrive at specific conclusions poses a barrier to their full acceptance in the medical community. This opacity often hinders the ability of clinicians to scrutinize or validate the algorithm's recommendations, thereby creating a potential roadblock in establishing trust in AI-assisted procedures.

Technical limitations also extend to the issue of interoperability. AI and robotic technologies frequently come from disparate vendors, each with its proprietary software and hardware configurations. This lack of standardization complicates the integration of these advanced tools into existing healthcare IT infrastructures, posing challenges in data exchange and potentially hampering patient care continuity.

Ethical considerations are no less significant [23]. The collection and utilization of patient data for AI algorithms raise concerns about data privacy and security. As these algorithms require access to extensive, sensitive patient information, the ethical implications of how this data is stored, accessed, and potentially misused cannot be ignored.

Equally compelling are questions surrounding responsibility and accountability [24], particularly as AI and robotics acquire increasingly autonomous functionalities. As these systems become more self-reliant, delineating the lines of responsibility between the human operators and the AI-robotic system becomes complex. In the unfortunate event of a medical error or adverse outcome, establishing culpability would be challenging, thereby complicating legal and ethical dimensions of medical malpractice.

From an economic standpoint, the adoption of AI and robotic technologies entails considerable initial investment [6]. The costs for hardware, software, and specialized training can be exorbitant, making it prohibitive for smaller healthcare institutions to adopt these advancements. This economic disparity could exacerbate existing inequalities in healthcare provision. Moreover, while these technologies promise long-term benefits in terms of operational efficiency and patient outcomes, these gains are often not immediately realized, necessitating a comprehensive cost-benefit analysis to justify the substantial financial outlays.

In conclusion, the integration of AI and robotics in orthopedics comes with many challenges, both technical and ethical. Addressing these concerns necessitates a multidisciplinary approach, involving clinicians, data scientists, ethicists, and policymakers. Despite these hurdles, the potential benefits in patient care and clinical outcomes cannot be overlooked. However, a cautious and informed approach is essential to navigate the complexities and ensure that the union of AI and robotics yields tangible, equitable improvements in orthopedic healthcare.

8.8 Conclusion

The aging global population, associated with a rise in musculoskeletal diseases, has created an urgent demand for innovative healthcare solutions. This urgency is particularly perceived in surgical settings, where there's a growing need for intelligent, efficient robotic assistance. This emergent need has been a catalyst for innovation, particularly among companies, leading to the creation of robotic systems with the capability to execute complex surgical tasks with a level of precision that was previously unattainable.

Initially, the healthcare industry was quick to embrace surgical robots primarily for their capacity to minimize surgical errors and thereby improve clinical outcomes. However, the expectations from these robotic systems have evolved significantly. Hospitals and healthcare providers now seek solutions that not only demonstrate clinical efficacy but are also ergonomic, have a degree of autonomy, and are economically sustainable. AI-driven surgical robotics aptly fulfills these diverse requirements. Surgeons, although initially hesitant, are gradually recognizing the indispensable nature of these advanced technologies. This perceptual shift is quantifiable, as evidenced by the 33% adoption rate of robotic systems among members of the American Association of Hip and Knee Surgeons (AAHKS) [25, 26], particularly for complex procedures like joint arthroplasty.

On the patient front, the ultimate beneficiaries of these cutting-edge surgical methodologies have expressed overwhelming support for robot-assisted surgeries. A substantial majority of individuals who underwent such advanced procedures have reported elevated levels of satisfaction and are inclined to recommend robot-assisted surgical approaches to others. However, it is crucial to acknowledge that the pathway to more widespread use of technology has several potential obstacles. Financial limitations, particularly in terms of high capital investments, pose a substantial challenge for many healthcare institutions. Additionally, the COVID-19 pandemic has exacerbated existing supply chain disruptions, affecting the timely procurement of essential robotic components, and thereby influencing sales and product delivery timelines.

Regulatory hurdles also persist, with the Food and Drug Administration (FDA) or the CE in Europe approval process remaining a significant bottleneck in the development and adoption of new robotic systems. This is exemplified by the case of Medtronik's Hugo robot [27], which has secured approval in multiple countries yet is still awaiting FDA clearance.

Despite these challenges, robotics in orthopedics is experiencing significant growth and presents big opportunities for both established medical technology conglomerates and agile startups. Positive market dynamics are leveling the competitive landscape, providing new entrants with an opportunity to effectively challenge the market dominion of established players. Concluding, the symbiosis between AI technologies and surgical robotics in orthopedics represents more than just an incremental technological advancement; it is a paradigm shift with the potential to revolutionize surgical practices and markedly improve patient outcomes. As we continue to navigate this rapidly evolving technological landscape, it becomes unequivocally clear that the marriage of AI and robotics in orthopedic surgery is not merely a futuristic concept but a clinical necessity that is already reshaping the healthcare industry.

References

1. Siebert W, Mai S, Kober R, Heeckt PF. Technique and first clinical results of robot-assisted total knee replacement. Knee. 2002;9(3):173–80. https://doi.org/10.1016/s0968-0160(02)00015-7. PMID: 12126674
2. Yu J, Wang Y, Li Y, Li X, Li C, Shen J. The safety and effectiveness of Da Vinci surgical system compared with open surgery and laparoscopic surgery: a rapid assessment. J Evid-Based Med. 2014;7(2):121–34.
3. Mayne A, Rajgor H, Munasinghe C, Agrawal Y, Pagkalos I, Davis E, et al. ROSA versus mako: comparing surgical accuracy in robotic total knee arthroplasty. Orthop Proc. 2023;105-B(SUPP_13):30.
4. D'Souza M, Gendreau J, Feng A, Kim LH, Ho AL, Veeravagu A. Robotic-assisted spine surgery: history, efficacy, cost, and future trends. Robot Surg Res Rev. 2019;6:9–23.
5. Alluri RK, Avrumova F, Sivaganesan A, Vaishnav AS, Lebl DR, Qureshi SA. Overview of robotic technology in spine surgery. HSS J® Musculoskelet J Hosp Spec Surg. 2021;17(3):308–16.
6. Childers CP, Maggard-Gibbons M. Estimation of the acquisition and operating costs for robotic surgery. JAMA. 2018;320(8):835.
7. Nogalo C, Meena A, Abermann E, Fink C. Complications and downsides of the robotic total knee arthroplasty: a systematic review. Knee Surg Sports Traumatol Arthrosc. 2023;31(3):736–50.
8. Kanji F, Catchpole K, Choi E, Alfred M, Cohen K, Shouhed D, et al. Work-system interventions in robotic-assisted surgery: a systematic review exploring the gap between challenges and solutions. Surg Endosc. 2021;35(5):1976–89.
9. Thomas TL, Goh GS, Nguyen MK, Lonner JH. Pin-related complications in computer navigated and robotic-assisted knee arthroplasty: a systematic review. J Arthroplast. 2022;37(11):2291–2307.e2.
10. Kort N, Stirling P, Pilot P, Müller JH. Robot-assisted knee arthroplasty improves component positioning and alignment, but results are inconclusive on whether it improves clinical scores or reduces complications and revisions: a systematic overview of meta-analyses. Knee Surg Sports Traumatol Arthrosc Off J ESSKA. 2022;30(8):2639–53.
11. Picard F, Deakin AH, Riches PE, Deep K, Baines J. Computer assisted orthopaedic surgery: past, present and future. Med Eng Phys. 2019 Oct;72:55–65.
12. Federer SJ, Jones GG. Artificial intelligence in orthopaedics: a scoping review. Gadekallu TR, editor. PLoS One. 2021;16(11):e0260471.
13. Leonard S, Wu KL, Kim Y, Krieger A, Kim PCW. Smart tissue anastomosis robot (STAR): a vision-guided robotics system for laparoscopic suturing. IEEE Trans Biomed Eng. 2014;61(4):1305–17.
14. Soldozy S, Young S, Yağmurlu K, Norat P, Sokolowski J, Park MS, et al. Transsphenoidal surgery using robotics to approach the Sella turcica: integrative use of artificial intelligence, realistic motion tracking and telesurgery. Clin Neurol Neurosurg. 2020;197:106152.
15. Batailler C, Hannouche D, Benazzo F, Parratte S. Concepts and techniques of a new robotically assisted technique for total knee arthroplasty: the ROSA knee system. Arch Orthop Trauma Surg. 2021;141(12):2049–58.
16. Hwang H, Choi JY, Yu HW, Moon JH, Kim JH, Lee EK, et al. Surgical outcomes in patients with low-risk papillary thyroid microcarcinoma from MAeSTro study: immediate operation versus delayed operation after active surveillanceA multicenter prospective cohort study. Ann Surg. 2023;278(5):e1087–95.
17. Shinozuka K, Turuda S, Fujinaga A, Nakanuma H, Kawamura M, Matsunobu Y, et al. Artificial intelligence software available for medical devices: surgical phase recognition in laparoscopic cholecystectomy. Surg Endosc. 2022;36(10):7444–52.
18. Suarez-Ahedo C, Lopez-Reyes A, Martinez-Armenta C, Martinez-Gomez LE, Martinez-Nava GA, Pineda C, et al. Revolutionizing orthopedics: a comprehensive review of robot-assisted surgery, clinical outcomes, and the future of patient care. J Robot Surg [Internet]. 2023 Aug 28 [cited 2023 Oct 18]. Available from https://doi.org/10.1007/s11701-023-01697-6
19. Ramkumar PN, Haeberle HS, Ramanathan D, Cantrell WA, Navarro SM, Mont MA, et al. Remote patient monitoring using mobile health for total knee arthroplasty: validation of a wearable and machine learning–based surveillance platform. J Arthroplast. 2019;34(10):2253–9.

20. Brown JD, O'Brien CE, Leung SC, Dumon KR, Lee DI, Kuchenbecker KJ. Using contact forces and robot arm accelerations to automatically rate surgeon skill at peg transfer. IEEE Trans Biomed Eng. 2017 Sep;64(9):2263–75.
21. Pedrett R, Mascagni P, Beldi G, Padoy N, Lavanchy JL. Technical skill assessment in minimally invasive surgery using artificial intelligence: a systematic review. Surg Endosc. 2023;37(10):7412–24.
22. Poon AIF, Sung JJY. Opening the black box of AI-medicine. J Gastroenterol Hepatol. 2021;36(3):581–4.
23. Kaya Bicer E, Fangerau H, Sur H. Artifical intelligence use in orthopedics: an ethical point of view. EFORT Open Rev. 2023;8(8):592–6.
24. Loftus TJ, Tighe PJ, Filiberto AC, Efron PA, Brakenridge SC, Mohr AM, et al. Artificial intelligence and surgical decision-making. JAMA Surg. 2020;155(2):148.
25. Sone K, Tanimoto S, Toyohara Y, Taguchi A, Miyamoto Y, Mori M, et al. Evolution of a surgical system using deep learning in minimally invasive surgery (review). Biomed Rep. 2023;19(1):45.
26. Sherman WF, Wu VJ. Robotic surgery in total joint arthroplasty: a survey of the AAHKS membership to understand the utilization, motivations, and perceptions of total joint surgeons. J Arthroplast. 2020;35(12):3474–3481.e2.
27. Cacciatore L, Costantini M, Tedesco F, Prata F, Machiella F, Iannuzzi A, et al. Robotic Medtronic Hugo™ RAS system is now reality: introduction to a new simulation platform for training residents. Sensors. 2023;23(17):7348.

9 Artificial Intelligence in Hip Arthroscopy

Kyle N. Kunze, Benedict U. Nwachukwu, Shane J. Nho, and Jorge Chahla

9.1 Introduction

Artificial intelligence (AI) has gained considerable recognition and interest for possessing capabilities that may soon transform healthcare logistics and patient care. Hip arthroscopy, like several other orthopedic specialties and subdisciplines, has been subjected to several applications of AI for research purposes. Although these investigations have yet to manifest as tangible, practice-changing applications, AI-derived tools in the hip arthroscopy literature withhold promise to confer clinical benefits.

Predominant applications of AI within the hip arthroscopy literature consist of machine learning and deep-learning models. Machine learning models for hip arthroscopy can be broadly classified into those pertaining to clinical outcome prediction, adverse event prediction, and resource utilization prediction. An indirect application of AI that impacts hip arthroscopy is the development of deep-learning models that can automate measurements of clinically relevant metrics utilized for surgical indications and planning, such as the lateral enter edge and alpha angles. Both of these domains of AI are rapidly evolving, with additional literature being published on a monthly basis.

This chapter will introduce the contemporary applications of AI surrounding the hip arthroscopy literature, highlighting several transformational investigations as they relate to the current understanding and capabilities of AI in this realm. An evidence-based discussion of these studies will be included, with expansion on how such studies may translate into tangible clinical benefits. Finally, the current state of AI in the hip arthroscopy literature will be critically examined to better understand the current limitations of this literature and the future directions for the field.

9.2 Artificial Intelligence for Predicting Clinical Outcome Achievement

Substantial attention has been devoted to understanding how applying machine learning methods to hip arthroscopy datasets may be leveraged to optimize predictions for clinical outcome achievement [1]. Under the categorization of clinical outcome achievement, primary outcomes

K. N. Kunze · B. U. Nwachukwu
Department of Orthopaedic Surgery, Hospital for Special Surgery, New York, NY, USA

Sports Medicine and Shoulder Service, Hospital for Special Surgery, New York, NY, USA

S. J. Nho · J. Chahla (✉)
Section of Young Adult Hip Surgery, Division of Sports Medicine, Department of Orthopaedic Surgery, Rush University Medical Center, Chicago, IL, USA

Midwest Orthopaedics at Rush, Chicago, IL, USA

F. Familiari et al. (eds.), *Artificial Intelligence in Orthopaedic Surgery Made Easy*,
https://doi.org/10.1007/978-3-031-70310-2_9

have included satisfaction metrics and patient-reported outcome measures and achievement of the minimal clinically important difference (MCID), patient acceptable symptom state (PASS), as well as substantial clinical benefit (SCB). Several different datasets, including both institutional and national or claims registries, in addition to varying subsets of these datasets, have been utilized to explore their ability to predict these outcomes (Table 9.1).

Kunze et al. [2] utilized a dataset derived from one large academic and three community hospitals over a five-year period to determine the ability to predict achievement of the MCID for the hip outcome score (HOS)—activities of daily living (ADL) at a minimum of two-years postoperatively. In this dataset of 818 patients comprising 21 unique candidate predictor variables, this group determined that the best-performing algorithm in terms of discrimination, calibration, Brier score, and decision-curve analysis was a stochastic gradient boosting algorithm. The most important features for making these predictions were: (1) body mass index, (2) age, (3) preoperative HOS-ADL score, (4) preoperative pain level, (5) patient sex, (6) Tönnis grade, (7) preoperative symptom duration, and (8) number of drug allergies. Furthermore, they utilized advanced coding

Table 9.1 Artificial intelligence-based studies in hip arthroscopy literature concerning prediction of clinical outcomes

Study	Patients	Primary outcomes	Algorithm performance	Predictive variables	External validation
Nwachukwu et al. 2020 [6]	1103	MCID for HOS-ADL, HOS-SS, mHHS	*AUROC*: HOS-ADL (0.89), HOS-SS (0.85), mHHS (0.84)	*HOS-ADL*: anxiety/depression, chronic symptoms, BMI, preoperative HOS-ADL, hip injections *HOS-SS*: anxiety/depression, chronic symptoms, preoperative HOS-SS, hip injections, running *mHHS*: anxiety/depression, preoperative mHHS, hip injections, female sex	No
Ramkumar et al. 2020 [7]	1735	MCID (1-Year) for mHHS, HOS-ADL, HOS-SS, IHOT-33 MCID (2-Year) for mHHS, HOS-ADL, HOS-SS, IHOT-33	*AUROC* (1-Year): mHHS (0.15–0.94), HOS-ADL (0.078–0.92), HOS-SS (0.25–0.84), IHOT-33 (0.21–0.41) *AUROC* (2-Year): mHHS (0.06–0.89), HOS-ADL (0.063–0.70), HOS-SS (0.058–0.63), (0.15–0.81)	Defined a priori: Alpha angle, lateral center-edge angle, femoral version angle, McKibbin index, hip impingement index	No
Kunze et al. 2021 [4]	935	MCID for VAS satisfaction	*AUROC:* 0.94 *Calibration slope*: 0.94 *Calibration intercept*: −0.43 *Brier sore*: 0.050	Anxiety/depression, lateral center-edge angle, chronic symptom duration, drug allergies, Workers compensation	No
Kunze et al. 2021 [2]	818	MCID for HOS-ADL	*AUROC:* 0.84 *Calibration slope*: 0.83 *Calibration intercept*: 0.20 *Brier sore*: 0.13	Age, BMI, sex, preoperative HOS-ADL, preoperative VAS pain, chronic symptom duration, drug allergies	No

(continued)

Table 9.1 (continued)

Study	Patients	Primary outcomes	Algorithm performance	Predictive variables	External validation
Kunze et al. 2021 [3]	1118	MCID for HOS-SS	*AUROC*: 0.77 *Calibration slope*: 1.22 *Calibration intercept*: 0.07 *Brier sore*: 0.14	Age, BMI, alpha angle, Tönnis grade and angle, preoperative HOS-SS	Yes
Kunze et al. 2022 [5]	859	MCID, PASS and SCB for IHOT-12	*MCID*: AUROC 0.78, calibration slope 0.85, calibration intercept 0.02, Brier score 0.14 *PASS*: AUROC 0.74, calibration slope 0.79, calibration intercept 0.03, Brier score 0.21 *SCB*: AUROC 0.71, calibration slope 0.95, calibration intercept −0.03, Brier score 0.22	*MCID*: history of back pain, anxiety depression, preoperative IHOT-12, BMI, preoperative HOS-ADL, alpha angle, preoperative HOS-SS *PASS*: chronic symptom duration, history of back pain, anxiety/depression, BMI, preoperative mHHS, age, preoperative HOS-ADL, preoperative IHOT-12 *SCB*: age, chronic symptom duration, history of back pain, hip injections, anxiety/depression, BMI, sports participation, preoperative HOS-ADL, preoperative mHHS, preoperative IHOT-12	No
Kunze et al. 2022 [8]	154	MCID for HOS-SS	*AUROC*: 0.80 *Calibration slope*: 1.16 *Calibration intercept*: 0.13 *Brier sore*: 0.15	Age, BMI, alpha angle, Tönnis grade and angle, preoperative HOS-SS	Not applicable

Metrics reported for best-performing model
Not applicable indicates the single study that was an external validation study
AUROC, area under the receiver operator curve; IHOT, international hip outcome tool; mHHS, modified Harris hip score; BMI, body mass index, HOS-ADL, hip outcome score—activities of daily living; HOS-SS, HOS-Sports Subscale; VAS, visual analog scale; MCID, minimal clinically important difference; PASS, patient acceptable symptom state; SCB, substantial clinical benefit

analytics to develop a provider-facing tool derived from this algorithm that performs real-time risk prediction at an open-source URL available on desktop and mobile devices. Such platforms help demonstrate the potential clinical utility of AI for direct patient care in terms of determining surgical candidacy and optimizing quality. This group has performed numerous analyses for other important and commonly used metrics used to assess outcome improvement after hip arthroscopy including the MCID for the HOS-sports subscale (SS) in athletes, [3] MCID visual analog scale (VAS) for satisfaction, [4] and the MCID, PASS, and SCB for the international hip outcome tool (IHOT)—12 item questionnaire [5].

Ramkumar et al. [7] Investigated whether a dataset restricted to features consisting of radiographic hip measurements could predict clinical outcomes when machine learning algorithms were applied. Specifically, outcome measures included the modified Harris hip score (mHHS), HOS-ADL, HOS-SS, and IHOT-33, while radiographic indices included the alpha angle, femoral version angle, lateral center-edge angle, McKibbin index, and hip impingement index. They reported that no combination of radiographic indices, nor any measurement in isolation, significantly predicted any of the outcome measures in their dataset, suggesting that clinical improvements may be achieved regardless of preoperative radiographic indices.

In the majority of published literature, the development and validation of machine learning algorithms for understanding the prediction of change in clinical outcomes after hip arthroscopy has demonstrated good to excellent performance [1]. Importantly, the reporting and transparency of these diagnostic and prognostic models are in accordance with recommended guidelines for such modeling. As with many fields, external and prospective validation efforts remain scarce, which precludes the use of these algorithms and related interactive tools in clinical practice as generalization to external populations cannot be confirmed at this time. This remains the major barrier to advancing the use of this statistical methodology and technology in a clinical manner. It is imperative that these efforts are pursued as the development of these algorithms remains academic practices and proof-of-concept without further validation.

9.3 Artificial Intelligence for Anticipating Adverse Events

Machine learning has also been applied to understand the risk of prolonged narcotic consumption, development of osteoarthritis of the hip, as well as revision hip arthroscopy (Table 9.2). These studies may have further implications in refining surgical candidates for arthroscopic hip preservation surgery. Furthermore, understanding the risk of adverse events may facilitate enhanced shared decision-making discussions and allow for targeted interventions of modifiable risk factors in order to decrease the incidence of additional episodes of care for unanticipated adverse events.

Haeberle et al. [10] studied a cohort of 3147 patients of whom 4.6% ($n = 171$) underwent subsequent hip surgery after primary hip arthroscopy. They developed several Random Forest models on their dataset to determine the performance for predicting several forms of subsequent hip surgery. For conversion to total hip arthroplasty (THA), the area under the receiver operator curve (AUROC) was 0.80, with 81% accuracy. For hip resurfacing arthroplasty (HRA), the AUROC was 0.62, with 69% accuracy. For revision hip arthroscopy, the AUROC was 0.77, with 76% accuracy. For periacetabular osteotomy (PAO), the AUROC was 0.76 with 74% accuracy. They reported that the most important factors in predicting the need for revision hip arthroscopy were higher body mass index and lower preoperative HOS-ADL, while THA factors included greater age and lower preoperative iHOT-33. For HRA, increased BMI was the most important factor, and for PAO, a larger neck-shaft angle and lower preoperative mHHS were the most important factors.

Martin et al. [16] queried the Danish Hip Arthroscopy Registry for patients who underwent primary hip arthroscopy to determine whether a machine learning algorithm could be developed to understand the probability of needing revision hip arthroscopy within 1, 2, and 5 years of the index primary hip arthroscopy. The authors developed four models (Cox elastic net, random survival forest, gradient-boosted regression, and super learner) and assessed performance based on the AUROC and calibration. Their models demonstrated fair discrimination using preoperatively available features (AUROC: 0.62–0.67) that were not improved by incorporating all available features in the registry (AUROC: 0.63–0.66). As such, the clinical usefulness and performance of their models was limited. This demonstrates an important point when considering the use of AI-based statistical approaches in that AI may not be appropriate to answer all scientific questions and traditional statistical methods may often be superior.

Kunze et al. [11] utilized an institutional dataset comprising 775 patients of which 18.2% ($n = 141$) experienced prolonged postoperative narcotic use after primary hip arthroscopy. The authors developed several machine learning algorithms on this dataset, finding that a stochastic gradient boosting method conferred the highest performance when determining which patients were at risk for prolonged opioid use. Furthermore, they determined that preoperative mHHS, age, body mass index, preoperative pain level, and workers' compensation status were the most important variables for predicting pro-

Table 9.2 Artificial intelligence-based studies in hip arthroscopy literature concerning the prediction of adverse events

Study	Patients	Primary outcomes	Algorithm performance	Predictive variables	External validation
Kunze et al. 2020 [9]	2113	Loss to follow-up	*AUROC*: 0.76	Male sex, non-white/Caucasian race, smoking, failure to provide phone number, preoperative IHOT-12, preoperative mHHS	No
Haeberle et al. 2021 [10]	3147	Revision hip arthroscopy, PAO, HRA, THA	*Revision hip arthroscopy*: AUROC (0.77), accuracy (76%) *PAO*: AUROC (0.76), accuracy (74%) *HRA*: AUROC (0.62), accuracy (69%) *THA*: AUROC (0.80), accuracy (81%)	*Revision hip arthroscopy*: BMI, preoperative HOS-ADL *PAO*: neck-shaft angle, preoperative mHHS *HRA*: BMI *THA*: Age, preoperative IHOT-33	No
Kunze et al. 2021 [11]	775	Prolonged postoperative opioid use	*AUROC*: 0.75 *Calibration slope*: −0.02 *Calibration intercept*: 0.88 *Brier score*: 0.13	Preoperative mHHS, age, BMI, preoperative VAS pain, Workers compensation	No
Ko et al. 2021 [12]	1071	Hip osteoarthritis development	Not applicable; statistically significant differences detected between patient clusters at $p < 0.05$ level	Age, sex, BMI, FAI-type, diabetes, internal rotation range of motion	No
Song et al. 2021 [13]	1276	Conversion to inpatient admission	*AUROC*: 0.71 *Calibration slope*: 0.99 *Calibration intercept*: 0.001 *Brier score*: 0.068	Operative time, general anesthesia, age extremes, male sex, BMI, ASA score > 1, abnormal sodium, platelet count, hematocrit, leukocyte count	No
Domb et al. 2022 [14]	2415	Revision hip arthroscopy, conversion to THA	*Revision hip arthroscopy*: AUROC (0.66) *THA*: AUROC (0.85)	Revision hip arthroscopy[a] THA[b]	No
Grazal et al. 2022 [15]	6760	Prolonged postoperative opioid use	*AUROC*: 0.71 *Brier score*: 0.21	Postoperative opioid use, age, preoperative opioid use, preoperative mental health comorbidity, preoperative substance abuse diagnosis	No
Martin et al. 2023 [16]	5581	Revision hip arthroscopy	*AUROC* (1-Year): 0.67 *Calibration statistic* (1-year): 2.32 *AUROC* (2-Year): 0.66 *Calibration statistic* (2-year): 0.28 *AUROC* (5-Year): 0.65 *Calibration statistic* (5-year): 1.13	Sex, preoperative HAGOS QoL score, preoperative NRS Activity score, preoperative HAGOS symptoms/sport scores	No

Metrics reported for best-performing model

AUROC, area under the receiver operator curve; IHOT, international hip outcome tool; mHHS, modified Harris hip score; BMI, body mass index, HOS-ADL, hip outcome score—activities of daily living; VAS, visual analog scale; HRA, hip resurfacing arthroplasty; PAO, periacetabular osteotomy; THA, total hip arthroplasty; FAI, femoroacetabular impingement; ASA, American Society of Anesthesiologists score; NRS, numeric rating scale; HAGOS, Copenhagen Hip and Groin Outcome Score

[a] Lower preoperative mHHS, female sex, workers' compensation, and increasing lateral joint space

[b] Higher preoperative NAHS, presence of crossover, and increasing degree of LCEA. Revision hip arthroscopy, MRI chondral damage, MRI subchondral cyst, increasing Tönnis grade, recreational/fitness sports level before surgery, increasing medial to lateral joint space ratio, increasing neck-shaft angle, increasing alpha angle on the radiograph, and antalgic gait or Trendelenburg

longed opioid use in this dataset. They went on to develop an interactive open-source application for office-based use to help assess individual patient risk of prolonged opioid use.

Other applications of AI pertaining to predicting the likelihood of adverse events include the long-term risk of hip osteoarthritis development and being lost to follow-up (Table 9.2), though several other complications and unanticipated events have yet to be studied. Prior to investigating additional primary outcomes, it is important for the researcher to consider whether the investigation is novel or whether the effort would simply be repackaging data. Furthermore, it is essential that answering the question is clinically important and should the analysis be pursued, that appropriate reporting guidelines are adhered to.

9.4 Artificial Intelligence for Estimating Resource Utilization

Few studies have examined the ability of datasets to predict the risk of an excessive episode of care costs and conversion of outpatient to inpatient admissions. These studies have important implications for payors and when considering surgical indications as unanticipated admissions or prolonged episodes of care inherently translate into additional costs to institutions and healthcare systems.

Song et al. [13] utilized a national surgical outcomes database to identify patients that underwent elective outpatient hip arthroscopy between 2006 and 2018. They developed and compared four machine learning algorithms to determine the predictive ability of this dataset on the primary outcome of overnight admissions that were unanticipated. Of 1276 patients, 8.5% (n = 109) were admitted overnight, with the most important features being increasing operative time, general anesthesia, age extremes, male sex, body mass index, American Society of Anesthesiologists classification exceeding one, and abnormal sodium, platelet, hematocrit, and leukocyte counts. They reported that their ensemble model (weighted ensemble of all four algorithms) performed best, conferring an AUROC of 0.71, calibration intercept of 0.001, calibration slope of 0.99, and a Brier score of 0.068.

In addition to excessive resource utilization and unanticipated events, total costs and drivers of these chargers have also been investigated utilizing machine learning. Lu et al. [17] queried the New York State Ambulatory Surgery and Services databases and identified 5121 patients who underwent elective primary hip arthroscopy. They reported that the median cost after hip arthroscopy was $19,720 and that a gradient-boosted ensemble model demonstrated the best performance. Major identified cost drivers included total hours in facility less than 12 or more than 15, operating room time exceeding 100 min, performance of a labral repair, age younger than 30 years, Elixhauser Comorbidity Index (ECI) of one or greater, African American race, residence in extreme urban and rural areas, and higher household and neighborhood income. These data may be useful for determining candidates for outpatient hip arthroscopy candidates for in adjusting reimbursement rates and facility costs for select patients or geographic areas.

9.5 Artificial Intelligence for Surgical Planning and Imaging-Based Analyses

Several recent studies have investigated the ability of deep learning, a computer-vision domain of artificial intelligence that utilizes imaging or video-based inputs to perform predictions, to automate the measurement of several clinically important measurements around the hip. Though these studies have largely focused on nonspecific patient populations with varying backgrounds and pathologies, such capabilities are directly relevant to preoperative planning and surgical indications for hip arthroscopy procedures. Furthermore, these capabilities may confer important time savings for providers by optimizing clinical workflow.

Mulford et al. [18] recently developed a deep-learning tool to automate clinically relevant anatomic landmark annotation on hip and pelvis radiographs. In their study, 1100 anteroposterior pelvic radiographs were manually annotated by three reviewers and they trained a convolutional neural network to segment 22 different structures (7 points, 6 lines, and 9 shapes around the pelvis). They reported good dice scores of 0.88 and 0.80 for shape and line structures, respectively. For point structures, average distances between real and automated annotations ranged between 1.9 and 5.6 mm. Identifying landmarks for planning may reduce variability across institutions and between research centers, and may aid in planning when image resolution, contrast, or orientation are suboptimal.

Stotter et al. [19] manually annotated 62 radiographs (124 hips) and used an AI-drive software created by ImageBiopsy Lab (Vienna, Austria) to measure radiologic parameters used in the diagnosis of femoroacetabular impingement and hip dysplasia. Measurements the femoral neck-shaft angle, lateral center-edge angle, acetabular index, femoral head extrusion index, and Sharp angle. The authors found that the software could be reliable for automating several measurements around the hip, though that on average most of the deviations from the median values were consistent across human readers and their algorithm. It is possible that with increased numbers of radiographs and additional training the performance of such software could outrank trained human observers consistently.

Substantial effort has also been devoted to utilizing landmarks and metrics around the hip and pelvis for other related purposes, including automating the measurement of acetabular inclination and version, leg-length discrepancies, limb alignment, and bone quality [20–25]. Further development and refinement of such tools hold promise to create an impact in the field of medicine and hip surgery and may also extend to intraoperative applications and real-time surgical feedback if integrated with operating room technology and augmented reality platforms.

9.6 Future of Artificial Intelligence in Hip Arthroscopy

The major limitation of AI-based hip arthroscopy literature, and a pervasive limitation among AI literature in general, remains a failure to externally validate models on independent datasets (Tables 9.1 and 9.2). To date, only one study group has externally validated a machine learning algorithm developed to predict clinically significant functional improvement after hip arthroscopy. Kunze et al. [8] investigated the propensity for a previously published machine learning algorithm utilized to predict likelihood of achieving the MCID for the HOS-SS in athletes undergoing hip arthroscopy to perform on an independent, external patient registry. They reported comparable improved performance in this independent population relative to the performance of the interval validation cohort, suggesting that it may be a reliable tool to predict functional improvement after hip arthroscopy. Such efforts represent an important step forward toward the introduction of such tools into clinical practice. Indeed, potential uses of this technology include integration into electronic medical records for automated and personalized risk prediction, optimization of surgical candidacy, and increased value of care rendered. However, as mentioned, studies performing external validation are unfortunately lacking.

9.7 Conclusion

The application of artificial intelligence within the hip arthroscopy literature has largely targeted the prediction of clinical outcomes and adverse events, with only one study attempting external validation to confirm the utility of their algorithm. Therefore, despite the existence of several potential clinical applications of these efforts, the utility of these models remains severely limited. Researchers must carefully select clinical questions and appropriately apply artificial intelligence only when warranted, be transparent with reporting of their methods, and take steps to validate models on external populations.

References

1. Kunze KN, Krivicich LM, Clapp IM, Bodendorfer BM, Nwachukwu BU, Chahla J, et al. Machine learning algorithms predict achievement of clinically significant outcomes after orthopaedic surgery: a systematic review. Arthroscopy. 2022;38(6):2090–105.
2. Kunze KN, Polce EM, Nwachukwu BU, Chahla J, Nho SJ. Development and internal validation of supervised machine learning algorithms for predicting clinically significant functional improvement in a mixed population of primary hip arthroscopy. Arthroscopy. 2021;37(5):1488–97.
3. Kunze KN, Polce EM, Clapp I, Nwachukwu BU, Chahla J, Nho SJ. Machine learning algorithms predict functional improvement after hip arthroscopy for femoroacetabular impingement syndrome in athletes. J Bone Joint Surg Am. 2021;103(12):1055–62.
4. Kunze KN, Polce EM, Rasio J, Nho SJ. Machine learning algorithms predict clinically significant improvements in satisfaction after hip arthroscopy. Arthroscopy. 2021;37(4):1143–51.
5. Kunze KN, Polce EM, Clapp IM, Alter T, Nho SJ. Association between preoperative patient factors and clinically meaningful outcomes after hip arthroscopy for femoroacetabular impingement syndrome: a machine learning analysis. Am J Sports Med. 2022;50(3):746–56.
6. Nwachukwu BU, Beck EC, Lee EK, Cancienne JM, Waterman BR, Paul K, et al. Application of machine learning for predicting clinically meaningful outcome after arthroscopic femoroacetabular impingement surgery. Am J Sports Med. 2020;48(2):415–23.
7. Ramkumar PN, Karnuta JM, Haeberle HS, Sullivan SW, Nawabi DH, Ranawat AS, et al. Radiographic indices are not predictive of clinical outcomes among 1735 patients indicated for hip arthroscopic surgery: a machine learning analysis. Am J Sports Med. 2020;48(12):2910–8.
8. Kunze KN, Kaidi A, Madjarova S, Polce EM, Ranawat AS, Nawabi DH, et al. External validation of a machine learning algorithm for predicting clinically meaningful functional improvement after arthroscopic hip preservation surgery. Am J Sports Med. 2022;50(13):3593–9.
9. Kunze KN, Burnett RA, Lee EK, Rasio JP, Nho SJ. Development of machine learning algorithms to predict being lost to follow-up after hip arthroscopy for femoroacetabular impingement syndrome. Arthrosc Sports Med Rehabil. 2020;2(5):e591–e8.
10. Haeberle HS, Ramkumar PN, Karnuta JM, Sullivan S, Sink EL, Kelly BT, et al. Predicting the risk of subsequent hip surgery before primary hip arthroscopy for femoroacetabular impingement syndrome: a machine learning analysis of preoperative risk factors in hip preservation. Am J Sports Med. 2021;49(10):2668–76.
11. Kunze KN, Polce EM, Alter TD, Nho SJ. Machine learning algorithms predict prolonged opioid use in opioid-naive primary hip arthroscopy patients. J Am Acad Orthop Surg Glob Res Rev. 2021;5(5):e21:00093–8.
12. Ko S, Pareek A, Jo C, Han HS, Lee MC, Krych AJ, et al. Automated risk stratification of hip osteoarthritis development in patients with femoroacetabular impingement using an unsupervised clustering algorithm: a study from the Rochester epidemiology project. Orthop J Sports Med. 2021;9(11):23259671211050613.
13. Song BM, Lu Y, Wilbur RR, Lavoie-Gagne O, Pareek A, Forsythe B, et al. Machine learning model identifies increased operative time and greater BMI as predictors for overnight admission after outpatient hip arthroscopy. Arthrosc Sports Med Rehabil. 2021;3(6):e1981–e90.
14. Domb BG, Ouyang VW, Go CC, Gornbein JA, Shapira J, Meghpara MB, et al. Personalized medicine using predictive analytics: a machine learning-based prognostic model for patients undergoing hip arthroscopy. Am J Sports Med. 2022;50(7):1900–8.
15. Grazal CF, Anderson AB, Booth GJ, Geiger PG, Forsberg JA, Balazs GC. A machine-learning algorithm to predict the likelihood of prolonged opioid use following arthroscopic hip surgery. Arthroscopy. 2022;38(3):839–47 e2.
16. Martin RK, Wastvedt S, Lange J, Pareek A, Wolfson J, Lund B. Limited clinical utility of a machine learning revision prediction model based on a national hip arthroscopy registry. Knee Surg Sports Traumatol Arthrosc. 2023;31(6):2079–89.
17. Lu Y, Lavoie-Gagne O, Forlenza EM, Pareek A, Kunze KN, Forsythe B, et al. Duration of care and operative time are the primary drivers of total charges after ambulatory hip arthroscopy: a machine learning analysis. Arthroscopy. 2022;38(7):2204–16 e3.
18. Mulford KL, Johnson QJ, Mujahed T, Khosravi B, Rouzrokh P, Mickley JP, et al. A deep learning tool for automated landmark annotation on hip and pelvis radiographs. J Arthroplasty. 2023.
19. Stotter C, Klestil T, Roder C, Reuter P, Chen K, Emprechtinger R, et al. Deep learning for fully automated radiographic measurements of the pelvis and hip. Diagnostics (Basel). 2023;13(3)
20. Jang SJ, Kunze KN, Bornes TD, Anderson CG, Mayman DJ, Jerabek SA, et al. Leg-length discrepancy variability on standard anteroposterior pelvis

radiographs: an analysis using deep learning measurements. J Arthroplast. 2023;38:2017.
21. Jang SJ, Fontana MA, Kunze KN, Anderson CG, Sculco TP, Mayman DJ, et al. An interpretable machine learning model for predicting 10-year Total hip arthroplasty risk. J Arthroplast 2023;38(7S):S44-S50 e6.
22. Uemura K, Otake Y, Takao M, Makino H, Soufi M, Iwasa M, et al. Development of an open-source measurement system to assess the areal bone mineral density of the proximal femur from clinical CT images. Arch Osteoporos. 2022;17(1):17.
23. Rouzrokh P, Wyles CC, Philbrick KA, Ramazanian T, Weston AD, Cai JC, et al. A deep learning tool for automated radiographic measurement of acetabular component inclination and version after Total hip arthroplasty. J Arthroplast. 2021;36(7):2510–7 e6.
24. Yamamoto N, Sukegawa S, Kitamura A, Goto R, Noda T, Nakano K, et al. Deep learning for osteoporosis classification using hip radiographs and patient clinical covariates. Biomol Ther. 2020;10(11)
25. Deng Y, Wang L, Zhao C, Tang S, Cheng X, Deng HW, et al. A deep learning-based approach to automatic proximal femur segmentation in quantitative CT images. Med Biol Eng Comput. 2022;60(5):1417–29.

Artificial Intelligence in Knee Arthroscopy

10

Luke V. Tollefson, Evan P. Shoemaker, Nicholas I. Kennedy, and Robert F. LaPrade

10.1 Introduction

Knee arthroscopy is a minimally invasive procedure that utilizes small incisions to insert an arthroscope and additional instruments to visualize the internal structures of the knee joint in real time. This can be done alone or in conjunction with more complex surgeries for better visualization of internal anatomy. This procedure can additionally be used as a diagnostic element in planning future procedures and once conservative treatment methods are no longer productive. Knee arthroscopic procedures are typically performed to assess and repair meniscus damage, reconstruct anterior cruciate ligament (ACL) and posterior cruciate ligament (PCL) tears, patellar misalignment, remove loose bodies of cartilage and bone within the synovium, and perform a chondroplasty on damaged cartilage. Due to the minimally invasive nature, arthroscopic procedures are commonly same-day outpatient procedures depending on the severity and complexity of the operation. Risks and complications associated with these procedures are relatively low and uncommon, albeit they do exist. Tissues and nerve damage may occur because of instrument movement within joints, blood clotting can occur with procedures that last longer than an hour, and a risk of infection as with any invasive procedure. Although these procedures are generally very streamlined, with the implementation of artificial intelligence (AI) there is a potential opportunity for improvement in many of the stages of treatment. There is an opportunity for AI to be implemented into healthcare to improve the efficacy and efficiency of patient treatment [1]. In the subsequent chapter, we will go in-depth into how AI implementation may improve diagnostics, predictive accuracy, operative advantage, and optimized rehabilitation, as well as possible problematic factors that may be encountered in both small to large-scale arthroscopic surgeries. AI has the potential to improve knee arthroscopic surgery in all facets of surgery from preoperative diagnosis and planning to postoperative rehabilitation and return to activities (Fig. 10.1).

L. V. Tollefson · E. P. Shoemaker · R. F. LaPrade (✉)
Twin Cities Orthopedics, Edina, MN, USA

N. I. Kennedy
Orthopedics Northwest, Yakima, WA, USA

F. Familiari et al. (eds.), *Artificial Intelligence in Orthopaedic Surgery Made Easy*,
https://doi.org/10.1007/978-3-031-70310-2_10

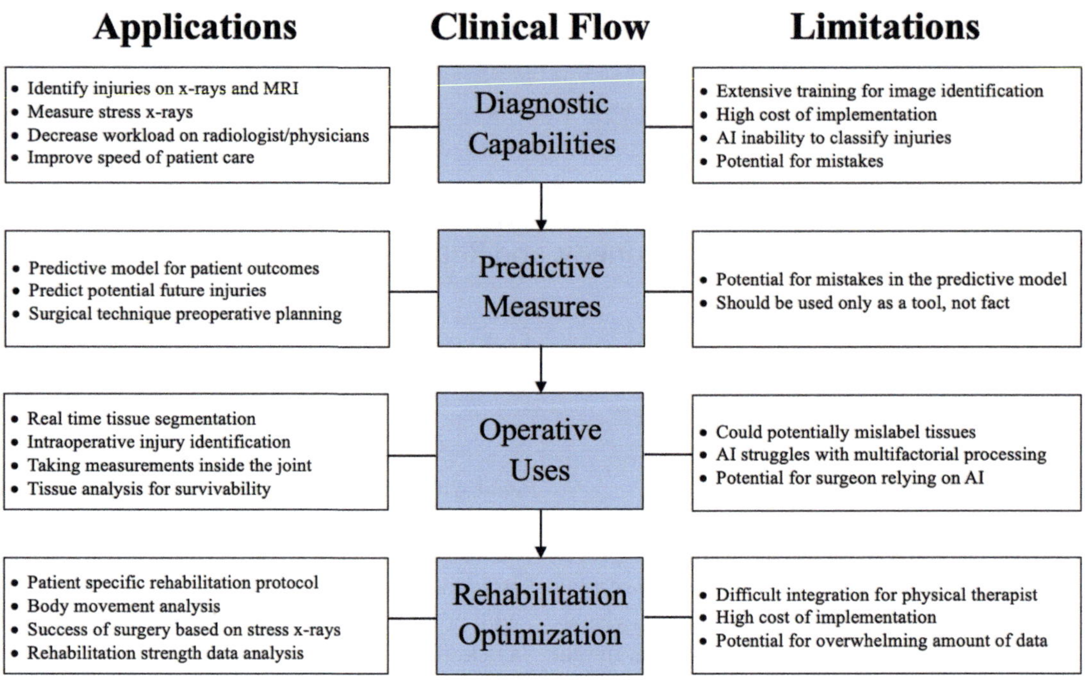

Fig. 10.1 Flowchart summarizing the clinical flow of using artificial intelligence in a clinical and surgical setting. The applications and limitations for each stage are listed and expanded upon in the rest of the chapter

10.2 Diagnostic

The first potential beneficial use of AI in knee arthroscopic surgery would be its potential as a diagnostic tool. AI could be used to supplement the diagnostic capabilities of radiologists and physicians in assessing knee injuries. The possibility of a symbiotic relationship exists between AI and radiologists, which could allow AI to reduce observer fatigue, improve efficiency, and improve overall diagnostic accuracy through error minimization. The radiologist would be able to analyze more images with better accuracy through the use and assistance of AI. Intelligent algorithms are applicable to various conditions including soft tissue injuries analyzed with MRI and bony tissue injuries like osteoarthritis, bone age and growth analysis, and complex fractures [2]. From an efficiency standpoint, the faster one can process diagnostic images, the quicker treatment can be provided which would support improved patient outcomes. The integration of these systems could provide significant benefits to front-line care settings (primary care clinicians and urgent cares) for proper diagnoses and supplying adequate information for suitable orthopedic referrals.

In relation to knee pathology diagnosis, studies have constructed a convolutional neural network (CNN) to identify various injuries from radiographs. CNNs are networks whose main objectives are to find pattern recognition in images and perform image manipulation (sharpening or blurring) of pixelation. Their secondary objective is geometric feature recognition (i.e., human eye aggregate features like ellipses or circles) for compilation and identification of defects [3]. Results compared the performance indicators of time and accuracy with reference to expert orthopedic physicians. The difference in the accuracy of the machines with respect to humans was not statistically significant, although time spent on average on each sample was 16 times faster on the machines [4]. Despite the results and advantages, they do come with a caveat. Machine learning and artificial intelligence need outlines for classification to make these applicable to the physical examination. Other limitations could be related to standardization of imaging that results in the inability of machine learning to identify anatomical abnormalities that lie outside of their significant parameter range. Unlike a physician, machines do not have the ability to use critical thinking to analyze an image that may look abnormal.

Using AI and CNNs, the identification of injuries via radiographs has already been utilized. Some groups have used these networks to diagnose tibial plateau fractures based on patient radiographs. Although AI technology is unable to classify these fractures, it does have the capability to identify them [4]. This could aid radiologists and physicians by using AI to first identify the fracture, and then having experts verify and classify the fracture that the AI system identified. Additionally, certain technologies have been used to determine the progression and diagnosis of osteoarthritis based on radiographic images [5]. The AI program was trained to identify bony defects related to the progression of osteoarthritis; the goal is to help physicians identify the progression of osteoarthritis early in the progression. These AI technologies have both been compared to board-certified physician evaluations of the same images and have shown that computer-aided diagnosis was not statistically different from the physician evaluation. Furthermore, with the explosion of AI evolution in the past decade, it would not be irrational to expect the capability of image analysis to exponentially increase as image quality and system complexity develop. In the future, AI could help to increase the agreement and reliability of diagnoses.

Another important diagnostic tool in orthopedic injury diagnosis is stress radiographs to determine the extent of a ligamentous injury. Common stress radiographs for knee injuries include ACL stress, PCL stress, and varus/valgus stress testing. These stress radiographs are performed bilaterally, and the injured side is often compared to the uninjured side. Based on previous research, for each specific stress radiograph technique, measurements can be taken of the movement or gapping. Comparing the difference between the injured side and the uninjured side can help determine the extent and likelihood that a ligamentous injury is present [6]. Additionally, these stress radiographs can help predict if other structures, like menisci or other concomitant ligaments, are injured as well. On some occasions, the measuring of the movement or gapping can be a bit subjective as no radiographic image is the same, and sometimes different orientations or rotations can cause the images to look different. AI could be useful to quickly analyze and measure specific movements or gapping, saving time for the surgeons in their analysis of images. AI could quickly identify specific landmarks, no matter the orientation of the image. The limitation with this would be the extensive time required to train the system. It would require a physician to verify thousands of radiographic images so the AI technology would be familiar with all orientations of the images. With training, the AI system could help physicians measure and analyze images faster than they would be able to without AI. However, like all other diagnostic uses for AI, this should never be used as a concrete diagnostic tool, verification should always be performed by the physician.

Artificial intelligence technology could also be beneficial in MRI analysis. Conventional MRI diagnostic accuracy is currently being tested against quantitative abbreviated MRI systems using prospective artificial intelligence image quality enhancement for arthroscopic procedures. Current methods of prospectively augmented MRIs with deep learning displayed strong inter-reader agreement with conventional MRIs and near-equivalent diagnostic arthroscopic performance. Various studies using AI to diagnose ACL injuries and meniscus injuries using MRI images are currently being evaluated. The preliminary data suggests that AI may be able to diagnose these types of injuries at the same level and accuracy as a human reader [7, 8]. Furthermore, some models have been trained to identify the type of ACL tear based on the location of the tear on MRI [9]. The ability of automatic generation of T2 mapping subsequently increases the imaging sensitivity for osteochondral abnormalities [10].

Concomitant with physicians' usage, AI-supplemented diagnostics have a promising future for the improvement of patient care.

One of the major limitations of current AI technology is the learning curve and time associated with teaching AI to properly identify images. Current technology requires AI to be told what something is, for example, identifying a torn ACL on MRI or identifying a tibial plateau fracture. This becomes problematic when one ACL tear MRI image looks different from another ACL tear MRI image. Some differences may be minute and something a physician might be able to pick up on, but an AI diagnostic tool might not be able to because of its strict rules related to reading an image. Additionally, AI has trouble classifying injuries like fractures; it may be able to identify a fracture but not tell what kind it is. Also, AI technology might struggle if it must rely on two images from different angles. Commonly, MRI or radiographic images must be viewed from various angles to determine the location and extent of an injury. Another deleterious limitation of AI technology is the inability of AI to perform a physical examination. After an acute injury, an MRI image is not always reliable. For example, the lateral meniscus root is notoriously difficult to diagnose on MRI due to the difficulties in visualizing the injury. AI might analyze an image of someone with a torn lateral meniscus root and determine they are injury-free. However, a physical examination of the patient's knee and an in-depth description of the patient's history can help to determine if an injury is present or not [11]. This difference between MRI or other injuries and the physical examination is especially evident in patients with chronic injuries. Someone who has a Baker's cyst in the back of their knee may not be symptomatic and thus does not require it to be drained. However, if AI saw an MRI image of someone with a Baker's cyst, it would most likely suggest draining the cyst. It is important to treat the patient, not their images, and unfortunately, AI can only treat the image.

Using AI in diagnostic capabilities of knee arthroscopic injuries could aid and supplement the diagnosis, but not replace all diagnostic tools. Physician physical examination, symptom gathering, and human interpretation of images are and will continue to be important in a patient's diagnosis. AI can aid in determining injuries on radiographs, making MRI images clearer, and identifying possible areas of injury or defect of the knee; however, a person will always be required to verify that the information is correct and classify different injury types.

10.3 Predictive

Prior to any surgical intervention, the operating physician evaluates the individual risk assessment of their patients to determine if the proposed procedure is the right choice for them. The goal is to maximize the benefits by reducing limiting aspects and coming to a consensual agreement for the "right" plan of action. Artificial intelligence can be utilized both pre- and post-operatively. These plans result from the analysis of patient BMI, age, genetics, lifestyle choices, and pre-existing comorbidities. The preceding directly affects risk of physiological complications like blood clotting during surgery, recovery time, and operation failure rates. Additionally, studies have already reported specific risk factors for extended opioid use after knee arthroscopic surgery. Some of the risk factors included preoperative patient-reported outcomes, symptom duration, and prior opioid use [12]. Knowing these factors and using these predictive models could help providers optimize treatment and care to decrease the chance of patients using opioids for an extended period. From an economic and lifestyle standpoint, artificial intelligence could implement analysis for anticipated hospital stays, receptivity to certain drugs, and the effects of continued postoperative opioid usage.

Artificial intelligence and machine learning also aid in the development of predictive models from the increasing availability of digital healthcare datasets. The models examine variables of patient-specific attributes, functional scores and preoperative pain, comorbidities, psychological features, socioeconomic indicators, and the influence on postoperative outcomes [13]. Furthermore, beyond the scope of data-model analysis, artificial intelligence aids in the construction of three-dimensional models of patient anatomy. These systems integrate preoperative imaging and surface mapping to provide physicians with tangible models prior to any cut being made. Physical models are beneficial in explaining minimally invasive procedures in depth to patients prior to and what to expect following their operation. All this in the compilation can provide patients with expected outcomes with remarkable accuracy to assist in their personal determination of care.

AI could also be used as a predictor of possible injuries in the future. Technology has already been used to determine which movement markers between sexes could be responsible for the increased prevalence of ACL injuries in females. By understanding what movement might lead to a higher chance of an ACL tear, movement modification can be done to help decrease the risk of an ACL injury. AI technology has also been used as a predictor for cartilage injury and degradation by using MRI images and T2 mapping. The ability to detect early cartilage damage would be beneficial to slow the progression to more severe cartilage damage. In the future, AI could be used to scan the body and analyze different movements to determine possible areas at risk for injury. This predictive model could help treat patients before an injury occurs, this could be in the form of activity modification, early surgical intervention, or physical therapy.

Potential issues with the implementation of artificial intelligence could pose a negative front to patients with significant comorbidities and create a disparity between those who receive affordable care. As the databases continue to grow and statistical evidence of predictive models becomes more accurate, insurance companies could utilize this significantly to determine if they should offer coverage to certain patients. If it is determined that a patient is at a high risk for surgery, AI should be used to deny them coverage of treatment or ability to proceed with the operation because they pose a liability to the hospital. Using artificial intelligence in predictive models must be done carefully and used only as a tool, and not facts or guarantees to ensure a detrimental gap will begin to expand for certain cohorts of patients. It is important to have predictive information on how patient outcomes might change based on patient dispositions, but this should only be used to ensure the physician, hospital, and anybody else associated is prepared. Just because AI determines a patient is high risk, does not mean the patient will have a poor outcome.

In addition to predictive patient outcomes, predictive technology could help surgeons determine how surgery should be performed before entering the operative room. AI can be used to create 3D models of a patient's knee based on MRI, CT, and radiographic images. Although the images are not always conclusive in terms of injury type and the extent of an injury, certain things can be predicted using AI. An osteotomy is a bony realignment surgery that cen be used to increase or decrease posterior tibial slope or correct varus or valgus malalignment. Although this surgery is not directly an arthroscopic surgery, it is often used in conjunction with arthroscopic surgery. AI could be used to predict what type of opening wedge or closing wedge osteotomy should be used to best correct any deformity of the knee. Having a plan going into surgery does not mean that plan will be used, but it could be beneficial to have more predictive tools at the disposal for the surgeons. Another useful application of 3D modeling could be the visualization of previously drilled ACL or PCL tunnels for a revision ACL or PCL surgery. Oftentimes these tunnels need to be bone grafted before a revision surgery can be performed. AI could be used to visualize these tunnels and predict how much bone graft will be needed for each tunnel.

10.4 Operative

The operative aspect of arthroscopy involves the most complexity and coordination. The integration of artificial intelligence into other procedural types may guide the implementation of arthroscopy. AI is already being used in other knee surgeries like arthroplasty, where AI is being used preoperatively and intraoperatively for surface mapping, specific bone landmarking, and ligament balancing [13]. Comparatively, arthroscopy is a surgery that provides less direct visualization but could still benefit from AI technology. In the future, AI may assist in introducing similar mapping elements for knee arthroscopy, tissue segmentation and identification, and intraoperative injury identification.

One potential benefit of AI in knee arthroscopic surgery is real-time segmentation of tissue. This technology is already being tested and developed to allow real-time labeling of different tissues and structures of the knee. The technology is currently limited and tissue identification is not very accurate, however, with more development, it could be a useful tool due to the difficulty in orientation and visualization in the knee [14, 15]. Although this technology should never be a replacement for in-depth knowledge of the various knee structures and possible deviations in the structures between patients, artificial intelligence could offer a secondary tool for surgeons to segment the different tissues in the knee. If used properly, AI could be used as a tool to confirm certain structures and map out the knee and the various injuries that might be present in that space. There is also the potential that this technology could be used with augmented reality to further enhance the interface for the surgeon. The segmentation and identification of the structures of the knee could be extremely beneficial for educational purposes. Oftentimes, using an arthroscopic camera in the knee joint and learning the identification of the structures of the knee can be very confusing. AI could help students properly identify the structures and diagnose injuries like meniscal or ligament tears.

The use of segmentation of tissues has been utilized in other procedures and structures, like laparoscopic procedures, with great success [16]. However, there are some limitations to consider when determining the transferability into arthroscopy. First, the anatomy of the knee: the joint space between the femoral condyles and the tibial plateau under flexion is typically only 10 mm in width, a menial space that decreases the overall field of view. Second, with minimal viewing exposure, loose bodies like fat or osteochondral debris may impede the ability to properly register anatomic structures. Finally, arthroscopic procedures typically require variable flexion positions to optimize exposure of key structures prompting shifting from origin positions. All of these in combination create additional impediments for an accurate segmentation system to be implemented. A lot of progress still needs to be made in using AI in knee arthroscopic surgeries, but it has the potential to help surgeons identify and diagnose various structures and injuries inside the knee joint.

Artificial intelligence also has the potential to be used intraoperatively for injury identification and surgical treatment suggestions. This technology for intraoperative diagnostic assessment is already being tested arthroscopically in the shoulder for the long head of the bicep (LHB) tendon. The technology is being utilized to determine the extent of an LHB tendon injury and then the AI technology can provide a recommendation for the subsequent surgical treatment [17]. Similar technology could eventually be used in the knee to determine the extent of certain injuries to ligament, meniscus, and cartilage. This could function as a secondary set of eyes to confirm a diagnosis and treatment options in surgery. Although it should not be used as a sole determinator for injury identification and surgery type, it could be a useful verification tool for surgeons.

Additionally, tissue analysis intraoperatively could assess the likely survivability of certain ligament grafting based on origin, construction, and anatomical fit after placement. A growing trend in orthopedic surgery has been the utilization of patient-specific implants that ensure superior outcomes. Machine learning systems created preoperative plans that guide construction and create the reduced need for surgeons to make intraoperative revisions. There have also been clear implications for revision surgery whereby these systems are able to accurately identify patient implants or hardware that may no longer be in routine use (up to 10% of implants are unable to be preoperatively identified) [18]. This is a critical part of the process for salvage option planning and future equipment ordering [19]. In association with artificial intelligence, revision procedures can become more cost-effective if most of the preoperative planning is conducted prior and procedural plans deviate less as a result equating to less time.

Artificial intelligence and machine learning could also be beneficial for taking measurements inside the joint. Measurement of different injuries, like the location and depth of a meniscal tear or the size of an osteochondral defect, could be useful for surgeons and for intraoperative surgical planning. This could also provide an improved method and system for classification of injuries. By having specific measurements and locations of various injuries, a more refined classification system could be developed for various knee injuries. Occasionally, determining the correct location for an ACL tunnel or how much of a meniscectomy should be performed can be difficult. AI technology could be utilized to provide surgeons with specific measurements and landmarks of the locations for repair sutures, tunnels, grafts, plates, and more based on 3D models of the joint.

One potential limitation of using AI in the operative setting is the limitations AI has with multifactorial processing. In the setting of knee arthroscopic surgery, many things are occurring at once with multiple different camera angles, instruments being used, and potential differences between the structures in someone's knee. Plus, in some cases, structures in the knee are not always as they seem in terms of diagnosis and required treatment. For example, an intact ACL might not actually be a functioning ACL. In many cases, revision ACL reconstruction needs to be done to fix a graft that has been stretched out and is nonfunctional. The graft may still be intact in the joint, but it might not be tight like it should be. It would be difficult for AI to diagnose a problem like this. AI technology needs to improve to be able to better understand the knee joint and be able to process multifactorial inputs.

10.5 Rehabilitation

During the postoperative rehabilitation stage of knee arthroscopic surgery, AI and machine learning can be used to improve the recovery of patients. The current technology allows physical therapists to analyze how their patients move through various exercises so they can then tailor their patients' rehabilitation to the results from their tests and the specific surgery they underwent. Baseline postoperative assessments are conducted via force plates, motion capture, and dynamometry technologies to track the body movements of patients as they perform various exercises including double-legged squats, single-leg squats, and single-leg jumps. In collaboration with machine learning systems, the data acquired from this testing can be used to determine how the rehabilitation should continue. This data can also be used in retrospective studies to track how different surgical and rehabilitation techniques affect patient outcomes. Additionally, as more information becomes available, AI will be able to determine the best path for patient rehabilitation to correct for any deficiencies in strength or function.

The frontal plane biomechanics of the knee are typically used as a predictive marker for injury risk [20]. For anterior cruciate ligament (ACL) reconstruction, it is well-established that malalignment and/or biomechanical alteration of the tibiofemoral and patellofemoral joint can lead to accelerated progression of osteoarthritis. More than 120,000 ACL injuries occur annually, and treatment typically (90%) proceeds with reconstruction followed by rehabilitation. For professional athletes, returning to play can take nearly 12 months following a continued rigorous rehabilitation program. More than 50% fail to return to pre-injury levels of functional performance and the development of osteoarthritis 5–10 years post-op occurs in 50–100%. With the utilization of inertial measurement unit sensors to assess joint angles, load acceleration, and velocity in functional movement tests, the overall risk of re-injury can be assessed, and rehabilitation programs can be optimized to prevent further degradation of the joint space [21]. With all these metrics, thousands of data points are compiled and an adaptive process that used to take weeks can begin immediately. This immediacy improves physical therapist efficiency and the opportunity to form adaptive plans based on the pace of progression for an individual.

Furthermore, the compilation of these metrics into easily discernible data using AI provides an easy medium for mental and physical reassurance in their return to daily norms, whether that is a high-athletic competition or casual daily activities. The quality of patient outcomes is highly dependent on understanding and adherence to recommended rehabilitation protocols. Nonadherence is a growing threat to overall health and well-being that can carry future appreciable economic weight. In some pathologic conditions, more than 40% of patients sustain substantial risk through misunderstanding, forgetting, or ignoring guidance from their healthcare professionals [22]. Although AI cannot solve nonadherence, it can hopefully allow providers to give the patients a better picture of their rehabilitation and how they should proceed. With scientifically backed data, it can be easier for patients to understand how they are progressing and can give them concrete examples of how they should proceed.

Another important part of the rehabilitation process is the measurement of the success of a surgery. Like measuring the movement and gapping in stress radiographs in a diagnostic setting, these measurements can also be used to determine the success of a surgery. Measuring the movement and gapping of the knee postoperative can help determine if the deficiency that was measured preoperatively was successfully corrected. This information is useful when comparing different surgical techniques and the success rate associated with the surgery. In the future, AI could be used in the research process to verify measurements and provide more accurate data to back up these studies.

The rehabilitation process is an integral part of the success of knee arthroscopic surgeries. Depending on the type of surgery, the rehabilitation process and protocols change. By incorporating AI into the rehabilitation process, the protocols could become even more refined and specific to each patient. Additionally, this process could become automated by AI allowing physical therapists to spend more time focusing on their patients and less time having to create plans for each individual patient. By having a better understanding of patient rehabilitation with specific measurements, body movement analysis, and statistics, physicians and physical therapists can obtain a better and deeper understanding of the success and effectiveness of different surgical and rehabilitation techniques.

10.6 Potential Problems

Artificial intelligence has a multitude of upsides that make implementation into medicine, orthopedics, and surgery seem advantageous, although it does not come without drawbacks. The first problem within machine learning and intelligence systems is that their evolution and ability rely heavily on large datasets. Bias is an issue with a small dataset and will affect future performance negatively [23]. Due to this issue, AI technology and machine learning require a huge amount of training. This training would require professionals in each field to train and verify the accuracy of the AI machine. Furthermore, generalization for AI machines is difficult and because of this, finding outliers or anomalies in imaging or the data AI is analyzing is nearly impossible. AI does not have the capability for critical thinking, so although it does a great job of identifying common and obvious deformities or injuries, it would struggle in situations in which an injury is abnormal or involves multiple structures.

An overarching problem with the age of digitalization is the issue of data security. With the increased conglomeration of data to assist in the development of machine models the risk of compromised exposure can happen. Of the existing machine learning and neural network technology that exists today, a large amount of them are owned or controlled by large corporations like Google, Microsoft, Apple, IBM, and many more

[24]. They can typically gain access to patient-protected health information (PHI) via muddled information-sharing agreements. In 2016, an example of poor privacy protection in one of these partnerships became relevant news. DeepMind, owned by Google, partnered with the Royal Free London NHS Foundation to implement machine learning into an acute kidney injury management study. From this partnership, Google obtained significant PHI on an "inappropriate legal basis" according to a senior advisor in the English Department of Health. There was a subsequent transfer of this PHI to storage in the United States that effectively annexed significant quantities of patient information outside of their personal jurisdiction to another [25]. As we have established, arthroscopic procedures can range in complexity which affects their significance to overall health and well-being. The availability of this information will change as the integration of artificial intelligence continues and its vulnerability may increase if precautionary measures are not taken to protect it.

Additionally, dependence is a double-edged sword. After the artificial intelligence technology has been implemented, the learning curve for certain procedures or image analysis would decrease, making them more accessible as the complexity increases. This could potentially improve patient treatment and help medical treatment occur more efficiently and promptly. But then a question arises, will surgeons become less qualified and more dependent on the technology? If adverse or abnormal conditions are present, will they be able to recognize it? These are difficult questions to answer currently, however, these are important considerations to keep in mind as AI technology continues to improve. With increased autonomy, there could become a shift in procedural responsibility from physicians to AI machines.

Another big problem could arise when patients do not trust AI or errors occur in the system. For example, patients might not agree to having AI be a part of their treatment and if so, this would seriously decrease the effectiveness of a practice if AI has already become a standard part of an orthopedic practice. Also, if AI makes a mistake, who is to blame? At this point, AI cannot run by itself and must be constantly monitored by a professional. However, the future of AI could involve autonomous regulation without constant supervision by real people. When we get to this point, what would the consequences and protocols be if AI makes a mistake in identifying an injury in patient imaging. Is the person in charge of the AI software to blame, or is the provider using the software to blame? This can quickly become a difficult situation for which we currently have no regulations or oversight. Before AI technology is fully implemented in orthopedic arthroscopic practice, questions like this need to be addressed.

Cost of implementation is an economic overarching issue, not just the monetary expense but also time taken to become effectively familiarized with these systems. Artificial intelligence equipment adapted for healthcare can range between \$20,000 and \$1,000,000 per system. For systems of minimal quality, the costs can range from \$8,000–\$15,000. Effective AI systems are not a one-stop off-the-shelf purchase, everything must be custom-built. This requires data scientists, AI and software engineers, and medical management oversight to prevent knowledge limitation which all accrues costs. Additionally, there is a cost to running the machines and maintaining the program. Then, the integration of systems into standard operating procedures may condense provider availability for extended periods of time due to training, increasing the opportunity cost of the complete implementation of these machines.

10.7 Conclusions

Artificial intelligence has the potential to be an important and useful part of knee arthroscopic surgery. It has potential uses in the diagnostic, predictive, operative, and rehabilitative settings of knee arthroscopic surgery. Uses in diagnostics can help to interpret and classify images like radiographs, CT, and MRI for diagnostics of injuries. It has the potential to aid hospitals and providers in their prediction of patient outcomes and needs before, during, and after surgery. It could help in the operative setting by aiding surgeons in surgical planning, tissue identification, and intraoperative measurements. Finally, it has the potential to improve the rehabilitation process for patients by gaining a deeper understanding of their specific strengths and weaknesses and helping them implement a personalized plan to maximize their recovery.

The future integration of artificial intelligence is imminent in many facets of medicine. How and why we utilize it are important factors to consider when weighing the pros and cons of the incorporation and adaptation of a new medical norm. As we have seen, the opportunities for improvement in efficiency and accuracy are readily available. Although some of the technology might not be there yet, soon it will be. Although these positives are not rendered without plausible consequences, the dispersion of information into machine learning systems increases the risk of dependency on AI, huge financial expenses, and rigorous testing and time taken to verify the reliability of the technology.

References

1. Sunarti S, Fadzlul Rahman F, Naufal M, Risky M, Febriyanto K, Masnina R. Artificial intelligence in healthcare: opportunities and risk for future. Gac Sanit. 2021;35(Suppl 1):S67–70. https://doi.org/10.1016/j.gaceta.2020.12.019.
2. Gyftopoulos S, Lin D, Knoll F, Doshi AM, Rodrigues TC, Recht MP. Artificial intelligence in musculoskeletal imaging: current status and future directions. AJR Am J Roentgenol. 2019;213(3):506–13. https://doi.org/10.2214/AJR.19.21117.
3. Innocenti B, Radyul Y, Bori E. The use of artificial intelligence in orthopedics: applications and limitations fo machine learning in diagnosis and prediction. Appl Sci. 2022;12(21) https://doi.org/10.3390/app122110775.
4. Liu PR, Zhang JY, Xue MD, Duan YY, Hu JL, Liu SX, et al. Artificial intelligence to diagnose Tibial plateau fractures: an intelligent assistant for orthopedic physicians. Curr Med Sci. 2021;41(6):1158–64. https://doi.org/10.1007/s11596-021-2501-4.
5. Smolle MA, Goetz C, Maurer D, Vielgut I, Novak M, Zier G, et al. Artificial intelligence-based computer-aided system for knee osteoarthritis assessment increases experienced orthopaedic surgeons' agreement rate and accuracy. Knee Surg Sports Traumatol Arthrosc. 2023;31(3):1053–62. https://doi.org/10.1007/s00167-022-07220-y.
6. LaPrade RF, Heikes C, Bakker AJ, Jakobsen RB. The reproducibility and repeatability of varus stress radiographs in the assessment of isolated fibular collateral ligament and grade-III posterolateral knee injuries. An in vitro biomechanical study. J Bone Joint Surg Am. 2008;90(10):2069–76. https://doi.org/10.2106/JBJS.G.00979.
7. Minamoto Y, Akagi R, Maki S, Shiko Y, Tozawa R, Kimura S, et al. Automated detection of anterior cruciate ligament tears using a deep convolutional neural network. BMC Musculoskelet Disord. 2022;23(1):577. https://doi.org/10.1186/s12891-022-05524-1.
8. Li Z, Ren S, Zhang X, Bai L, Jiang C, Wu J, Zhang W. Deep learning-based image feature with arthroscopy-aided early diagnosis and treatment of meniscus injury of knee joint. J Healthc Eng. 2021;2021:2254594. https://doi.org/10.1155/2021/2254594.
9. Qu C, Yang H, Wang C, Wang C, Ying M, Chen Z, et al. A deep learning approach for anterior cruciate ligament rupture localization on knee MR images. Front Bioeng Biotechnol. 2022;10:1024527. https://doi.org/10.3389/fbioe.2022.1024527.
10. Chaudhari AS, Grissom MJ, Fang Z, Sveinsson B, Lee JH, Gold GE, et al. Diagnostic accuracy of quantitative multicontrast 5-minute knee MRI using prospective artificial intelligence image quality enhancement. AJR Am J Roentgenol. 2021;216(6):1614–25. https://doi.org/10.2214/AJR.20.24172.
11. Bhatia S, LaPrade CM, Ellman MB, LaPrade RF. Meniscal root tears: significance, diagnosis, and treatment. Am J Sports Med. 2014;42(12):3016–30. https://doi.org/10.1177/0363546514524162.
12. Lu Y, Forlenza E, Wilbur RR, Lavoie-Gagne O, Fu MC, Yanke AB, et al. Machine-learning model successfully predicts patients at risk for prolonged postoperative opioid use following elective knee arthroscopy. Knee Surg Sports Traumatol Arthrosc. 2022;30(3):762–72. https://doi.org/10.1007/s00167-020-06421-7.
13. Batailler C, Shatrov J, Sappey-Marinier E, Servien E, Parratte S, Lustig S. Artificial intelligence in knee arthroplasty: current concept of the available clinical applications. Arthroplasty. 2022;4(1):17. https://doi.org/10.1186/s42836-022-00119-6.
14. Ali S, Jonmohamadi Y, Fontanarosa D, Crawford R, Pandey AK. One step surgical scene restoration for robot assisted minimally invasive surgery. Sci Rep. 2023;13(1):3127. https://doi.org/10.1038/s41598-022-26647-4.
15. Jonmohamadi Y, Takeda Y, Liu F, Sasazawa F, Maicas G, Crawford R, et al. Automatic segmentation of multiple structures in knee arthroscopy using deep learning. IEEE Access. 2020;8:51853–61. https://doi.org/10.1109/ACCESS.2020.2980025.
16. Park SH, Park HM, Baek KR, Ahn HM, Lee IY, Son GM. Artificial intelligence based real-time microcirculation analysis system for laparoscopic colorectal

surgery. World J Gastroenterol. 2020;26(44):6945–62. https://doi.org/10.3748/wjg.v26.i44.6945.
17. Benhenneda R, Brouard T, Dordain F, Gadea F, Charousset C, Berhouet J, Francophone Arthroscopy S. Can artificial intelligence help decision-making in arthroscopy? Part 1: use of a standardized analysis protocol improves inter-observer agreement of arthroscopic diagnostic assessments of the long head of biceps tendon in small rotator cuff tears. Orthop Traumatol Surg Res. 2023;109:103648. https://doi.org/10.1016/j.otsr.2023.103648.
18. Wilson NA, Jehn M, York S, Davis CM 3rd. Revision total hip and knee arthroplasty implant identification: implications for use of unique device identification 2012 AAHKS member survey results. J Arthroplast. 2014;29(2):251–5. https://doi.org/10.1016/j.arth.2013.06.027.
19. Kurmis AP, Ianunzio JR. Artificial intelligence in orthopedic surgery: evolution, current state and future directions. Arthroplasty. 2022;4(1):9. https://doi.org/10.1186/s42836-022-00112-z.
20. Culvenor AG, Schache AG, Vicenzino B, Pandy MG, Collins NJ, Cook JL, Crossley KM. Are knee biomechanics different in those with and without patellofemoral osteoarthritis after anterior cruciate ligament reconstruction? Arthritis Care Res (Hoboken). 2014;66(10):1566–70. https://doi.org/10.1002/acr.22313.
21. Kianifar R, Lee A, Raina S, Kulic D. Automated assessment of dynamic knee valgus and risk of knee injury during the single leg squat. IEEE J Transl Eng Health Med. 2017;5:2100213. https://doi.org/10.1109/JTEHM.2017.2736559.
22. Martin LR, Williams SL, Haskard KB, Dimatteo MR. The challenge of patient adherence. Ther Clin Risk Manag. 2005;1(3):189–99.
23. Lee LS, Chan PK, Wen C, Fung WC, Cheung A, Chan VWK, et al. Artificial intelligence in diagnosis of knee osteoarthritis and prediction of arthroplasty outcomes: a review. Arthroplasty. 2022;4(1):16. https://doi.org/10.1186/s42836-022-00118-7.
24. Powles J, Hodson H. Google DeepMind and healthcare in an age of algorithms. Health Technol (Berl). 2017;7(4):351–67. https://doi.org/10.1007/s12553-017-0179-1.
25. Murdoch B. Privacy and artificial intelligence: challenges for protecting health information in a new era. BMC Med Ethics. 2021;22(1):122. https://doi.org/10.1186/s12910-021-00687-3.

11 Artificial Intelligence in Shoulder Arthroscopy

Marco-Christopher Rupp, Annabel R. Geissbuhler, Grant Dornan, Jonas Pogorzelski, and Peter J. Millett

11.1 Introduction

As of 2023, technological advancements in artificial intelligence (AI) have reached a tipping point leading to substantial public awareness of the significant potential of this technology [1]. AI offers orthopedic surgeons the opportunity to explore the potential applications to their specific areas of expertise, including shoulder arthroscopy.

In general, AI is defined as the ability of machines to solve problems that traditionally require human intelligence, such as visual perception, speech recognition, and decision-making [2]. This technology has, in the last 10–20 years, started to be leveraged in medicine across different specialties to both automate clinical tasks and augment clinicians' abilities [3]. The development of AI in health care is largely due to increasingly accessible computing power, dramatic technological advancements in the various aspects of AI (machine-learning (ML), deep learning (DL), computer vision and natural language processing (NLP)), sharply increasing health care system costs, and the exponential availability of digital data [4].

While fields relying heavily on data, such as radiology, pathology, and oncology, were at the forefront of this development [5], the capabilities of AI to analyze enormous data sets in real-time have most recently been deployed to various aspects of shoulder surgery and sports medicine. AI can enable preoperative risk stratification, prediction of clinically relevant outcome improvement, interpretation of X-rays and advanced musculoskeletal imaging, and automation of administrative tasks such as medical record keeping and billing.

The adoption of AI heralds the potential to improve the accuracy and speed of diagnosis and treatment, to analyze large amounts of data for insight into disease and injury patterns and their prognosis, and to evaluate comprehensively advanced imaging. For orthopedic surgeons, these features allow for better individualization of treatment plans based on patient-specific factors [4]. Thus, AI may be part of the answer to the current sentiment of "insufficient time", "insufficient context", and "insufficient presence" in healthcare systems across the globe [6].

M.-C. Rupp
Steadman Philippon Research Institute, Vail, CO, USA

Department of Orthopaedic Sports Medicine, Technical University of Munich, Munich, Germany

A. R. Geissbuhler · G. Dornan
Steadman Philippon Research Institute, Vail, CO, USA

J. Pogorzelski
Department of Orthopaedic Sports Medicine, Technical University of Munich, Munich, Germany

P. J. Millett (✉)
Steadman Philippon Research Institute, Vail, CO, USA

The Steadman Clinic, Vail, CO, USA
e-mail: drmillett@thesteadmanclinic.com

F. Familiari et al. (eds.), *Artificial Intelligence in Orthopaedic Surgery Made Easy*, https://doi.org/10.1007/978-3-031-70310-2_11

The aim of this chapter is to comprehensively review the AI solutions already available specific to shoulder arthroscopy and to explore potential avenues for the successful future implementation of this technology to increase the capabilities of shoulder arthroscopists.

11.2 Clinical Areas of Use of AI in Shoulder Arthroscopy

The potential use of AI along the continuum of care in shoulder arthroscopy is visualized in Fig. 11.1.

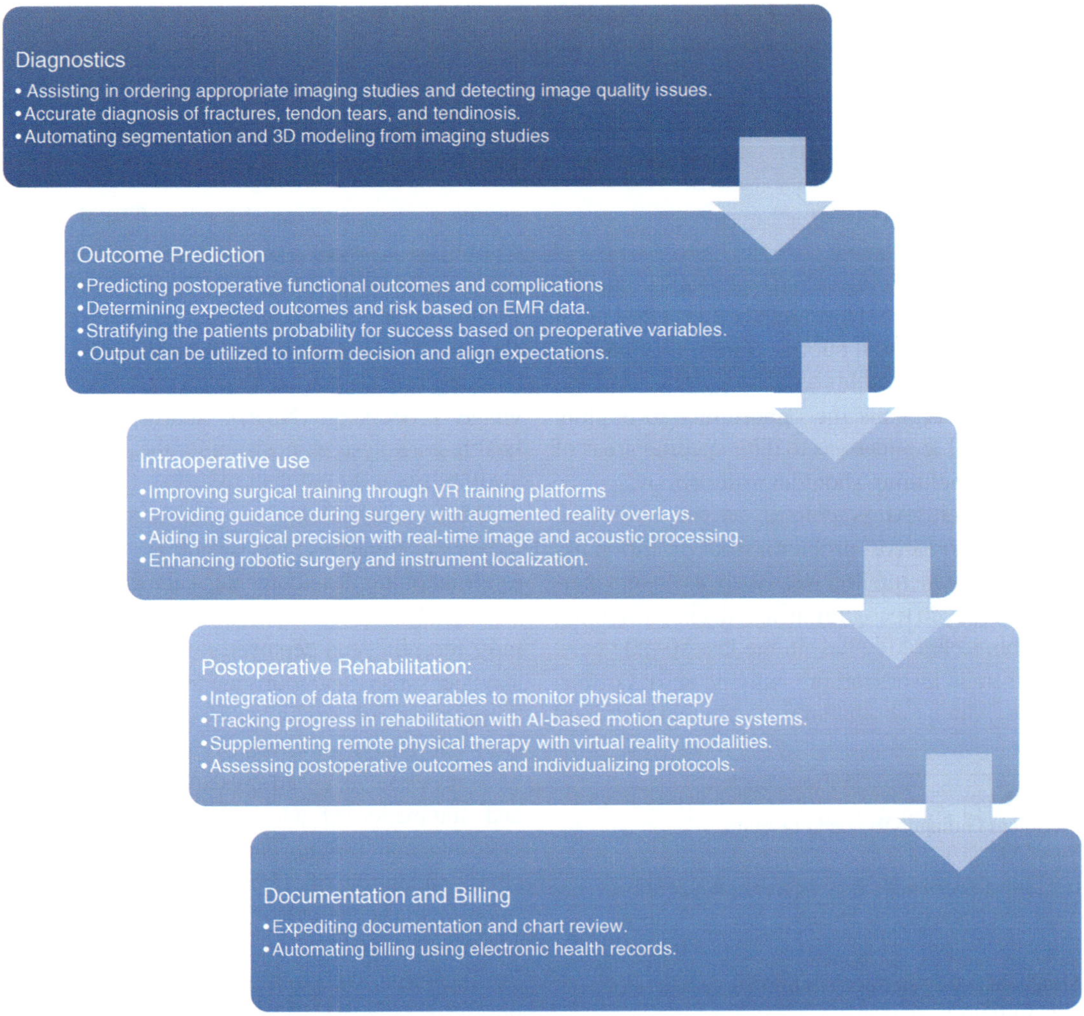

Fig. 11.1 Clinical use cases of AI across the continuum of care in shoulder arthroscopy

11.3 Diagnostics

AI has the potential to transform all aspects of the shoulder-specific radiographic value chain; from optimizing the ordering of imaging studies to analyzing and interpreting images [7]. Starting with the ordering of imaging, AI solutions can integrate information from electronic medical records (EMR) to assist physicians in ordering appropriate imaging in a targeted fashion [8]. Since the overutilization of advanced imaging may lead to increased clinical workload, as well as posing unnecessary financial costs and radiation exposure for patients, the use of AI support tools in ordering imaging has the potential to increase efficiency in outpatient consultations that include imaging acquisition [7]. For shoulder arthroscopy, this may reduce the amount of preoperative standard X-rays obtained and allow for preemptive capacity allocation of advanced imaging in cases such as shoulder instability.

AI-based technology also has the capacity to optimize the time spent conducting advanced imaging and decrease the likelihood of patient recall for repeated imaging. For example, Hahn et al. have developed a deep-learning algorithm for shoulder MRIs, decreasing the scan time by 67% without affecting image quality, artifacts, or diagnostic performance [9]. Further, 93.7% accuracy was found using an ML algorithm to identify MRI images of unacceptable quality [10], which may be particularly relevant for identifying shoulder MRIs impacted by motion artifacts.

The analysis of imaging in orthopedics often requires a specialist human rater and can still be both time-consuming and prone to error. Thus, many AI systems have been created to decrease the clinical burden of image interpretation, with great success in detecting both fractures [11] and soft tissue injuries [12]. A systematic review of AI detection of fractures found that AI was able to detect fractures at a comparable diagnostic quality to clinicians [11]. Specifically in shoulders, AI has been used to accurately diagnose proximal humerus fractures [13], rotator cuff tears [14], and biceps tendinosis [15]. A recent study even suggests that algorithms can detect radiographic patterns typically unseen by expert human raters. In this study, subscapularis tendon tears were identified by a machine-learning algorithm with moderate accuracy using only axillary radiographs by noticing minute changes in the lesser tuberosity [16].

In addition, the past 10 years have seen the emergence of MRI/CT segmentation for quantification of pathologies such as rotator cuff atrophy and 3D reconstruction of joints for preoperative planning. Both processes can be very time-consuming and thus are out-of-reach for many practices, but AI-based tools show substantial promise in automating both segmentation and the creation of 3D models from imaging studies. A recent study by Medina et al. found that a ML algorithm had over 95% accuracy in segmenting the muscles of the rotator cuff [17]. Further, Ro et al. found that AI was able to accurately evaluate the fatty infiltration of the rotator cuff [18]. Given that 3D quantification of fatty infiltration has been shown to be superior to the classic 2D classification according to Goutallier [19], the use of AI algorithms for segmentation has the potential to improve the preoperative analysis of muscle quality in rotator cuff tears [20]. Segmentation of the rotator cuff has even been performed using a deep-learning model applied to ultrasound imaging [21]. Due to the widespread availability and low cost of ultrasounds in comparison to other advanced imaging modalities, the development of AI tools to improve the diagnostic quality of ultrasounds could transform the diagnosis of rotator cuff tears.

AI algorithms have also been applied to 3-dimensional modeling for surgical planning. A review article by Samim et al. found that artificial intelligence-assisted postprocessing models were reliably able to produce 3D models of shoulder from MRIs, providing a comprehensive evaluation of osseous morphology with only one preoperative imaging study [22]. AI algorithms have also been able to produce 3D models from only 2-dimensional radiographs, providing 3D bone reconstructions similar to a CT scan model at a fraction of the time and cost [23].

11.4 Outcome Prediction

AI also shows substantial promise in predicting patient outcomes to assist in both physician and patient-informed decision-making and align patient expectations to reality [24]. Advanced statistical models have already been developed to predict outcomes after shoulder surgery, such as prognostic monograms developed at our practice to assist in patient selection for arthroscopic rotator cuff repair [25]. Machine-learning algorithms can be expected to build upon the prognostic abilities of these statistical models, and automize the process of creating predictive models. In the field of arthroscopic shoulder surgery, multiple studies have shown that ML algorithms can accurately predict postoperative functional outcomes. Potty et al. utilized ML and predictive analytics to accurately predict ASES scores after rotator cuff repair [26]. Similarly, Kumar et al. utilized a database of anatomic and reverse total shoulder arthroplasty cases to train three different ML algorithms, finding that all three algorithms were able to accurately predict postoperative ASES scores, UCLA scores, constant scores, global shoulder function scores, VAS pain scores, and postoperative range of motion [27].

Machine-learning models have also demonstrated their potential to predict complications after shoulder surgery [28–30]. Karnuta et al. developed an artificial neural network model to predict the length of stay, discharge disposition, and inpatient charges for total shoulder arthroplasty and hemiarthroplasty with good accuracy and reliability [30]. Lopez et al. also developed a similar model with a specific focus on non-home discharge after total shoulder arthroplasty [28]. These AI models show high accuracy in predicting complications that would elongate inpatient recovery, helping shoulder surgeons accurately predict the costs [31] associated with shoulder replacement and managing postoperative expectations. Currently, models are in development for predicting the probability of retear after rotator cuff repair [32] and instability after Bankart repair [29], showing investment in the potential of AI to predict complications and risk of revision operations after arthroscopic shoulder surgery.

AI also has the ability to automatically determine expected patient outcomes and risk for complications based on information contained in EMRs [33–35]. In a technical feasibility study, Twick et al. developed a highly accurate ML algorithm for the purpose of determining patients at risk of surgical site infection and anastomosis leak complications after general surgery utilizing exclusively EMR-contained patient data [35]. Taneja et al. [34] and Desai et al. [33] were able to create similar, EMR-based complication and outcome prediction ML models for sepsis and heart failure, demonstrating an ability for widespread utilization of EMR-based machine-learning models. It can be expected that in the future, machine-learning models will be applied to shoulder arthroscopy to automatically assess expected patient outcomes and risk of complications by incorporating information already contained in EMR.

The culmination of functional outcomes and complication prediction is the ability to stratify patients by their propensity to achieve favorable outcomes at a low complication rate. For example, Kunze et al.'s systematic review found that outcome-prediction ML models were reliably able to risk-stratify patients based on whether they were expected to achieve a clinically meaningful improvement postoperatively, providing guidance to both patients and physicians on whether surgery is the optimal strategy at that point in time [24]. This process will allow shoulder surgeons to provide highly personalized treatment plans to individual patients, including a modification of the surgical technique, or modulation of physical therapy and return-to-sport timelines based on an individual's personalized prediction of postoperative success or failure [29, 32]. Overall, it can be expected in the future that surgeons will be able to utilize ML models to preoperatively provide patients with a full personalized picture of their expected recovery timeline, likely complications, monetary cost of surgery, and postoperative outcomes, allowing patients to make an informed decision and hold realistic expectations postoperatively.

11.5 Intraoperative Use

Augmented reality and virtual overlays are already being used in shoulder surgery for preoperative planning and training, and this trend is only expected to grow over time. Due to the steep learning curve associated with arthroscopic surgery, virtual reality (VR) simulations show promise in being utilized for training of resident physicians [36]. Systematic reviews by Vaughan et al. and Berthold et al. of virtual reality-based training platforms for orthopedic surgery demonstrated that residents trained with shoulder arthroscopy VR performed more quickly and made fewer mistakes than residents trained with conventional methods [37, 38]. VR training platforms also avoid the need for cadavers or animals to be used for surgical training purposes, while still providing trainees surgical practice before operating on actual patients [38]. VR training platforms are currently limited by availability and high monetary cost but are expected to be a vital tool in surgical training and preoperative planning in the future [38].

Intraoperatively, AI will play a vital role in orthopedic surgery error prevention via augmented reality overlays, real-time image and sound processing, robotic surgery, and intelligent instruments. Augmented reality overlays provide surgeons with the ability to place virtual information onto their surgical field, to provide intuitive guidance while still having a vision of the real world [39]. Due to the technical challenge of properly placing the glenoid component in rTSA, virtual overlays have already been developed to assist in placing glenoid guide pins, with promising results [39]. Intuitively, the development of augmented reality overlays for shoulder arthroscopic surgery has lagged behind open surgery due to more limited intraoperative visibility and the challenges associated with repairing soft tissue structures, but it can be expected that similar platforms will be developed for shoulder arthroscopy in the future.

Real-time processing of both surgical images and sound also shows promise in limiting errors in shoulder arthroscopy. In a study by Seibold et al., a deep-learning algorithm was developed to detect acoustic changes associated with drill breakthrough events in hip cadaver surgery and was able to detect breakthrough events many times more quickly than a surgeon's reaction time [40]. In shoulder procedures such as sternoclavicular reconstruction or clavicular fracture fixation where drill accuracy is vital, AI acoustic processing could help surgeons optimize drill hole placement and react quickly when a breakthrough event occurs. Furthermore, real-time image processing may be a tool in the future of shoulder arthroscopy. In other specialties, algorithms have been developed to detect landmarks in real time to help direct surgeons [41]. Similar systems are being developed to detect landmarks in knee arthroscopy, and it can be expected that similar algorithms will be used in the future of shoulder arthroscopy.

AI algorithms also can address some of the issues that have made robotic shoulder arthroscopy challenging. In a study performed by Bozkurt et al., the da Vinci robotic surgical system was able to perform shoulder arthroscopy in both the beach chair and lateral decubitus position. However, the surgery was challenged by the large size of the machine, obstruction of camera view by fluid and pressure, and an inability to obtain 3D visualization during close views [42]. Thus, the use of AI to help guide the machine to landmarks, enhance intraoperative images, and produce models for enhanced preoperative planning would help increase the feasibility of robotic arthroscopic surgery. Intelligent surgical tools have also been developed for other specialties that could become highly useful in shoulder arthroscopy. Cho et al. developed a surgical instrument for endoscopic spine surgery that can intelligently detect the tip of the instrument and help the surgeon localize it to a desired point from the video input [43]. A tool of this type would be utilized in shoulder arthroscopy, assisting surgeons in localizing their instruments to difficult-to-reach areas seen through the scope, such as inferior humeral osteophytes in the CAM procedure [44]. Overall, AI will play a role in the future of shoulder arthroscopy, through virtual reality surgical training and augmented reality intraoperative overlays, real-time image and acoustic processing, and intelligent instruments.

11.6 Postoperative Rehabilitation

Among many other disruptive healthcare changes, the coronavirus pandemic has highlighted the necessity of high quality, remote postoperative rehabilitation programs, a problem which AI is well-equipped to handle [45]. In home-based rehabilitation, patient-monitoring techniques such as phone or video calls with a therapist often lack the ability to reliably track progress in strength and range of motion [45]. Other challenges arise with at-home therapy including decreased patient compliance and the risk of overexertion or inadequate effort [45]. To address these challenges, virtual rehabilitation platforms have been developed using AI-powered motion capture systems that are compatible with mobile and wearable devices, which could be utilized in the rehabilitation following shoulder arthroscopy [45]. These AI algorithms provide patients instantaneous feedback on their exercises and provide accountability for patients with monitoring of daily progress [45]. Smartwatches have also been leveraged to develop an ML algorithm that can identify seven different shoulder exercises, illustrating a capacity for remote monitoring of the frequency, duration, and biomechanics of motions that construct a physical therapy regimen after arthroscopic shoulder surgery [46]. Similarly, virtual reality modalities have been used to supplement remote physical therapy. A study conducted by Pekyavas et al. utilized Wii Fit virtual reality exercises for patients with subacromial impingement syndrome and found that these patients had better range of motion and less pain than patients treated with a traditional home exercise programs [47].

Overall, AI has the capacity to transform postoperative rehabilitation through increasing the quality of remote rehabilitation, tracking patient progress and outcomes, and individualizing rehabilitation protocols.

11.7 Documentation and Billing

Lastly, AI-based technology has the opportunity to expedite documentation and coding. It is estimated that clinical documentation and chart review can consume up to 34% to 55% of a physician's workday and has been identified as one of the leading causes of lost physician productivity [48]. To address this challenge, a proof-of-concept study by Klann et al. found that an AI algorithm was able to use voice recognition to accurately identify and place single- and multi-word phrases extracted from a patient-physician interaction into note format, and this algorithm plans to also integrate NLP to extract clinical meaning from narrative medical text in the future [49]. A study by Deliberato et al. found that AI was able to extract and organize clinical information from previous imaging reports, clinical notes, and laboratory results more quickly than a human, showing that AI has the potential to greatly reduce the time that physicians spend reviewing patient records [50]. Further, it can be anticipated that outcome prediction algorithms, like those discussed in previous sections, can be automatically integrated into chart review algorithms, and thus automatically calculated in the process of note creation [48].

In addition, AI algorithms have shown the capacity to automate billing using only electronic health records. An algorithm combining both ML and NLP was developed by Kim et al. to automatically generate CPT codes from physician-dictated operative reports with 87% accuracy [51]. Specifically in orthopedics, a similar algorithm was used by Zaidat et al. to generate CPT codes from spine surgery operative notes, with a maximal accuracy of 88% [52]. With many companies such as Deloitte, Optum, and Capita all racing to create the first autonomous clinical coding system, it can be expected that automated coding will be commonplace within the next 10 years [53]. Overall, AI shows great promise in automating pre-visit chart review, documentation, coding, and billing, decreasing physician workload, and improving clinical efficiency.

11.8 Considerations and Repercussions for Clinical Application

11.8.1 Limitations of AI in Shoulder Arthroscopy

Although many AI algorithms have been created for experimental use, the lengthy approval process for AI algorithms as well as monetary and indirect costs serve as a roadblock for more widespread use. In the United States, AI algorithms are regulated by the Food and Drug Administration (FDA), where it is considered Software as a Medical Device (SAMD) [54]. It is estimated that the average medical device takes a total from 3 to 7 years to take to the market from inception [55]. On top of the 3–7 years necessary to gain FDA approval, it can be expected that new devices will need even more time to become available in a widespread fashion and integrated into healthcare systems.

Beyond the time-consuming approval process and indirect costs of implementation, there are also direct monetary costs to purchasing AI algorithms and associated hardware. Virtual reality training modules and augmented reality overlays are prime examples, with the headsets needed to utilize the software costing thousands of dollars per headpiece. Thus, even though this chapter describes many AI algorithms that could have a substantial impact on the efficiency and efficacy of shoulder arthroscopy, it is not likely that this technology will experience widespread implementation until efforts are made to safely expedite approval of new algorithms, improve indirect costs to clinical workflow, and reduce monetary costs.

Further, studies suggest that AI implementation can lead to unintended consequences such as alert fatigue, disruption of patient-physician communication styles, and creation of new hazards that take even more vigilance to detect [56]. For example, a study by Dratsch et al. found that AI false negatives on breast mammograms led to radiologists having less accurate reads on the same mammogram than if the radiologist had read the mammogram without AI assistance [56].

Other limitations to a successful implementation of AI in the workplace include bias, in part due to limits on data sharing and patient hesitancy. Bias in AI can stem from many different sources, such as biased samples, data gaps, societal prejudices, and training bias [57]. For example, melanoma detection AI algorithms have been found to have half the diagnostic accuracy on Black patients in comparison to white patients, in part because less than 10% of the datasets used to train the algorithm were of Black patients [58]. Thus, it is important to continually train AI algorithms on large, diverse patient populations, as could easily be achieved through data sharing. However, our healthcare environment in the US currently has no method of incentivizing the sharing of data [59]. If anything, measures in place to protect PHI such as HIPAA, disincentivize the sharing of even deidentified patient data, for fears of legal repercussions of accidental privacy breach [54]. Thus, it will be important to promote data sharing in AI algorithm development to ensure that these algorithms can be used accurately on all patients.

In addition, patient hesitancy toward AI serves as a barrier to increasing both sample populations for AI algorithm creation and adoption of AI in clinical practices. A systematic review by Young et al. found that many participants were concerned about risks to privacy, including the release of PHI by hackers or technical malfunction, thus limiting the number of patients willing to consent to having their health information used for the creation of AI algorithms [60]. Patient fears such as inaccurate diagnosis and depersonalization of care will also limit the number of patients willing to receive care from entities that utilize AI for healthcare [60]. In general, patients are most amenable to the use of AI as a system to assist, and not replace, physicians [60]. Young et al. also noted that patients reacted most favorably toward AI after being counseled on the exact use and effectiveness of the algorithm, suggesting that increased education on the use and scope of AI is the first step toward improving public perception [60]. Overall, adoption of AI is currently limited by the lengthy approval process, direct and indirect costs to the healthcare system, bias of algorithms, and patient hesitancy.

11.8.2 Advantages of AI in Shoulder Arthroscopy

The advantages of clinically implementing will likely capitalize across the entire continuum of care in shoulder arthroscopy (Fig. 11.2).

The first advantage of AI in shoulder arthroscopy is improved diagnostic and treatment accuracy. As discussed previously, AI has been shown to have similar diagnostic accuracy as radiologists in detecting many different pathologies, sometimes even showing diagnostic capabilities beyond that of humans. Regarding treatment accuracy, AI provides physicians with new tools to promote the selection of the most efficacious treatment plan through outcomes prediction and helps physicians accurately carry out this plan with advanced image segmentation, improved surgical training, and intraoperative guidance. Even postoperatively, AI algorithms have the potential to optimize patient rehabilitation to assist patients in safely returning to their preferred activities.

Another advantage of AI in shoulder arthroscopy is the optimization of clinical processes. AI has the potential to ensure the proper ordering of advanced imaging, expedite MRIs, immediately recognize imaging errors, and improve the diagnostic abilities of less expensive and more readily available imaging sources (such as ultrasound and plain radiographs) to increase clinical efficiency while decreasing demand for unnecessary imaging studies. AI can also reduce the administrative burden on providers by automating billing and documentation. Postoperatively, remote monitoring of patients has the potential to decrease the demand for in-person rehabilitation and the frequency of postoperative return visits. Through the automatization and/or expedition of clinical processes, AI can decrease the inundation of healthcare systems and promote reallocation of resources to where they are needed most.

AI also has the capacity to increase consistency in treatment across practices. Widespread utilization of different machine-learning algorithms to diagnose and treat patients will ensure that all physicians are prescribing similar care to patients with the same conditions, reducing inequity in care due to differences in resources or physician bias. Especially once the technology becomes more affordable, AI can provide lower-budget hospitals with resources that normally would be too expen-

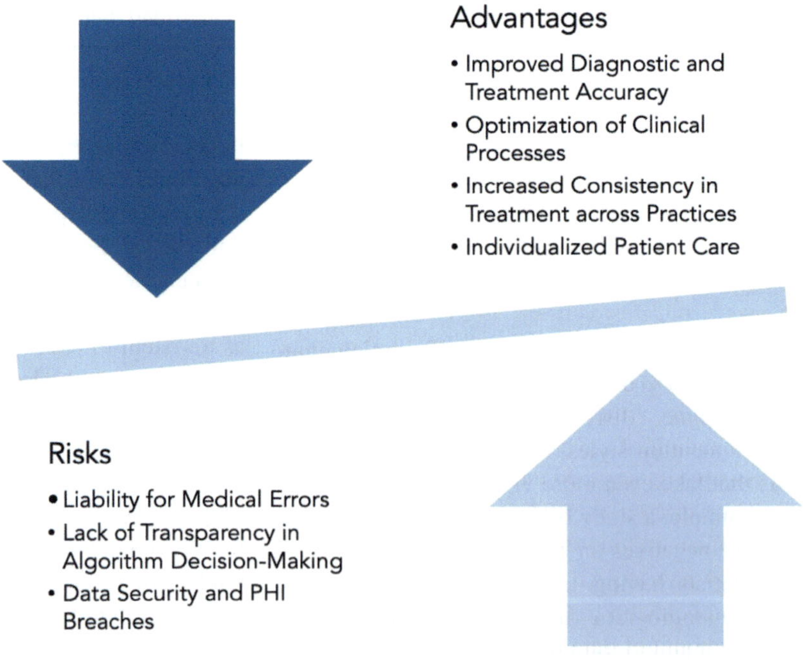

Fig. 11.2 Schematic depiction of potential advantages and risks for the implementation of AI in shoulder surgery

sive or time-consuming, such as preoperative 3D modeling, segmentation, and augmented reality intraoperative guides. Overall, AI has the potential to be a powerful tool in promoting equitable treatment and outcomes across our healthcare system.

Lastly, AI provides the opportunity for treatment to be individualized to the needs of the patient. Before a patient even sees a physician, outcomes prediction algorithms can be seamlessly integrated into the EHR to predict the outcomes of the patient after treatment. This would allow the physician to tailor care directly to the patient and their functional demands, choosing the most efficacious treatment. In patients deemed high risk for complications, the physician can then alter their postoperative care, such as extending physical therapy or delaying return-to-sport, to limit these risks.

Overall, these advantages are expected to confer an increase in clinical efficiency and patient outcomes, while reducing physician workloads and burnout.

11.8.3 Risks of AI Implementation

Some of the risks of AI implementation include liability, lack of transparency in algorithm decision-making, and data security (Fig. 11.2).

Liability for physician decision-making with AI guidance is complicated, as it is unclear whether the physician and/or the creator of the algorithm should be held responsible for misdiagnosis or other errors [54, 61]. In the future, legislation needs to be constructed to clearly address who is liable for medical errors that are a result of using AI algorithms, and/or liability could be inferred from third parties such as insurers [54]. In the meantime, physicians can and should be held accountable for any medical errors made in their practice, and thus should have a sound understanding of any algorithm they use to treat patients [61].

However, this is complicated by the "black box" effect, the idea that it is difficult to know precisely how an AI algorithm arrives at a particular conclusion [61]. AI algorithms often take a vast amount of data into account when coming to a treatment decision, but it is often unclear how different pieces of information are weighed in the decision-making process. Thus, it can be difficult for a physician to verify that the decision made by the algorithm is correct. Since AI algorithm decision-making often lacks transparency and physicians can ultimately be held liable for any medical error made in their care, many physicians may find the use of AI algorithms too risky to implement into clinical practice.

Another risk of implementing AI is data security. PHI data breaches are all too common, with a total of 3822 PHI breaches affecting over 283,335,803 people occurring between 2011 and 2021 [62]. Widespread implementation of AI algorithms is only expected to increase the number of PHI breaches, as in the lifetime of any given algorithm, a significant amount of personal health information will be accessed and utilized. Although measures such as patient deidentification and regular privacy audits can limit the risk of data breach, the risk can never be fully eliminated [54]. In the future, it will be necessary for those creating and overseeing AI algorithms to be vigilant and continuously improve their methods of data protection and deidentification to reduce the risk of harmful PHI breaches.

11.8.4 Considerations for Clinical Practice Implementation

Some considerations for the implementation of AI into clinical practice include the level of expertise required for successful implementation. As discussed above, since ultimately a physician can be held liable for any medical errors in their care, physicians should have at the minimum an understanding of the workings of any AI algorithm they plan to use to assist in their medical decision-making in shoulder arthroscopy. Further expertise would also be required by any practice looking to develop their own algorithm. In addition, not all algorithms may not immediately be compatible with a particular practice as the correct input must be available for an algorithm to work correctly. For example, in Kang et al.'s ML algorithm developed for the detection of subscapularis tears on axillary radiographs, 118 patients were excluded simply because their radiographs or MRIs were of insufficient quality, or they had incomplete clinical history [16]. Algorithms relying on automatic input from medical records would also require a compatible EHR. Thus, not all algorithms will be easily integrated into clinical practice and may require practices to implement additional training for healthcare providers or alter their standard of care.

Further, healthcare providers will need to comply with various regulations and standards when implementing AI in clinical practice. As discussed in the limitations section, AI algorithms must undergo a lengthy approval process to be released on the market. After approval, currently, the only regulations and standards in place for AI use in clinical practice are confidentiality guidelines put forward by HIPAA and cybersecurity regulations managed by the FDA [54]. As new regulations emerge to promote the safe use of AI in healthcare, it will be important for practices to consider how they will stay up to date with emerging regulations and ensure their compliance.

11.8.5 Status Quo and Future Directions

To date, a substantial amount of AI-based solutions has been developed for clinical use cases in different specialties, that are not directly related to shoulder arthroscopy, but from a technological and clinical perspective may be suitable for clinical implementation in shoulder arthroscopy.

Currently, the most scientific evidence as well as the most advanced and complete AI solutions around prediction models have been generated to predict clinical outcomes [26, 28] as well as diagnostic as imaging [11, 13–15] in shoulder surgery. The solutions developed for these use cases can already be utilized today. Most likely, the next area ripe for augmentation by AI solutions in shoulder arthroscopy will be the quantitative preoperative analysis of advanced imaging prior to shoulder arthroscopy, which will provide shoulder surgeons with more accurate and clinically relevant information prior to surgery (i.e. muscle quality in RCT) and increase the feasibility of 3D planning (i.e. for bone block reconstruction in shoulder instability). On a 1–5 year horizon, AI technology may likely advance predictive imaging possibilities, which will allow for the detection of shoulder pathology in a stage where lifestyle modification and non-invasive treatments will be effective, as well as the first applications of VR in shoulder arthroscopy. On a 5–10 year horizon, we predict the use of AI technology to leverage the information contained in the EMR to optimize clinical processes such as image acquisition, but also the automated use of this information to predict complications, outcomes, and costs. It is likely that in this time frame, AI algorithms will be employed to unburden administrative tasks related to documentation as well as billing. We also predict that AI technology will be integrated into wearables to optimize and personalize postoperative rehabilitation during this time. On a 10–20 year horizon, we predict that real-time processing of arthroscopic imaging, tactile, and audiovisual information will be integrated into the development of smart instruments and surgical suites. Finally, in this timeframe, there will likely be the first attempts to automate certain steps of arthroscopic procedures, given a successful parallel development of robotic capabilities (Fig. 11.3). However, comprehensive regulation as well as successful integration of shoulder surgeons into the development of those solutions be pivotal in determining, whether the organic integration of AI technology will enhance orthopedic surgeons' capabilities to new levels of capabilities or lower degrees of acceptance result in the perception of AI technology as an adversary.

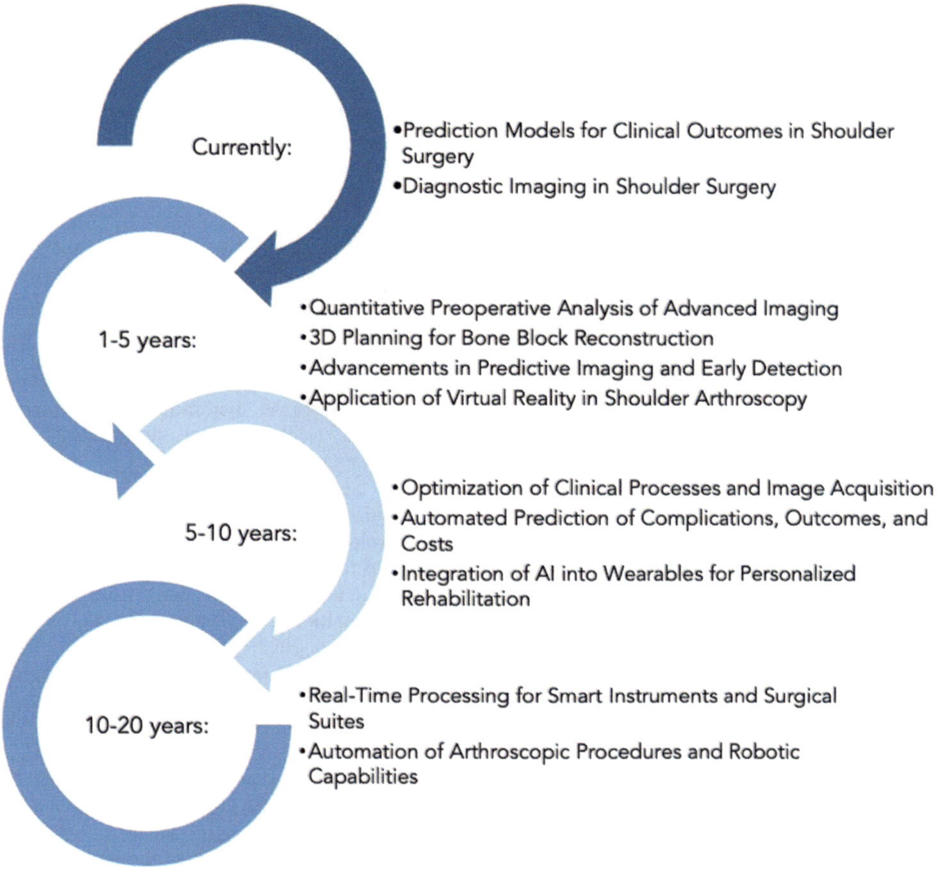

Fig. 11.3 Prediction of a potential timeline of implementation of AI in shoulder arthroscopy

References

1. Sanderson K. GPT-4 is here: what scientists think. Nature. 2023;615(7954):773.
2. Hashimoto DA, Rosman G, Rus D, Meireles OR. Artificial intelligence in surgery: promises and perils. Ann Surg. 2018;268(1):70–6.
3. Xiang Y, Zhao L, Liu Z, Wu X, Chen J, Long E, et al. Implementation of artificial intelligence in medicine: status analysis and development suggestions. Artif Intell Med. 2020;102:101780.
4. Ramkumar PN, Kunze KN, Haeberle HS, Karnuta JM, Luu BC, Nwachukwu BU, et al. Clinical and research medical applications of artificial intelligence. Arthroscopy. 2021;37(5):1694–7.
5. Liu PR, Lu L, Zhang JY, Huo TT, Liu SX, Ye ZW. Application of artificial intelligence in medicine: an overview. Curr Med Sci. 2021;41(6):1105–15.
6. Topol EJ. High-performance medicine: the convergence of human and artificial intelligence. Nat Med. 2019;25(1):44–56.
7. Gorelik N, Gyftopoulos S. Applications of artificial intelligence in musculoskeletal imaging: from the request to the report. Can Assoc Radiol J. 2021;72(1):45–59.
8. Gyftopoulos S, Lin D, Knoll F, Doshi AM, Rodrigues TC, Recht MP. Artificial intelligence in musculoskeletal imaging: current status and future directions. AJR Am J Roentgenol. 2019;213(3):506–13.
9. Hahn S, Yi J, Lee HJ, Lee Y, Lim YJ, Bang JY, et al. Image quality and diagnostic performance of accelerated shoulder MRI with deep learning-based reconstruction. AJR Am J Roentgenol. 2022;218(3):506–16.
10. Küstner T, Gatidis S, Liebgott A, Schwartz M, Mauch L, Martirosian P, et al. A machine-learning framework for automatic reference-free quality assessment in MRI. Magn Reson Imaging. 2018;53:134–47.
11. Kuo RYL, Harrison C, Curran TA, Jones B, Freethy A, Cussons D, et al. Artificial intelligence in fracture detection: a systematic review and meta-analysis. Radiology. 2022;304(1):50–62.
12. Kunze KN, Rossi DM, White GM, Karhade AV, Deng J, Williams BT, et al. Diagnostic performance of

artificial intelligence for detection of anterior cruciate ligament and meniscus tears: a systematic review. Arthroscopy. 2021;37(2):771–81.
13. Chung SW, Han SS, Lee JW, Oh KS, Kim NR, Yoon JP, et al. Automated detection and classification of the proximal humerus fracture by using deep learning algorithm. Acta Orthop. 2018;89(4):468–73.
14. Lin DJ, Schwier M, Geiger B, Raithel E, von Busch H, Fritz J, et al. Deep learning diagnosis and classification of rotator cuff tears on shoulder MRI. Investig Radiol. 2023;58(6):405–12.
15. Key S, Demir S, Gurger M, Yilmaz E, Barua PD, Dogan S, et al. ViVGG19: novel exemplar deep feature extraction-based shoulder rotator cuff tear and biceps tendinosis detection using magnetic resonance images. Med Eng Phys. 2022;110:103864.
16. Kang Y, Choi D, Lee KJ, Oh JH, Kim BR, Ahn JM. Evaluating subscapularis tendon tears on axillary lateral radiographs using deep learning. Eur Radiol. 2021;31(12):9408–17.
17. Medina G, Buckless CG, Thomasson E, Oh LS, Torriani M. Deep learning method for segmentation of rotator cuff muscles on MR images. Skeletal Radiol. 2021;50(4):683–92.
18. Ro K, Kim JY, Park H, Cho BH, Kim IY, Shim SB, et al. Deep-learning framework and computer assisted fatty infiltration analysis for the supraspinatus muscle in MRI. Sci Rep. 2021;11(1):15065.
19. Fuchs B, Weishaupt D, Zanetti M, Hodler J, Gerber C. Fatty degeneration of the muscles of the rotator cuff: assessment by computed tomography versus magnetic resonance imaging. J Shoulder Elb Surg. 1999;8(6):599–605.
20. Kim H, Shin K, Kim H, Lee ES, Chung SW, Koh KH, et al. Can deep learning reduce the time and effort required for manual segmentation in 3D reconstruction of MRI in rotator cuff tears? PLoS One. 2022;17(10):e0274075.
21. Familiari F, Galasso O, Massazza F, Mercurio M, Fox H, Srikumaran U, et al. Artificial intelligence in the management of rotator cuff tears. Int J Environ Res Public Health. 2022;19(24):16779.
22. Samim M. 3D MRI models of the musculoskeletal system. Semin Musculoskelet Radiol. 2021;25(3):388–96.
23. Fernandes LR, Arce C, Martinho G, Campos JP, Meneghini RM. Accuracy, reliability, and repeatability of a novel artificial intelligence algorithm converting two-dimensional radiographs to three-dimensional bone models for total knee arthroplasty. J Arthroplast. 2022.
24. Kunze KN, Krivicich LM, Clapp IM, Bodendorfer BM, Nwachukwu BU, Chahla J, et al. Machine learning algorithms predict achievement of clinically significant outcomes after orthopaedic surgery: a systematic review. Arthroscopy. 2022;38(6):2090–105.
25. Frangiamore S, Dornan GJ, Horan MP, Mannava S, Fritz EM, Hussain ZB, et al. Predictive modeling to determine functional outcomes after arthroscopic rotator cuff repair. Am J Sports Med. 2020;48(7):1559–67.
26. Potty AG, Potty ASR, Maffulli N, Blumenschein LA, Ganta D, Mistovich RJ, et al. Approaching artificial intelligence in orthopaedics: predictive analytics and machine learning to prognosticate arthroscopic rotator cuff surgical outcomes. J Clin Med. 2023;12(6):2369.
27. Kumar V, Roche C, Overman S, Simovitch R, Flurin PH, Wright T, et al. What is the accuracy of three different machine learning techniques to predict clinical outcomes after shoulder arthroplasty? Clin Orthop Relat Res. 2020;478(10):2351–63.
28. Lopez CD, Constant M, Anderson MJJ, Confino JE, Heffernan JT, Jobin CM. Using machine learning methods to predict nonhome discharge after elective total shoulder arthroplasty. JSES Int. 2021;5(4):692–8.
29. van Spanning SH, Verweij LPE, Allaart LJH, Hendrickx LAM, Doornberg JN, Athwal GS, et al. Development and training of a machine learning algorithm to identify patients at risk for recurrence following an arthroscopic Bankart repair (CLEARER): protocol for a retrospective, multicentre, cohort study. BMJ Open. 2022;12(9):e055346.
30. Karnuta JM, Churchill JL, Haeberle HS, Nwachukwu BU, Taylor SA, Ricchetti ET, et al. The value of artificial neural networks for predicting length of stay, discharge disposition, and inpatient costs after anatomic and reverse shoulder arthroplasty. J Shoulder Elb Surg. 2020;29(11):2385–94.
31. Gowd AK, Agarwalla A, Beck EC, Rosas S, Waterman BR, Romeo AA, et al. Prediction of total healthcare cost following total shoulder arthroplasty utilizing machine learning. J Shoulder Elb Surg. 2022;31(12):2449–56.
32. Allaart LJH, Spanning SV, Lafosse L, Lafosse T, Ladermann A, Athwal GS, et al. Developing a machine learning algorithm to predict probability of retear and functional outcomes in patients undergoing rotator cuff repair surgery: protocol for a retrospective, multicentre study. BMJ Open. 2023;13(2):e063673.
33. Desai RJ, Wang SV, Vaduganathan M, Evers T, Schneeweiss S. Comparison of machine learning methods with traditional models for use of administrative claims with electronic medical records to predict heart failure outcomes. JAMA Netw Open. 2020;3(1):e1918962.
34. Taneja I, Damhorst GL, Lopez-Espina C, Zhao SD, Zhu R, Khan S, et al. Diagnostic and prognostic capabilities of a biomarker and EMR-based machine learning algorithm for sepsis. Clin Transl Sci. 2021;14(4):1578–89.
35. Twick I, Zahavi G, Benvenisti H, Rubinstein R, Woods MS, Berkenstadt H, et al. Towards interpretable, medically grounded, EMR-based risk prediction models. Sci Rep. 2022;12(1):9990.
36. Verhey JT, Haglin JM, Verhey EM, Hartigan DE. Virtual, augmented, and mixed reality appli-

cations in orthopedic surgery. Int J Med Robot. 2020;16(2):e2067.
37. Berthold DP, Muench LN, Rupp MC, Siebenlist S, Cote MP, Mazzocca AD, et al. Head-mounted display virtual reality is effective in orthopaedic training: a systematic review. Arthrosc Sports Med Rehabil. 2022;4(5):e1843–e9.
38. Vaughan N, Dubey VN, Wainwright TW, Middleton RG. A review of virtual reality based training simulators for orthopaedic surgery. Med Eng Phys. 2016;38(2):59–71.
39. Schlueter-Brust K, Henckel J, Katinakis F, Buken C, Opt-Eynde J, Pofahl T, et al. Augmented-reality-assisted K-wire placement for glenoid component positioning in reversed shoulder arthroplasty: a proof-of-concept study. J Pers Med. 2021;11(8):777.
40. Seibold M, Maurer S, Hoch A, Zingg P, Farshad M, Navab N, et al. Real-time acoustic sensing and artificial intelligence for error prevention in orthopedic surgery. Sci Rep. 2021;11(1):3993.
41. Sato K, Fujita T, Matsuzaki H, Takeshita N, Fujiwara H, Mitsunaga S, et al. Real-time detection of the recurrent laryngeal nerve in thoracoscopic esophagectomy using artificial intelligence. Surg Endosc. 2022;36(7):5531–9.
42. Bozkurt M, Apaydin N, Işik C, Bilgetekin YG, Acar HI, Elhan A. Robotic arthroscopic surgery: a new challenge in arthroscopic surgery Part-I: Robotic shoulder arthroscopy; a cadaveric feasibility study. Int J Med Robot. 2011;7(4):496–500.
43. Cho SM, Kim YG, Jeong J, Kim I, Lee HJ, Kim N. Automatic tip detection of surgical instruments in biportal endoscopic spine surgery. Comput Biol Med. 2021;133:104384.
44. Millett PJ, Fritz EM, Frangiamore SJ, Mannava S. Arthroscopic management of glenohumeral arthritis: a joint preservation approach. J Am Acad Orthop Surg. 2018;26(21):745–52.
45. Erickson BJ, Shishani Y, Gobezie R. Remote patient monitoring of postoperative rehabilitation. Phys Med Rehabil Clin N Am. 2023;34(2):489–97.
46. Burns DM, Leung N, Hardisty M, Whyne CM, Henry P, McLachlin S. Shoulder physiotherapy exercise recognition: machine learning the inertial signals from a smartwatch. Physiol Meas. 2018;39(7):075007.
47. Pekyavas NO, Ergun N. Comparison of virtual reality exergaming and home exercise programs in patients with subacromial impingement syndrome and scapular dyskinesis: short term effect. Acta Orthop Traumatol Turc. 2017;51(3):238–42.
48. Lin SY, Shanafelt TD, Asch SM. Reimagining clinical documentation with artificial intelligence. Mayo Clin Proc. 2018;93(5):563–5.
49. Klann JG, Szolovits P. An intelligent listening framework for capturing encounter notes from a doctor-patient dialog. BMC Med Inform Decis Mak. 2009;9(Suppl 1):S3.
50. Deliberato RO, Celi LA, Stone DJ. Clinical note creation, binning, and artificial intelligence. JMIR Med Inform. 2017;5(3):e24.
51. Kim JS, Vivas A, Arvind V, Lombardi J, Reidler J, Zuckerman SL, et al. Can natural language processing and artificial intelligence automate the generation of billing codes from operative note dictations? Global Spine J. 2022:21925682211062831.
52. Zaidat B, Tang J, Arvind V, Geng EA, Cho B, Duey AH, et al. Can a novel natural language processing model and artificial intelligence automatically generate billing codes from spine surgical operative notes? Global Spine J. 2023:21925682231164935.
53. Venkatesh KP, Raza MM, Kvedar JC. Automating the overburdened clinical coding system: challenges and next steps. NPJ Digit Med. 2023;6(1):16.
54. Abdullah YI, Schuman JS, Shabsigh R, Caplan A, Al-Aswad LA. Ethics of artificial intelligence in medicine and ophthalmology. Asia Pac J Ophthalmol (Phila). 2021;10(3):289–98.
55. Van Norman GA. Drugs, devices, and the FDA: Part 2: an overview of approval processes: FDA approval of medical devices. JACC Basic Transl Sci. 2016;1(4):277–87.
56. Yu KH, Beam AL, Kohane IS. Artificial intelligence in healthcare. Nat Biomed Eng. 2018;2(10):719–31.
57. Norori N, Hu Q, Aellen FM, Faraci FD, Tzovara A. Addressing bias in big data and AI for health care: a call for open science. Patterns (NY). 2021;2(10):100347.
58. Kamulegeya LH, Okello M, Bwanika JM, Musinguzi D, Lubega W, Rusoke D, et al. Using artificial intelligence on dermatology conditions in Uganda: a case for diversity in training data sets for machine learning. BioRxiv 2019:826057.
59. Jiang F, Jiang Y, Zhi H, Dong Y, Li H, Ma S, et al. Artificial intelligence in healthcare: past, present and future. Stroke Vasc Neurol. 2017;2(4):230–43.
60. Young AT, Amara D, Bhattacharya A, Wei ML. Patient and general public attitudes towards clinical artificial intelligence: a mixed methods systematic review. Lancet Digit Health. 2021;3(9):e599–611.
61. Smith M, Heath Jeffery RC. Addressing the challenges of artificial intelligence in medicine. Intern Med J. 2020;50(10):1278–81.
62. Tin D, Hata R, Granholm F, Ciottone RG, Staynings R, Ciottone GR. Cyberthreats: a primer for healthcare professionals. Am J Emerg Med. 2023;68:179–85.

12 Artificial Intelligence in Sports Medicine

Mohamad Y. Fares, Peter Boufadel,
Amar S. Vadhera, and Joseph A. Abboud

12.1 Introduction

Amidst the current advances in technology and digitalization that are witnessed worldwide, artificial intelligence (AI) is rising as a highly promising field with numerous potential applications in many different domains [1]. Even though the use of AI in medicine was implied more than 60 years ago, practical applications in diagnosing, managing, and preventing pathologies have only emerged recently [2]. Research in this field is still growing, and there is a lot more to learn about the use of AI in different medical domains [1]. A cardiovascular study once showed that AI-derived technology can exceed the accuracy of predicting cardiovascular risk in patients when compared to established medical guidelines [3]. AI has also been involved in evaluating dermatologic images and analyzing radiological results, and in many cases, was able to achieve results that were deemed comparable to humans [4, 5]. While numerous medical applications of AI have been described, the relative novelty implies a need for further research efforts and initiatives.

Sports medicine is considered a large field of medicine that involves huge financial investments [6, 7]. An estimated 8.6 million sports-related injuries are annually reported in the United States, and this entails the prominence of this field and its significance on national health expenditures [6, 7]. That being said, the use of AI in the field of sports medicine may provide assistance to the diagnosis, management, and prevention of sports injuries, as well as help study its trends and patterns [1, 6]. Research exploring the use of AI in the field of sports medicine has been generally limited in literature. As such, the aim of this chapter is to explore the potential applications of AI in the field of sports medicine, while focusing on its potential use in injury risk prediction and prophylaxis, biomechanical and biomotion analysis, diagnostic accuracy enhancement, surgical assistance, and research applications, using a comprehensive literature review.

12.2 Injury Risk Prediction and Prophylaxis

The involvement of AI in professional sports comes as no surprise, given the magnanimous financial investments allocated in that industry [6, 7]. The maintenance of athlete health is pivotal for the industry, and this involves dietitians, physical therapists, trainers, and sports physicians, all of whom cater to the optimization of

Mohamad Y. Fares and Peter Boufadel contributed equally and are co-first authors.

M. Y. Fares · P. Boufadel · A. S. Vadhera ·
J. A. Abboud (✉)
Division of Shoulder and Elbow Surgery, Rothman Orthopaedic Institute, Philadelphia, PA, USA

F. Familiari et al. (eds.), *Artificial Intelligence in Orthopaedic Surgery Made Easy*,
https://doi.org/10.1007/978-3-031-70310-2_12

athletic health and performance. Sports injuries constitute a huge financial loss to clubs and leagues alike. In the 2014–2015 season, the National Basketball Association reported a 344 million USD loss due to player injuries, and in the 2019–2020 season, the National Football League reported a 521 million USD loss due to player injuries [8, 9]. As a result, efforts to predict injury and potentially extrapolate prevention plans have emerged across different sports and have manifested in the development of wearable health technologies that monitor performance, and the establishment of large injury registries and research databases [1]. These efforts paved the way for numerous AI applications for monitoring performance, predicting injury, and estimating injury risk.

The wearable health technology industry has risen in popularity in recent years, with a market size of around 19 million USD in 2019 [10]. Athletes, both amateur and professional, can use straps, watches, or bands that can monitor their performance and provide data on their health and fitness [1, 11]. This gives athletes a chance to improve and optimize training, and consequently, enhance their performance [1, 11].

On a more systematic and professional front, machine learning laboratories have been established in an attempt to explore possible applications of AI in arthroplasty and sports medicine. Several studies from the Machine Learning Arthroplasty Laboratory at the Cleveland Clinic explored the Major League Baseball and National Hockey League injury data to predict injury risk using machine learning models [12, 13]. One of these studies by Luu et al. screened annual hockey injury data along with player-specific characteristics, and used machine learning training and algorithms to predict next season injury trends and patterns [13]. The best-performing machine learning algorithm showcased good to excellent reliability and outperformed logistic regression analysis [13]. Similarly, in another study for baseball players, data on position players and pitchers were compiled, and when machine learning algorithms were tested for prediction of next season injury risk, the best-performing algorithm had an accuracy rate of 70%, outperforming logistic regression and demonstrating fair reliability [12]. These studies displayed the potential carried by AI applications in injury risk prediction and demonstrated the prowess of machine learning when compared to logistic regression for the prediction of injury patterns and trends [12, 13]. Using more granular data with more insight into injury mechanisms would allow specialists to come up with better machine learning algorithms and more reliable injury-predicting models.

12.3 Biomechanics and Motion Analyses

Studying the biomechanics of human movement has long been explored in the field of sports medicine [14]. Motion analysis often includes a descriptive assessment and analysis of human movement, as well as the kinematics of motion and performance [14]. The field of biomechanics and motion analyses can provide immense insight into factors that can affect performance and impact injury risk [14]. Through studying motion patterns in the field, scientists can predict movements or techniques that may result in injury and monitor movements or techniques that result in enhanced performance. While many previous studies used to depend on descriptive observations and measuring tools, modern technology, manifested in the use of wearable sensors and video cameras, can provide more accurate and detailed information and can pave the way for applying AI in this field.

A biomechanics motion capture lab conducted a study to explore the kinematic sequence of baseball pitching, with an aim to improve performance and minimize injury risk [15]. A motion capture system that incorporated advanced cameras, trackers, and reflective markers was used to create a 15-segment model of every included pitcher [15]. Pitchers were then asked to throw pitches of different intensity and using different approaches [15]. After collecting the data, the authors showed that the kinematic sequence used by baseball pitchers from the windup or from the stretch is similar [15]. They also noted that the kinematic sequence places more stress on the shoulder and elbow joints than the pitching approach [15]. This led them to the conclusion that ideal kinematic sequences should be prioritized for the sake of avoiding injury [15]. The same research group used the same technology in another study to identify which throwing patterns is the most superior with regards to safety and effectiveness [16]. The authors identified a total of 17 different throwing sequences and were able to note which of the sequences were safe and effective, and which ones placed the joints at a higher risk for injury [16]. These detailed analyses on the kinematic sequences of throwing represent one facet of how advanced technology may be able to help in improving performance and safety in the field of sports medicine [16]. One can imagine that these studies can be emulated in different sports like soccer, basketball, and football, where one can study motion sequences of different athletic movements and motions. Hence, the applications for advanced technology and AI in this field remain boundless, with numerous potential benefits that can be reaped.

12.4 Enhancing Diagnostic Modalities

The expanding landscape of AI and machine learning (ML) presents promising opportunities to optimize both clinical and radiographic diagnoses of orthopedic injuries. Given the significant reliance on radiological imaging in orthopedic surgery, AI and ML applications have largely focused on enhancing efficiency in musculoskeletal radiology for diverse tasks and automating workflow. Such tasks that can potentially be improved include designing imaging protocols, reducing image acquisition and processing time, automatic image correction for images with noise or poor quality, automatic identification of features within images, automated diagnostic inputs and inferences, as well as radiological pattern recognition and integration with other sources of information [17]. In the field of sports medicine, a growing number of deep learning–based methods with powerful pattern recognition capabilities have been developed that utilize medical imaging for diagnosing anterior cruciate ligament (ACL) tears, meniscus tears, rotator cuff tears, and Achilles tendinopathy.

Several applications for the diagnosis of ACL and meniscus tears are reported in the literature. In one study demonstrating the use of AI in the clinical assessment of ACL tears, Labbe et al. developed an SVM-based algorithm to objectively grade the pivot shift test using sensors and recorded knee joint kinematics in 107 different knees [18]. The developed model was found to be in substantial agreement with orthopedic surgeons in the grading of the test using the International Knee Documentation Committee criteria, with 66% having the same grade and 96% within one grade. Moreover, AI technology can analyze morphological characteristics on MR images and detect structures and abnormalities. In the aim of aiding the diagnosis process, Štajduhara et al. trained SVM and random forest ML models on 917 sagittal plane MR images of the knee to detect both milder ACL injuries and complete ACL ruptures [19]. The SVM model was found to have an area under the curve (AUC) of 0.894 for detecting ACL injuries and 0.943 for detecting complete rupture. Similar results have also been achieved using convolutional neural networks (CNN) [20–22]. CNNs are a type of deep learning model that can automatically recognize and extract patterns from images without any explicit human programming, making them appropriate for tasks including image classification and object detection. Bien et al. developed a CNN model trained on a dataset of 1370 knee MRIs capable of detecting ACL tears, meniscal tears, and general abnormalities with comparable performance to that of general radiologists, with AUC values of 0.937, 0.965, and 0.847, respectively [20]. While the model had a lower sensitivity compared to general radiologists in detecting both ACL and meniscal tears, the use of the model predictions to assist in diagnosis was found to significantly increase clinical experts' specificity in identifying ACL tears [20]. The model also demonstrated the potential of AI to reduce processing time and improve efficiency [20]. When tasked to classify a dataset of 120 images, the model completed it in two minutes versus over three hours on average for the general radiologists. Similar models have been built to diagnose meniscal injuries [20, 23–25]. For example, Roblot et al. built and assessed a high-performance CNN algorithm trained on a dataset of 1123 MR images of the knee to detect the position of the two meniscal horns, the presence of a meniscal tear, and the orientation of the tear, with an overall AUC value of 0.90 [23].

While the majority of diagnostic applications within sports medicine have been focused on the knee, similar techniques have more recently been introduced for detecting soft tissue injuries in other body parts, such as the shoulder and ankle. In a comprehensive systematic review by Zhan et al., it was found that AI models of diverse ML techniques, trained on distinct diagnostic modalities encompassing ultrasound images, MRIs and radiographs, exhibit significant potential in facilitating the detection of rotator cuff pathologies [26]. Overall, the algorithmic model AUC values to detect rotator cuff pathology from ultrasound images, MRIs, and radiographic series ranged from 0.789 to 0.950, 0.844 to 0.943, and 0.820 to 0.830, respectively. In addition, AI models demonstrated impressive feats in diagnosing rotator cuff pathology in comparison to clinical physicians. Horng and Chen developed an AI model highly proficient in assessing rotator cuff pathology into four categories using ultrasound images: normal, tendon inflammation, calcific tendonitis, and rotator cuff tear [27]. The model performed similarly to musculoskeletal radiologists in terms of accuracy, sensitivity, and specificity. In fact, Shim et al. developed a CNN model that even outperformed orthopedic experts in diagnosing rotator cuff tears using MR images, exhibiting significantly higher levels of accuracy and specificity compared to both experienced and general orthopedic surgeons, although no difference in sensitivity [28]. AI applications in diagnosing Achilles tendinopathy have also been performed. Wang et al. devised several ML models using ultrasonographic images of 88 feet in skiers and attained excellent results, with an AUC value of 0.99, sensitivity of 90% and specificity of 100% [29]. Kapiński et al. similarly achieved 97.6% accuracy, 98.3% sensitivity, and 99.45% specificity in classifying Achilles tendons from MRI images as injured or healthy [30].

In summary, AI and ML applications have proven to be effective tools with significant potential in enhancing orthopedic diagnosis, particularly in sports medicine. While AI can improve the efficiency and accuracy of detecting various musculoskeletal pathologies on multiple imaging modalities, further research and validation of AI models are necessary to ensure their reliability and widespread applicability in clinical practice.

12.5 Intraoperative Utilization

The incorporation of AI into intraoperative procedures within sports medicine has been scarcely explored in research, and significant applications have yet to be seen. In contrast, AI has demonstrated notable achievements intraoperatively in other surgical disciplines and orthopedic subspecialties, such as distinguishing similarly appearing structures as well as healthy and diseased tissues [31–35]; identifying anatomical landmarks and safe sites for dissection (20); providing navigational assistance using augmented and mixed reality for more precise orthopedic implant fixations [36]; and multidisciplinary use of robotic-assisted surgery including arthroplasty and spine [37–39].

To date, applications of AI and deep learning intraoperatively within the realm of sports medicine are limited to a single CNN model developed for automatic segmentation of multiple knee arthroscopy structures into four classes: the femur, the ACL, the tibia, and the meniscus [40]. The model was trained on 3868 images collected from four cadaveric experiments and five knees, and it performed favorably with mean Dice similarity coefficients for the femur, ACL, tibia, and meniscus of 0.78, 0.41, 0.50, and 0.43, respectively. By offering real-time instance-based identification of structures during surgery, this technology may enhance the surgical team's insight and may have implications for both human surgical training and the advancement of medical robotic arthroscopy [40]. Future advancements with a greater emphasis on AI-driven data have the potential to optimize intraoperative ACL or meniscal repairs. For instance, the use of a head-up display could enable AI-generated guidance on precise locations for re-inserting the ACL or repairing the meniscus [41]. This application could be extended to other injuries as well, including rotator cuff tears and Achilles rupture repairs.

Advancements in technology and the continuous search for more efficient and minimally invasive techniques to provide optimal care to patients have driven investigations of robotic surgery use in arthroscopy. Kather et al. performed two hip arthroscopies in human cadavers using the da Vinci surgical system demonstrating its feasibility with successful introduction of cameras and working instruments, docking of the robotic system, and instrument manipulation [42]. Likewise, Bozkurt et al. showed manipulation within the shoulder joint to be possible with a good range of motion of articulation [43]. The authors showed adequate arthroscopic control of the biceps tendon, glenoid labrum, rotator cuff muscles, rotator interval, glenohumeral ligament, and the coracoid process in both beach chair and lateral decubitus positions [43]. While robotic surgery may be advantageous in enabling more complex and precise tasks in restricted spaces, at this time, there are significant limitations. The large size of the robot body, robot arms, and current laparoscopic instruments may limit many arthroscopic manipulations, signifying the need for new and flexible robotic platforms and more specific instruments to be developed prior to any human clinical trials [42, 43]. This may also allow for applications in joints with more restricted spaces, such as the knee, wrist, and ankle. Although still in its early phases, the use of AI-driven data holds promise for various surgical opportunities in the future.

12.6 Patient-Reported and Objective Outcomes

With several different techniques and the ability to analyze large sets of data, AI and ML may provide exciting insight into how patients fare with different treatment options for their respective pathologies. Knowledge of the risks, potential side-effects, and outcomes related to various treatment approaches, including conservative management, surgical options, and if patient forgoes treatment, is essential in guiding decision-making and providing patients with the most accurate information regarding their prognosis. In fact, Potty et al. sought to prognosticate outcomes of arthroscopic rotator cuff repair using an ML algorithm [44]. Preoperative and 3-month, 6-month, and 12-month postoperative American Shoulder and Elbow Surgeons (ASES) scores of 631 patients were used to train the model whereby it would generate an expected postoperative score for each patient and calculate the change between preoperative and postoperative scores [44]. While not exact, the model performed well and demonstrated improvement in mean ASES scores by 12 months similar to reported trends in the literature, with 67% of patients within the minimal clinically significant difference (MCID) threshold and 84% within the substantial clinical benefit (SCB) threshold [44]. The authors were also able to identify predictive factors for postoperative outcomes, finding preoperative ASES score, preoperative pain score, body mass index, age, and tendon quality to be the variables most relied on by the model during prediction [44].

Similar ML applications have been developed for predicting patient-reported outcome measures for other sports medicine-related pathologies. Another example included an ML model developed by Nwachukwu et al. for the prediction of clinically meaningful outcomes after arthroscopic femoroacetabular impingement surgery [45]. The model was trained on data consisting of reported two-year outcomes of 898 patients and showed 74%, 73.5%, and 79.9% of patients achieved the MCID in the Hip Outcome Score–

Activities of Daily Living (HOS-ADL), HOS–Sport Specific (HOS-SS), and modified Harris Hip Score (mHHS) scores, respectively [45]. Anxiety/depression, symptom duration of greater than two years, preoperative intra-articular injection, and high preoperative outcome scores were all found to be predictive for not attaining MCID across the three hip outcome scores [45].

ML holds significant potential in uncovering more information about patient-reported and functional outcomes associated with different treatments. Knowledge of the factors predictive of favorable or unfavorable outcomes can assist in better understanding patient prognoses. This can additionally complement preoperative counseling, planning, and allocation of resources [44].

12.7 Improving Patient Experience

The vast applications of AI have immense potential beyond clinical management, diagnosis, and intraoperative assistance [46–48]. AI can and has been used as a means to improve patient experience during the management of different orthopedic procedures. These applications have taken numerous forms, including monitoring prognosis through sophisticated technology and aiding patient education through publicly available chatbots [46–48].

Using AI to aid patient management and monitoring has gained prominent attention in recent years. Applications for smart devices have been developed to act as management platforms that monitor recovery and help connect the physician and the patient in a digital space, facilitating communication and education [46, 47]. These mobile health solutions have been described and used in different medical fields and can provide a great tool for orthopedics and sports medicine [46, 47, 49]. A study by Lonner et al. described the use of such applications for managing patients who underwent robotic-assisted total knee arthroplasty [47]. The application incorporated wearable sensing technology to passively collect continuous data, both preoperatively and postoperatively, that is indicative of the patient's progress [47]. These include a range of motion, level of daily activity, overall health, and patient-reported outcomes [47]. Aside from monitoring surgical progress, these applications provide ample information that can be used for research purposes later [47]. The authors of the mentioned study concluded that the application can be integrated with robotic total knee arthroplasty to allow for a more holistic management approach [47]. Similar results have been noted for other medical and surgical specialties [50–52]. Considering the importance of follow-up and management in athletes, and the significance of monitoring not only healing and recovery but also level of performance, one can understand the vast benefits that can be reaped from these AI applications in the field of sports medicine.

In addition, in the digitalized world we live in today, access to well-trusted medical information may be limited, as physicians are not always available to answer patient queries should any arise. As such, AI chatbots may provide solutions to many patients and may help provide evidence-based education to concurrent and prospective patients. Research exploring the utility of chatbots in diagnosing and managing different medical conditions have shown promising results, and highlighted the potential benefits of such technology [48, 53, 54]. Nevertheless, considering the lack of empathy or intuition that is exhibited by chatbots, it is hard to conceive that they will act as replacement for physicians in the future [54]. Instead, these can serve as tools that supplement the management process and help aid patients through their recovery [54]. In the world of sports medicine, where injured athletes may have numerous questions about recovery and health, the utility of such chatbots may serve a great purpose and provide much benefit.

12.8 Conclusion

In the highly digitalized world of today, AI acts as a domain that can serve purpose in numerous fields, especially medicine. Sports medicine deals with the management of amateur and professional athletes, and as such is highly reliant on the health of the athletes in order to achieve optimal performance. The large amount of money invested in this field renders the need for continuous technological advancements necessary and pivotal for proper growth. As such, AI may offer numerous applications that can help sports physicians, physical therapists, trainers, and patients go through the management process in an easy and smooth way. These applications can take place on the research and performance front, and may include helping in predicting injury risk patterns, extrapolating preventive techniques, and conducting biomotion analyses. Other utilities can also involve the clinical front, where AI can help with diagnosis, operative management, research, and improving overall patient experience. While the potential of AI in medicine is still budding, current evidence suggests many possible benefits that can prove helpful to sports medicine professionals in managing athletes and improving their performance.

Competing Interests
JAA would like to disclose: Royalties from a company or supplier; Disclosures; OSTEOCENTRIC TECHNOLOGIES, ENOVIS, ZIMMER-BIOMET, STRYKER, GLOBUS MEDICAL, INC. Stocks in: SHOULDER JAM, AEVUMED, OBERD, OTS MEDICAL, ORTHOBULLETS, ATREON, RESTORE 3D. Research support from a company or supplier as a PI; Disclosures; ENOVIS, ARTHREX. Royalties, financial or material support from publishers; Disclosures; WOLTERS KLUWER, SLACK ORTHOPAEDICS, ELSEVIER. Board member/committee appointments for a society; Disclosures; AMERICAN SHOULDER AND ELBOW SOCIETY, MID ATLANTIC SHOULDER AND ELBOW SOCIETY, SHOULDER 360, PACIRA.

Funding
None.

References

1. Ramkumar PN, Luu BC, Haeberle HS, Karnuta JM, Nwachukwu BU, Williams RJ. Sports medicine and artificial intelligence: a primer. Am J Sports Med. 2022;50:1166–74.
2. McCarthy J, Minsky ML, Rochester N, Shannon CE. A proposal for the dartmouth summer research project on artificial intelligence, august 31, 1955. AI Mag. 2006;27:12.
3. Weng SF, Reps J, Kai J, Garibaldi JM, Qureshi N. Can machine-learning improve cardiovascular risk prediction using routine clinical data? PLoS One. 2017;12:e0174944.
4. Olczak J, Fahlberg N, Maki A, et al. Artificial intelligence for analyzing orthopedic trauma radiographs: deep learning algorithms—are they on par with humans for diagnosing fractures? Acta Orthop. 2017;88:581–6.
5. Haenssle HA, Fink C, Schneiderbauer R, et al. Man against machine: diagnostic performance of a deep learning convolutional neural network for dermoscopic melanoma recognition in comparison to 58 dermatologists. Ann Oncol. 2018;29:1836–42.
6. Rigamonti L, Estel K, Gehlen T, Wolfarth B, Lawrence JB, Back DA. Use of artificial intelligence in sports medicine: a report of 5 fictional cases. BMC Sports Sci Med Rehabil. 2021;13:1–7.
7. Sheu Y, Chen L-H, Hedegaard H. Sports-and recreation-related injury episodes in the United States, 2011–2014. Natl Health Stat Rep. 2016:1–12.
8. Lewis M. It's a hard-knock life: game load, fatigue, and injury risk in the national basketball association. J Athl Train. 2018;53:503–9.
9. Surgery HfS. Injuries cost NFL teams over $500 million in 20192020.
10. Research GV. Wearable medical device market size, industry report, 2027. 2020.
11. Chidambaram S, Maheswaran Y, Patel K, et al. Using artificial intelligence-enhanced sensing and wearable technology in sports medicine and performance optimisation. Sensors (Basel). 2022;22:6920.
12. Karnuta JM, Luu BC, Haeberle HS, et al. Machine learning outperforms regression analysis to predict next-season Major League Baseball player injuries: epidemiology and validation of 13,982 player-years from performance and injury profile trends, 2000–2017. Orthop J Sports Med. 2020;8:2325967120963046.
13. Luu BC, Wright AL, Haeberle HS, et al. Machine learning outperforms logistic regression analysis to predict next-season NHL player injury: an analysis of 2322 players from 2007 to 2017. Orthop J Sports Med. 2020;8:2325967120953404.
14. Zheng N, Barrentine SW. Biomechanics and motion analysis applied to sports. Phys Med Rehabil Clin N Am. 2000;11:309–22.

15. Scarborough DM, Leonard NK, Mayer LW, Oh LS, Berkson EM. The association of baseball pitch delivery and kinematic sequence on stresses at the shoulder and elbow joints. J Sports Sci Med. 2021;20:94.
16. Scarborough DM, Linderman SE, Sanchez JE, Berkson EM. Kinematic sequence classification and the relationship to pitching limb torques. Med Sci Sports Exerc. 2021;53:351–9.
17. Román-Belmonte JM, De la Corte-Rodríguez H, Rodríguez-Damiani BA, Rodríguez-Merchán EC. Artificial intelligence in musculoskeletal conditions. 2023.
18. Labbe DR, de Guise JA, Mezghani N, et al. Objective grading of the pivot shift phenomenon using a support vector machine approach. J Biomech. 2011;44:1–5.
19. Štajduhar I, Mamula M, Miletić D, Ünal G. Semi-automated detection of anterior cruciate ligament injury from MRI. Comput Methods Prog Biomed. 2017;140:151–64.
20. Bien N, Rajpurkar P, Ball RL, et al. Deep-learning-assisted diagnosis for knee magnetic resonance imaging: development and retrospective validation of MRNet. PLoS Med. 2018;15:e1002699.
21. Chang PD, Wong TT, Rasiej MJ. Deep learning for detection of complete anterior cruciate ligament tear. J Digit Imaging. 2019;32:980–6.
22. Liu F, Guan B, Zhou Z, et al. Fully automated diagnosis of anterior cruciate ligament tears on knee MR images by using deep learning. Radiol Artif Intell. 2019;1:180091.
23. Roblot V, Giret Y, Bou Antoun M, et al. Artificial intelligence to diagnose meniscus tears on MRI. Diagn Interv Imaging. 2019;100:243–9.
24. Fritz B, Marbach G, Civardi F, Fucentese SF, Pfirrmann CWA. Deep convolutional neural network-based detection of meniscus tears: comparison with radiologists and surgery as standard of reference. Skeletal Radiol. 2020;49:1207–17.
25. Rizk B, Brat H, Zille P, et al. Meniscal lesion detection and characterization in adult knee MRI: a deep learning model approach with external validation. Phys Med. 2021;83:64–71.
26. Zhan H, Teng F, Liu Z, et al. Artificial intelligence aids detection of rotator cuff pathology: a systematic review. Arthroscopy J Arthrosc Relat Surg. 2023.
27. Horng M-H. Texture classification of the ultrasonic images of rotator cuff diseases based on radial basis function network. 2008 IEEE International Joint Conference on Neural Networks (IEEE World Congress on Computational Intelligence): IEEE; 2008.
28. Shim E, Kim JY, Yoon JP, et al. Automated rotator cuff tear classification using 3D convolutional neural network. Sci Rep. 2020;10:15632.
29. Wang L, Wen D, Yin Y, et al. Musculoskeletal ultrasound image-based radiomics for the diagnosis of achilles tendinopathy in skiers. J Ultrasound Med. 2023;42:363–71.
30. Kapiński N, Zieliński J, Borucki BA, et al. Monitoring of the Achilles tendon healing process: can artificial intelligence be helpful? Acta Bioeng Biomech. 2019;21:103–11.
31. Harangi B, Hajdu A, Lampe R, Torok P. Recognizing ureter and uterine artery in endoscopic images using a convolutional neural network. 2017 IEEE 30th International Symposium on Computer-Based Medical Systems (CBMS): IEEE; 2017.
32. Barash Y, Klang E, Lux A, et al. Artificial intelligence for identification of focal lesions in intraoperative liver ultrasonography. Langenbeck's Arch Surg. 2022;407:3553–60.
33. Halicek M, Little JV, Wang X, et al. Optical biopsy of head and neck cancer using hyperspectral imaging and convolutional neural networks. Proc SPIE Int Soc Opt Eng. 2018;10469:104690X.
34. Halicek M, Lu G, Little JV, et al. Deep convolutional neural networks for classifying head and neck cancer using hyperspectral imaging. J Biomed Opt. 2017;22:60503.
35. Hou F, Liang Y, Yang Z, Gu W, Yu Y. Automatic identification of metastatic lymph nodes in OCT images. Optical Coherence Tomography and Coherence Domain Optical Methods in Biomedicine XXIII: SPIE; 2019.
36. Verhey JT, Haglin JM, Verhey EM, Hartigan DE. Virtual, augmented, and mixed reality applications in orthopedic surgery. Int J Med Robot Comput Assist Surg. 2020;16:e2067.
37. Lang JE, Mannava S, Floyd AJ, et al. Robotic systems in orthopaedic surgery. J Bone Joint Surg Br. 2011;93-B:1296–9.
38. Bautista M, Manrique J, Hozack WJ. Robotics in total knee arthroplasty. J Knee Surg. 2019;32:600–6.
39. D'Souza M, Gendreau J, Feng A, Kim LH, Ho AL, Veeravagu A. Robotic-assisted spine surgery: history, efficacy, cost, and future trends. Robot Surg. 2019;6:9–23.
40. Jonmohamadi Y, Takeda Y, Liu F, et al. Automatic segmentation of multiple structures in knee arthroscopy using deep learning. IEEE Access. 2020;8:51853–61.
41. Familiari F, Hochreiter B, Gerber C. Unacceptable failure of osteochondral glenoid allograft for biologic resurfacing of the glenoid. J Exp Orthop. 2021;8:111.
42. Kather J, Hagen ME, Morel P, Fasel J, Markar S, Schueler M. Robotic hip arthroscopy in human anatomy. Int J Med Robot Comput Assist Surg. 2010;6:301–5.
43. Bozkurt M, Apaydin N, Işik Ç, Bilgetekin YG, Acar HI, Elhan A. Robotic arthroscopic surgery: a new challenge in arthroscopic surgery Part-I: Robotic shoulder arthroscopy; a cadaveric feasibility study. Int J Med Robot Comput Assist Surg. 2011;7:496–500.
44. Potty AG, Potty ASR, Maffulli N, et al. Approaching artificial intelligence in orthopaedics: predictive analytics and machine learning to prognosticate arthroscopic rotator cuff surgical outcomes. J Clin Med. 2023;12:2369.
45. Nwachukwu BU, Beck EC, Lee EK, et al. Application of machine learning for predicting clinically

meaningful outcome after arthroscopic femoroacetabular impingement surgery. Am J Sports Med. 2019;48:415–23.

46. Christensen JC, Blackburn BE, Anderson LA, et al. Recovery curve for patient reported outcomes and objective physical activity after primary total knee arthroplasty-a multicenter study using wearable technology. J Arthroplast. 2023;38:S94–s102.
47. Lonner JH, Anderson MB, Redfern RE, Van Andel D, Ballard JC, Parratte S. An orthopaedic intelligence application successfully integrates data from a smartphone-based care management platform and a robotic knee system using a commercial database. Int Orthop. 2023;47:485–94.
48. Fayed AM, Mansur NSB, de Carvalho KA, Behrens A, D'Hooghe P, de Cesar NC. Artificial intelligence and ChatGPT in Orthopaedics and sports medicine. J Exp Orthop. 2023;10:74.
49. Bonn SE, Hult M, Spetz K, et al. Effect of a smartphone application on physical activity and weight loss after bariatric surgery-results from a randomized controlled trial. Obes Surg. 2023;33(9):2841–50.
50. Knight SR, Ng N, Tsanas A, Mclean K, Pagliari C, Harrison EM. Mobile devices and wearable technology for measuring patient outcomes after surgery: a systematic review. NPJ Digit Med. 2021;4:157.
51. Patel B, Thind A. Usability of mobile health apps for postoperative care: systematic review. JMIR Perioper Med. 2020;3:e19099.
52. Crawford DA, Duwelius PJ, Sneller MA, et al. 2021 Mark Coventry Award: use of a smartphone-based care platform after primary partial and total knee arthroplasty: a prospective randomized controlled trial. Bone Joint J. 2021;103:3–12.
53. Schukow C, Smith SC, Landgrebe E, et al. Application of ChatGPT in routine diagnostic pathology: promises, pitfalls, and potential future directions. Adv Anat Pathol. 2023;31(1):15–21.
54. Altamimi I, Altamimi A, Alhumimidi AS, Altamimi A, Temsah MH. Artificial Intelligence (AI) chatbots in medicine: a supplement, not a substitute. Cureus. 2023;15:e40922.

13 Artificial Intelligence in Hand Surgery

Niyathi Prasad, Giorgio Pajardi, Raffaella Russo, and Dawn LaPorte

13.1 Introduction

Artificial intelligence (AI) is a technology that replicates intelligent human thought, actions, or tasks through the use of a machine or digital platforms [1]. AI falls into two categories: machine learning and deep learning. Briefly, machine learning can change and learn as it is exposed to new data, while deep learning involves autodidactic neural networks to process large volumes of data, similar to the human brain [1]. Rapidly over the past decade, AI has become a part of our daily lives. Beyond healthcare, it has found its use in creating social media content, risk assessment by finance and banking platforms, self-driving cars, and sports teams to analyze players' performance [1]. Within orthopedic surgery, common applications of AI include image recognition, preoperative risk assessment, clinical decision making, or evaluating probabilities of certain outcomes after treatment [2]. While not as advanced as other subspecialties in orthopedic surgery, AI in hand surgery is an emerging field that will likely play a large and meaningful role in the future care of our patients. The purpose of this chapter is to summarize some of the recent developments in hand surgery and possibilities for the future.

N. Prasad · D. LaPorte (✉)
Johns Hopkins University School of Medicine
Baltimore, Baltimore, MD, USA
e-mail: Nprasad6@jhmi.edu; dlaport1@jhmi.edu

G. Pajardi
University of Milan, Milan, Italy
e-mail: gpajardi@centrostudimano.it

R. Russo
University of Catanzaro, Catanzaro, Italy

13.2 Diagnosis of Hand Pathology

Radiology and image recognition are the most advanced areas of AI within orthopedic surgery in general. Within hand surgery, significant work has been done to assist in the detection of scaphoid fractures, one of the most frequently missed fractures on X-ray in the ED [3, 4]. Yoon et al. utilized a deep learning network that can reliably detect scaphoids with fractures from those without fractures with an overall sensitivity of 87.1% and specificity of 92.1% and an area under the curve (AUC) of 0.955 [5]. Other studies have taken it a step further and compared the performance of the AI models to healthcare workers [6, 7]. Langerhuizen et al. compared a deep learning algorithm to the performance of five orthopedic surgeons in detecting scaphoid fractures using a set of four different radiographic views. The algorithm was 75% accurate, 84% sensitive, and 60% specific, while the orthopedic surgeons had a better specificity (93%), and similar accuracy (84%) and sensitivity (76%) to the algorithm. Additionally, the deep learning model was able to detect 5 out of 6 occult scaphoid fractures but

F. Familiari et al. (eds.), *Artificial Intelligence in Orthopaedic Surgery Made Easy*,
https://doi.org/10.1007/978-3-031-70310-2_13

made 13 false positive suggestions that were correctly identified by the surgeons [6]. In a similar article, Ozkaya et al. compared a deep learning algorithm to an emergency department provider and two orthopedic surgeons of differing experience levels in detecting scaphoid fractures on AP wrist radiographs. The deep learning algorithm was 76% sensitive and 92% specific. The more experienced orthopedic surgeon performed better than the algorithm, while the less experienced surgeon performed similarly and the emergency department provider showed the worst diagnostic performance [7]. Not all AI algorithms for scaphoid fractures rely on imaging. Bulstra et al. tested five machine learning algorithms in predicting scaphoid fracture probability using demographics, mechanism of injury, and exam maneuvers and designed a decision rule to initiate advanced imaging in high-risk patients [8]. Their study found that pain over the scaphoid on ulnar deviation, sex, age, and mechanism of injury were most associated with scaphoid fracture. The best-performing machine learning algorithm had an area under the curve of 0.77. A decision-making tool was proposed to initiate advanced imaging in patients with radial-sided wrist pain, negative radiographs, and a fracture probability >10% based on this machine learning algorithm. This yielded a 100% sensitivity and 38% specificity with a reduced number of patients undergoing advanced imaging by 36% without missing a fracture [8]. Beyond scaphoid fractures, AI has been used to help flag hand and wrist fractures within the emergency room [9, 10]. Tecle et al. presented the use of a deep learning network that used the cortical thickness of the second metacarpal bone on an AP radiograph of the hand to diagnose osteoporosis [11]. Additionally, outside of X-ray imaging, Kuock et al. developed a computer-aided soft tissue segmentation method with a deep learning algorithm to help distinguish tendon tissue from synovial sheath tissue on ultrasound, which can be used to help guide the treatment of trigger fingers [12]. Furthermore, one study has looked at AI and infrared thermography to help diagnose carpal tunnel syndrome, but the authors concluded that it cannot be recommended as an adequate diagnostic tool but rather a screening tool for severe cases [13]. These various tools can help decrease the burden of the emergency department for binary decisions (fracture or no fracture), reducing the rate of missed fractures, streamlining referrals to orthopedic surgeons, and facilitating appropriate ordering of advanced imaging. However, the big downside of these tools is that they are not externally validated and are unable to flag other associated pathologies like arthritis or bone tumors. It is likely these technologies will assist clinicians in their decision making and not replace them.

13.3 Applications in the Clinical Setting

Patient reported outcome measures (PROMs) are increasingly collected to measure healthcare quality and value before and after hand surgery [1]. Machine learning can prove to be a powerful tool to help predict injury and expected functional improvement after surgery based on demographic factors and help patients and clinicians with shared decision making. Studies have shown that a patient's expectation and knowledge before surgery influences postoperative satisfaction [1, 14, 15]. Two studies from the Hand and Wrist study group in the Netherlands used machine learning to develop and test algorithms that can calculate the probability of clinically relevant symptom improvement after carpal tunnel release [16] and functional improvement after surgery for thumb carpometacarpal osteoarthritis [17]. In a more general sense, Mahajan et al. developed and validated a machine learning model to identify patients before surgery who are high risk for postoperative adverse events [18]. With a dataset of 1,477,561 patients undergoing surgical procedures, the study developed an algorithm that had an area under the receiver operating curve of 0.956 for mortality, 0.923 for cardiac events, and 0.899 for cerebrovascular accidents. This outperformed the National Surgical Quality Improvement Program (NSQIP) surgical risk calculator which is currently the most widely used [18]. This model was accurate in identifying patients undergoing surgery who were at high risk of adverse outcomes using only preoperative variables that were available in the electronic medical record. This allows any surgeon, including hand surgeons who perform primarily elective cases, to provide individualized perioperative care, which may be associated with improved outcomes.

AI has also been developed to help physicians be more efficient during their clinical encounters. A hand surgery team at Thomas Jefferson University compared the quality and time spent documenting common orthopedic encounters in hand surgery during a clinic visit using either an AI-based virtual scribe service, an in-person medical scribe, a transcription service, and a voice recognition mobile application [19]. With ten standardized patients with prewritten clinical vignettes, 118 clinical encounters were created and equally split among the documentation services. Analysis of the AI-based service notes found that the formulation of the final plan was incorrect and needed a manual edit, and the transcription service and voice recognition services required substantial time compared to the AI-based notes. The study concluded, however, that AI-based notes overall decreased documentation burden without significantly lowering the quality of documentation compared to transcription and voice recognition software services [19].

13.4 Applications in Patient Education

Open AI platforms like Chat Generative Pre-Trained Transformer (ChatGPT) have become very popular in their use and patients may turn to it to learn more about their symptoms and possible treatment options. Seth et al. looked at the role of ChatGPT in the management of scaphoid fractures and found that it provided quick, user-friendly clinically validated information and medical advice [20]. However, the authors found that the diagnostic pathway was often inconsistent and had erroneous references and lacked consistency with medical advice [20]. Another article analyzed the quality and readability of the information on the ChatGPT platform for common hand conditions like carpal tunnel syndrome, trigger finger, and distal radius fractures, and compared it with corresponding articles in the American Society for the Surgery of the Hand (ASSH) HandCare website [21]. They found that ChatGPT provided high-quality answers to frequently asked questions. However, it was unclear where the answers came from as there were no citations. Furthermore, answers were written at a college reading level, compared to the ASSH website, which is at an eighth-grade reading level [21]. To ChatGPT's credit, every article about medical advice in both studies stressed the need to discuss all symptoms and possible treatment options with a surgeon [20, 21].

13.5 Future Directions

Technology using AI is a rapidly developing field and we have only scratched the surface of its potential uses in healthcare. Using multiple AI tools at the same time to automatically characterize specific elements of X-rays for common conditions on a large scale may allow increased diagnostic value per scan, which would substantially decrease the time burden for clinicians and reduce the level of expertise needed for review. For example, one model could grade osteopenia, assess radiocarpal and midcarpal arthritis and intercarpal alignment, and highlight joint incongruities with a series of radiographs [1]. Another possible application of AI technology is three-dimensional technology in creating patient-specific operation guides and three-dimensional printed plates [1, 22, 23]. To create these custom implants and jigs, detailed preoperative imaging with bony alignment planning must be performed which is often labor intensive. Machine learning algorithms can help speed up this process and revolutionize reconstructive surgery and fracture surgery by making custom implants more widely available. Ultimately, combining different AI techniques integrated into daily clinical workflow will be the most powerful. A model that could integrate radiological findings with information from clinic notes, demographics, and examination findings may allow AI to provide outcome predictions and suggest optimal treatment options, and even lead to the likelihood of improved PROMs [1].

13.6 Conclusion

In conclusion, AI is the fourth industrial revolution still in its infancy but with remarkable potential. Combining different types of AI in the future can help target-specific aspects and challenges within hand surgery, such as diagnosis, PROMs, surgical planning, and individualized care and management recommendations. The goal is to have systems that integrate naturally within clinical workflows that are accountable ethically, externally validated, and monitored after deployment. Ultimately in general healthcare AI models need to be transparent. The inner workings should be understood by the clinicians who use them so they can properly be interpreted and any discordance between the AI and clinician can be resolved. Furthermore, there must be patient buy-in and trust in the system to work. Regardless, AI is the future of healthcare and will be a valuable tool as the surgeon's "third eye" in clinical decision making.

References

1. Miller R, Farnebo S, Horwitz MD. Insights and trends review: artificial intelligence in hand surgery. J Hand Surg Eur. 2023;48(5):396–403.
2. Keller M, Guebeli A, Thieringer F, Honigmann P. Artificial intelligence in patient-specific hand surgery: a scoping review of literature. Int J Comput Assist Radiol Surg. 2023;18(8):1393–403.
3. Hendrix N, Scholten E, Vernhout B, Bruijnen S, Maresch B, de Jong M, et al. Development and validation of a convolutional neural network for automated detection of scaphoid fractures on conventional radiographs. Radiol Artif Intell. 2021;3(4):e200260.
4. Yoon AP, Lee YL, Kane RL, Kuo CF, Lin C, Chung KC. Development and validation of a deep learning model using convolutional neural networks to identify scaphoid fractures in radiographs. JAMA Netw Open. 2021;4(5):e216096.
5. Yoon AP, Chung KC. Application of deep learning: detection of obsolete scaphoid fractures with artificial neural networks. J Hand Surg Eur. 2021;46(8):914–6.
6. Langerhuizen DWG, Janssen SJ, Mallee WH, van den Bekerom MPJ, Ring D, Kerkhoffs GMMJ, et al. What are the applications and limitations of artificial intelligence for fracture detection and classification in orthopaedic trauma imaging? A systematic review. Clin Orthop. 2019;477(11):2482–91.
7. Ozkaya E, Topal FE, Bulut T, Gursoy M, Ozuysal M, Karakaya Z. Evaluation of an artificial intelligence system for diagnosing scaphoid fracture on direct radiography. Eur J Trauma Emerg Surg Off Publ Eur Trauma Soc. 2022;48(1):585–92.
8. AEJ B, Machine Learning Consortium. A machine learning algorithm to estimate the probability of a true scaphoid fracture after wrist trauma. J Hand Surg. 2022;47(8):709–18.
9. Reichert G, Bellamine A, Fontaine M, Naipeanu B, Altar A, Mejean E, et al. How can a deep learning algorithm improve fracture detection on X-rays in the emergency room? J Imaging. 2021;7(7):105.
10. Gan K, Xu D, Lin Y, Shen Y, Zhang T, Hu K, et al. Artificial intelligence detection of distal radius fractures: a comparison between the convolutional neural network and professional assessments. Acta Orthop. 2019;90(4):394–400.
11. Tecle N, Teitel J, Morris MR, Sani N, Mitten D, Hammert WC. Convolutional neural network for second metacarpal radiographic osteoporosis screening. J Hand Surg. 2020;45(3):175–81.
12. Kuok CP, Yang TH, Tsai BS, Jou IM, Horng MH, Su FC, et al. Segmentation of finger tendon and synovial sheath in ultrasound image using deep convolutional neural network. Biomed Eng Online. 2020;19(1):24.
13. Papež BJ, Palfy M, Mertik M, Turk Z. Infrared thermography based on artificial intelligence as a screening method for carpal tunnel syndrome diagnosis. J Int Med Res. 2009;37(3):779–90.
14. Krist AH, Tong ST, Aycock RA, Longo DR. Engaging patients in decision-making and behavior change to promote prevention. Stud Health Technol Inform. 2017;240:284–302.
15. Waljee J, McGlinn EP, Sears ED, Chung KC. Patient expectations and patient-reported outcomes in surgery: a systematic review. Surgery. 2014;155(5):799–808.
16. Hoogendam L, Bakx JAC, Souer JS, Slijper HP, Andrinopoulou ER, Selles RW, et al. Predicting clinically relevant patient-reported symptom improvement after carpal tunnel release: a machine learning approach. Neurosurgery. 2022;90(1):106–13.
17. Loos NL, Hoogendam L, Souer JS, Slijper HP, Andrinopoulou ER, Coppieters MW, et al. Machine learning can be used to predict function but not pain after surgery for thumb carpometacarpal osteoarthritis. Clin Orthop. 2022;480(7):1271–84.
18. Mahajan A, Esper S, Oo TH, McKibben J, Garver M, Artman J, et al. Development and validation of a machine learning model to identify patients before surgery at high risk for postoperative adverse events. JAMA Netw Open. 2023;6(7):e2322285.

19. PRNewswire [Internet]. 2023. Artificial intelligence proves to be an effective tool for documenting orthopaedic encounters in hand surgery. Available from: https://www.prnewswire.com/news-releases/artificial-intelligence-proves-to-be-an-effective-tool-for-documenting-orthopaedic-encounters-in-hand-surgery-301764164.html
20. Seth I, Lim B, Xie Y, Hunter-Smith DJ, Rozen WM. Exploring the role of artificial intelligence chatbot on the management of scaphoid fractures. J Hand Surg Eur. 2023;48(8):814–8.
21. Crook BS, Park CN, Hurley ET, Richard MJ, Pidgeon TS. Evaluation of online artificial intelligence-generated information on common hand procedures. J Hand Surg. 2023;48(11):1122–7.
22. Kabelitz M, Furrer PR, Hodel S, Canonica S, Schweizer A. 3D planning and patient specific instrumentation for intraarticular corrective osteotomy of trapeziometacarpal-, metacarpal and finger joints. BMC Musculoskelet Disord. 2022;23(1):965.
23. Dobbe JGG, Peymani A, Roos HAL, Beerens M, Streekstra GJ, Strackee SD. Patient-specific plate for navigation and fixation of the distal radius: a case series. Int J Comput Assist Radiol Surg. 2021;16(3):515–24.

14 Artificial Intelligence in Foot and Ankle Surgery

Emanuel Cortesão Seiça, Daniel Mendes, Manuel Resende Sousa, and João Vide

Key Points

- Image interpretation systems for foot and ankle (FA) surgery demonstrate commendable results in fracture identification, occult lesion prediction, and pathological classification, ensuring accurate diagnoses and informed treatment decisions.
- While clinical prediction models exhibit promising potential, ongoing development, and validation efforts are crucial. Continued refinement is essential to harness their full predictive power in FA surgery.
- Robotic technology in FA surgery not only enhances research endeavors but also fosters a deeper understanding of FA biomechanics. Dynamic robotic simulators play a pivotal role, facilitating comprehensive exploration and comprehension of intricate biomechanical processes.
- Artificial intelligence (AI) proves invaluable in surgical navigation, particularly in minimally invasive procedures common to FA surgery. Its precision and efficiency significantly contribute to enhancing surgical outcomes and patient recovery.
- Patient-specific instrumentation (PSI) systems for total ankle arthroplasty (TAA) hold promise. However, recent data underline the necessity for further improvement. Current findings suggest comparable patient outcomes with traditional TAA, necessitating continued research to unlock additional benefits.
- AI-powered orthosis revolutionizes the rehabilitation landscape. These innovations serve as invaluable emulators, enabling patients to explore various options before selecting a prosthesis or orthosis. Additionally, they guide gait and movement rehabilitation training, ensuring personalized and effective recovery journeys.

14.1 Introduction

The field of orthopedics is increasingly embracing artificial intelligence (AI), encompassing mathematical machine learning (ML) and deep learning (DL). AI, essentially mimicking human-like intelligence and critical thinking through complex models

E. C. Seiça (✉)
Hospital Beatriz Ângelo, Lisbon, Portugal

Hospital Particular do Algarve, Gambelas, Portugal

D. Mendes
Hospital CUF Tejo, Lisbon, Portugal

M. R. Sousa
Hospital da Luz, Lisbon, Portugal

Sport Lisboa e Benfica, Lisbon, Portugal

J. Vide
Hospital Particular do Algarve, Gambelas, Portugal

Hospital da Luz, Lisbon, Portugal

F. Familiari et al. (eds.), *Artificial Intelligence in Orthopaedic Surgery Made Easy*,
https://doi.org/10.1007/978-3-031-70310-2_14

and algorithms, stands poised to revolutionize the medical field, with data as its driving force.

AI's potential applications in foot and ankle (FA) surgery are vast: it can automate image interpretation from diverse sources (radiographic, macroscopic, microscopic, etc.), predict bone implants, recognize implants, conduct personalized multivariate risk analysis, optimize healthcare delivery, analyze biomechanics, forecast surgical outcomes and injury risks, enhance surgical precision and arthroscopy, and minimize errors in patient care. In the realm of FA surgery, particularly in minimally invasive procedures where extensive exposure of structures is challenging or poses a higher risk of complications, AI could prove invaluable in surgical navigation. Additionally, AI can play a significant role in the rehabilitation process, a critical aspect of FA surgery outcomes, where early range of motion and proper rehabilitation are pivotal. Therefore, harnessing the potential of AI and robotics in FA surgery is essential to advancing patient care and outcomes [1, 2].

The utilization of AI models and robotic technology has been extensively documented across various orthopedic specialties. However, FA surgery has lagged behind other orthopedic fields like knee and hip surgery in adopting this technology. Consequently, there's a growing urgency to explore and implement AI and robotics more comprehensively in FA surgery. These technologies have the potential to transform primary care, hospitals, and clinics by enhancing the efficiency and accuracy of FA pathology diagnoses, surgeries, and rehabilitation processes. Therefore, it's crucial for FA surgical professionals to stay updated on the latest advancements, enabling them to provide the best possible care to their patients. This chapter underscores the pivotal role of AI in FA surgery, addressing ethical concerns, cost implications, limitations, and both current and future perspectives in the field.

14.2 Role in Traumatology, Sports Injuries, and Orthopedics

Numerous authors have discussed the use of AI models in diagnosing conditions, assisting in management, and predicting clinical outcomes or associated issues. However, these models are mostly validated internally, emphasizing the need for further research before AI-based clinical applications can be widely implemented. The lack of external validation highlights the importance of conducting more thorough studies to evaluate the effectiveness of AI models in real clinical scenarios. Therefore, it's essential to be cautious about adopting these models until they have undergone rigorous external validation [2]. AI can serve as a valuable tool in motion analysis, seamlessly integrating visual data obtained through motion cameras with the dynamic distribution of plantar pressure from force platforms (Fig. 14.1).

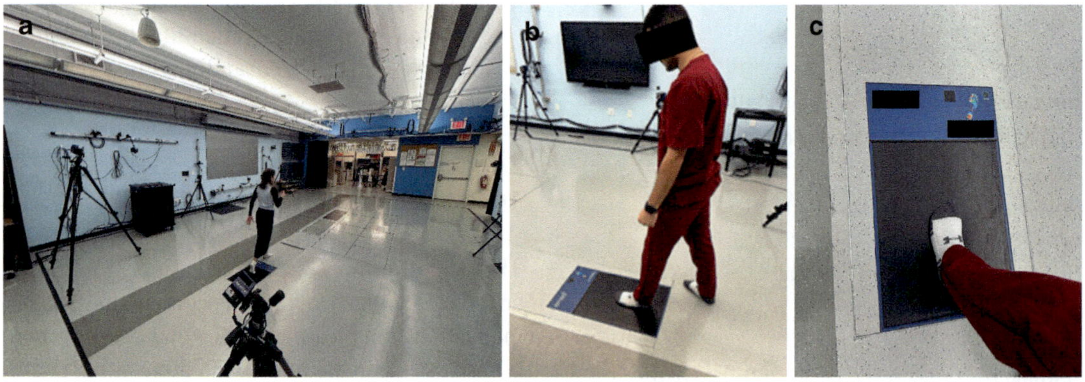

Fig. 14.1 Motion and plantar pressure analysis: (**a**) Visual data capturing the patient's walking motion through motion cameras; (**b**, **c**) Plantar pressure data recorded via a force platform. (Courtesy of Leon Root MD, Motion Analysis Laboratory (LRMALab), Dr. Scott Ellis, Dr. Howard Hillstrom, Dr. Grace DiGiovanni, and Dr. Seif El Masry)

14.2.1 Artificial Intelligence as a Diagnostic Tool: Image Interpretation

In orthopedic care, accurate interpretation of medical images is vital. Artificial intelligence and DL techniques can significantly expedite the diagnostic process while maintaining or enhancing accuracy. This involves recognizing visual patterns in image pixels through convolutional neural networks (CNNs), specialized deep neural networks used in image and video recognition tasks. CNNs automatically learn spatial features from input images, applying filters through layers to extract crucial details. They show promise in autonomous outcome prediction and are currently applied in fracture detection. Optimizing CNNs for diverse clinical settings presents ample opportunities for research and development. These advanced CNNs can perform tasks in both 2D and 3D computed tomography (CT) imaging, making them particularly valuable in regions and medical facilities where initial imaging interpretation is done by nonorthopedic professionals [3]. Furthermore, AI can ease the workload of orthopedic specialists and contribute to quicker and more precise diagnoses, even when they are the initial observers.

Guermazi et al. internally validated a DL model for detecting fractures in FA plain radiographs, achieving an impressive area under the curve (AUC) of 0.97, along with a sensitivity and specificity of 93%. AUC is a key metric in assessing ML and AI models, measuring their ability to distinguish between positive and negative cases. The high AUC in this study underscores the DL model's accuracy in detecting fractures in FA radiographs [4]. Several studies have investigated the effectiveness of different CNNs in detecting ankle fractures using similar approaches. These studies consistently showed comparable performance, with the AUC ranging from 0.81 to 0.99. These results indicate that CNNs hold great promise for accurately identifying ankle fractures and could be valuable in clinical applications [5–7].

Advanced medical systems can meticulously analyze subtle instability patterns or fractures visible on radiographs, allowing the detection of intricate injuries like Lisfranc injury or joint subluxation. Ashkani-Esfahani and colleagues have created and internally validated two deep convolutional neural network (DCNN) models capable of identifying Lisfranc instability from both single-view (anteroposterior) and 3-view radiographs (anteroposterior, lateral, and oblique), achieving AUCs ranging from 0.925 to 0.994 [8]. Wang et al. conducted internal and external validation of a DL system designed to detect and grade fatigue fractures from plain radiographs. The system showed outstanding performance in identifying fatigue fractures in foot images, achieving an AUC of 0.911 and a sensitivity of 90.8%. In the case of tibia and fibula images, the system performed reasonably well, with an AUC of 0.877 and a sensitivity of 85.5%. However, the DL system's external validity for grading fatigue fractures was not confirmed, displaying poor performance. Its overall accuracy for tibiofibular images was only 62.9%, and for foot images, it was 61.1%. These results indicate the potential effectiveness of the DL system in detecting fatigue fractures, but further research and development are essential to enhance its accuracy in grading such fractures [9]. Shin and colleagues have introduced a diagnostic model utilizing ankle radiographs to identify osteochondral lesions of the talus (OLT). Their model, based on a CNN, achieved a test data performance with an AUC of 0.774 (95% CI, 0.673–0.875), an accuracy of 81.58% (95% CI, 0.729–0.903), a positive predictive value of 80.95% (95% CI, 0.773–0.846), and a negative predictive value of 81.82% (95% CI, 0.804–0.832). These results indicate the model's ability to provide accurate and reliable diagnoses of OLTs using ankle radiographs, showcasing the significant potential to enhance the efficiency and efficacy of OLT diagnoses, which is of great interest to clinicians, researchers, and stakeholders in the medical diagnostics field [10].

Several studies have confirmed the effectiveness of machine learning (ML) and deep learning (DL) models in detecting and diagnosing hallux valgus. Hida et al. created an ML model capable of distinguishing between normal foot images and those displaying hallux valgus. The model exhibited a high accuracy range of 0.77 to 0.96 and holds potential for early and straightforward screening of hallux valgus [11]. Li T and colleagues validated a DL model capable of detecting 18 anatomical landmarks from weight-bearing radiographs, including crucial angles like hallux valgus angle (HVA), hallux interphalangeal angle (HIA), first-second intermetatarsal angle (IMA), and distal metatarsal articular angle (DMAA). The model's predictions demonstrated a strong correlation with manually observed values, with intraclass correlation scores ranging from 0.89 to 0.96 and R-values ranging from 0.81 to 0.97 [12]. Day et al. tested an AI-based software that automatically measures the M1–M2 IMA from weight-bearing cone-beam computed tomography (WBCT) scans in patients with hallux valgus. The software performed measurements faster than manual methods, correlated well with manual measurements, and had nearly perfect test-retest reliability [13]. Wang and colleagues validated a support vector machine model capable of classifying patients with symptomatic hallux valgus using HVA, IMA, and DMAA with an accuracy of 76.4%. These studies offer compelling evidence for the effectiveness of machine and DL models as valuable tools in detecting and diagnosing hallux valgus and other deformities [14] (Fig. 14.2).

In cases of flatfoot condition, Ryu and colleagues' recent study endeavors to create a DL model using CNNs to automate angle measurements for diagnosing flatfoot. This innovative approach involves landmark detection, reducing inconsistencies between different observers. Through rigorous internal and external validation, the model exhibited notably enhanced accuracy and reliability when compared to human observers. These findings hold practical significance for flatfoot diagnosis, potentially leading to a more standardized and objective diagnostic process [15].

CNNs have the capability to detect, pinpoint, and categorize fractures in plain radiographs. Olczak and team conducted an internal validation of neural network models designed to classify ankle fractures from radiographs according to the AO Foundation/Orthopaedic Trauma Association (AO/OTA) 2018 classification. The results revealed that the models demonstrated varying degrees of performance, ranging from fair to excellent, with AUC values spanning from 0.79 to 0.99 when classifying AO types [16].

Prijs and colleagues conducted both internal and external validations of a DL model tailored for detecting, classifying, and pinpointing ankle fractures from plain radiographs. Their model achieved outstanding results, boasting an impressive AUC of 0.92 and a remarkable accuracy rate of 99% during external validation [17].

In addition to plain radiographs, AI models can analyze CT and MRI images as well as ultra-

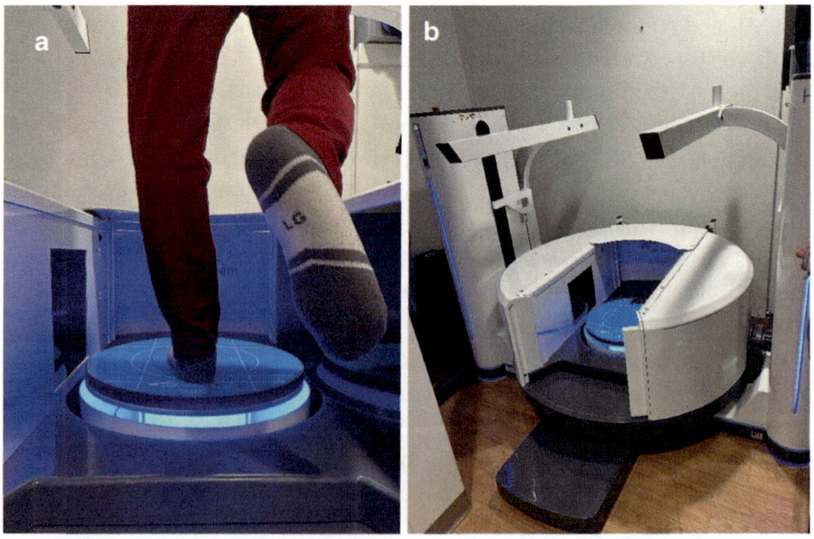

Fig. 14.2 Weight-bearing cone-beam computed tomography (WBCT): (**a**) Patient positioning for ankle and foot scans involves the patient standing at the center of the apparatus, with the X-ray source and image detector located at opposing sides. (**b**) The tube-detector system performs a singular rotation around the patient. (Courtesy of Dr. Scott Ellis, Dr. Grace DiGiovanni, and Dr. Seif El Masry)

sonography. Pranata et al. conducted an internal validation of two separate DCNN models for detecting the presence or absence of calcaneal fractures on CT images, achieving an excellent accuracy of 98% [18]. Aghnia Farda et al. also conducted an internal validation of a CNN model for classifying calcaneal fractures on CT images into the Sanders system, which exhibited a classification accuracy of nearly 72% after augmenting the data [19].

In ultrasonography, utilizing dynamic imaging or incorporating various images is recommended for optimal results. Wang and colleagues internally validated several radiomics-based ML models for diagnosing Achilles tendinopathy from ultrasonographic images in skiers. They achieved an impressive AUC of 0.99, 90% sensitivity, and 100% specificity [20].

Kawanishi et al. recently developed an artificial intelligence model using CNNs to estimate and assess the tension of the tibial nerve through ultrasound imaging analysis in different ankle positions. They reported a mean accuracy of over 0.77 using five-fold cross-validation [21].

Additionally, Kapiński and team conducted an internal validation of several DL models to classify Achilles tendon injuries and monitor tendon healing on MRI scans. They achieved a maximum accuracy of 97.6%, a sensitivity of 98.3%, and a specificity of 99.45% [22].

Furthermore, artificial intelligence has the capability to predict the presence of hidden lesions in additional fractures by analyzing the fracture pattern and trauma mechanism. Studies conducted by Hendrickx et al. and Oosterhoff et al. validated multiple ML and DL models for predicting patients with tibial shaft fractures and associated concealed posterior malleolar fractures, achieving AUC values ranging from 0.81 to 0.89 [23, 24].

In summary, artificial intelligence, particularly through advanced techniques like CNNs, significantly enhances orthopedic care by swiftly and accurately interpreting medical images. These AI models, as demonstrated in numerous aforementioned studies, offer exceptional precision in diagnosing fractures, complex injuries, and various orthopedic conditions from multiple imaging modalities, including radiographs, CT scans, MRI images, and ultrasonography. The implementation of AI not only expedites diagnoses but also ensures standardized and objective assessments, proving especially valuable in countries where initial imaging interpretation is done by non-specialists or even in scenarios involving orthopedic specialists. It relieves their workload and ensures swifter and more precise diagnoses, marking a significant advancement in orthopedic care.

14.2.2 Predictions, Clinical, and Performance Analysis

DL and ML are invaluable for analyzing and predicting clinical outcomes and performance, as well as guiding diagnoses based on patient records. By harnessing AI's capacity to process vast amounts of data and images, healthcare professionals and researchers can extract valuable insights to inform decision-making and enhance patient outcomes. A crucial application of AI is in the analysis of clinical data and images. This approach involves employing advanced algorithms and ML techniques to identify patterns and trends in the data. By leveraging this information, healthcare professionals can predict future outcomes. Comparing these predictions with outcome reports and existing literature provides a deeper understanding of common outcomes, enabling the development of more effective treatment plans. Another vital use of AI is in performance prediction. This entails utilizing data and images to forecast the likely effectiveness of a specific treatment or intervention. By analyzing this data and comparing it with past outcomes, healthcare professionals gain valuable insights into the efficacy of different treatments, enabling them to make more informed decisions about patient care. Several studies have utilized ML and DL models to predict various FA-related conditions. For instance, Keijsers et al. validated a neural network model that differentiated patients with forefoot pain from those without, utilizing plantar pressure data and achieving an accuracy of 70.4% [25]. Ardhianto and colleagues utilized DL to automate the measurement of the foot progression angle (FPA) from plantar pressure images, aiding clinicians in assessing gait abnormalities [26]. Likewise, Merrill and colleagues created logistic regression and gradient-boosting models to forecast short-term complications in patients undergoing open reduction and internal fixation (ORIF) for acute ankle fractures. Both models demonstrated strong performance, achieving AUCs ranging from 0.6979 to 0.7583 [27].

Lu and colleagues validated multiple ML models to predict lower extremity muscle strains in elite basketball players. Among these models, the XGBoost model achieved the highest AUC of 0.840 [28]. On the contrary, Jauhiainen and the team developed ML models to predict moderate and severe knee and ankle injuries in young basketball and floorball players. However, these models exhibited poor performance, achieving only AUCs of 0.63 and 0.65, respectively [29]. Ruiz-Pérez and colleagues validated numerous ML models to predict lower extremity noncontact soft tissue injuries in professional futsal players. The most effective model achieved an AUC of 0.767 [30].

Kwon and colleagues developed wearable monitoring sensors designed to track Achilles tendon loading and walking speed during ambulation in an immobilizing boot. This innovative technology serves as a clinically implementable strategy for monitoring patient loading and activity while recovering from Achilles tendon injuries [31]. Zhao and collaborators introduced a state-of-the-art DL multilabel classification model, utilizing ResNet-50, that excels in detecting flat foot types. This model proves valuable in assessing the clinical rehabilitation status of patients with abnormal foot types and various foot pathologies [32].

Diniz and colleagues created a ML model to forecast whether soccer players would recover to similar performance levels after an Achilles tendon rupture, achieving a commendable AUC of 0.81 [33]. Yin and collaborators designed a neural network model to anticipate patients who would attain the minimum clinically successful therapy (a decrease in the visual analog score, VAS, by 60% or more from baseline) at 6 months following extracorporeal shock wave therapy (ESWT) for chronic plantar fasciitis [34].

Mousa and colleagues developed an artificial intelligence-based artificial neural network and decision tree algorithms to predict diabetic foot ulcers, utilizing medical history and ML analysis of foot images [35]. In a recent study, Chauhan and colleagues tested ML models to enhance current diagnostic methods for diabetic ulcers in diabetic foot patients, achieving accuracies between 94% and 100% [36].

Lastly, Pakhomov and his team employed ML to automate the identification and classification of foot examination findings from clinical notes, achieving overall accuracies ranging from 81% to 87% [37].

14.2.3 Surgery

In the realm of surgical assistance, the availability of thoroughly tested and precise options remains limited. The prevailing solutions mainly revolve around navigation and assistance systems. Progress in this field is imperative to enhance the efficiency of surgical procedures and elevate patient outcomes. Computer-assisted surgery (CAS) can be executed using O-arm™ CTs or mobile 3D C-arm systems, which capture 3D fluoroscopic images through a 190-degree orbital rotation. The former furnishes real-time navigational guidance through a reference frame affixed to the patient's bone, leveraging the initial 3D CT reconstruction. This enables real-time instrumented navigation, refining the trajectory of surgical instruments and implants, thereby enhancing surgical control. The latter system upgrades 2D fluoroscopy to offer 3D imaging, facilitating intraoperative assessment of anatomical reduction and optimal implant placement. Both systems amalgamate multiplanar imaging, 3D reconstruction, and real-time navigation. They prove invaluable in interventions involving intricate anatomical areas, necessitating a 3D understanding of the treated segment and benefiting from high precision, particularly in minimally invasive procedures [38–41] (Fig. 14.3).

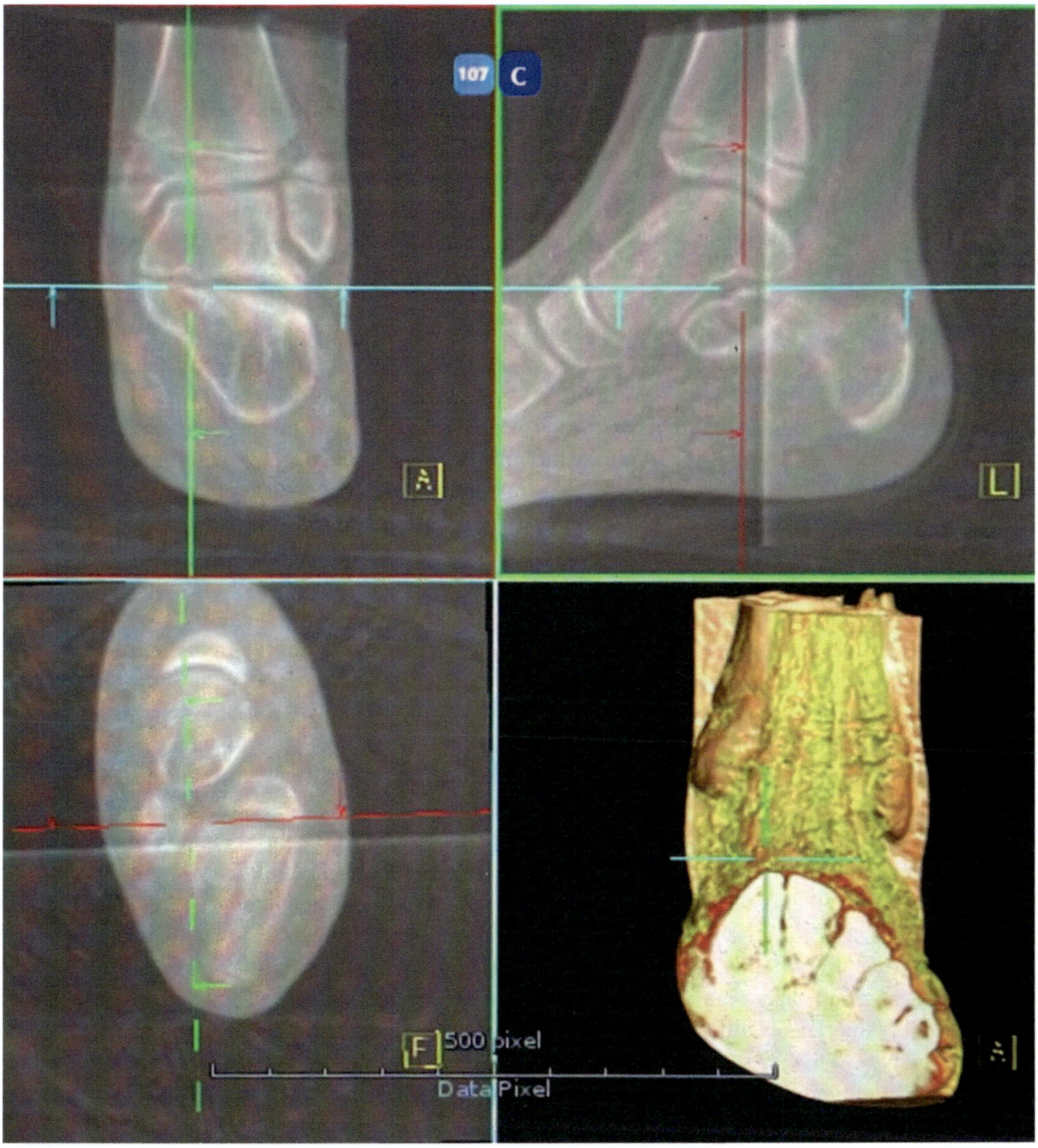

Fig. 14.3 Talocalcaneal coalition. Intraoperative three-dimensional views of the coalition using a mobile 3D C-arm. (Courtesy of Dr. Manuel Cassiano Neves)

The O-arm^{tm} performs an intraoperative scan of the specific anatomical area. A reference frame, fixed with two K-wires in the area of interest and spheres attached to these reference points, is crucial in this process. This reference frame, facing a recognition camera, serves as the foundation for the subsequent steps. After ensuring the satisfactory position and fixation of the reference frame, an intraoperative scan is acquired. The patient's anatomy is automatically registered using the reference frame, and surgical instruments are tracked through emitted infrared light and reflective spheres. This innovative method allows for real-time 3D triangulation of the instruments' relative positions.

Several systems incorporating similar principles are available in the market. These systems find valuable applications in various surgical scenarios, such as minimally invasive surgery for calcaneal fractures (especially in tongue-type fractures), where precise subchondral screw placement is crucial. They are also essential in pilon fractures, guiding the placement of screws in subchondral areas. Correction of malunions through osteotomy procedures benefits from these systems, aiding in guiding rotational and angular alignment. Additionally, these systems prove invaluable in arthrodesis procedures, whether involving subtalar, midfoot, or total ankle fusion. They also play a vital role in the management of tarsal coalitions and osteochondral lesions, opening avenues for guided retrograde curettage and grafting procedures. This advanced technology significantly enhances the precision and efficacy of these intricate surgical interventions [38, 42].

Yuan and colleagues conducted a study evaluating the safety and efficacy of assisted percutaneous screw placement combined with tarsal sinus incisions for treating calcaneal fractures. The study concluded that there were no differences in postoperative radiological measurements and fracture healing time between the groups. However, in the robot-assisted group, the intraoperative C-arm fluoroscopy dose was significantly lower. Importantly, patients in the robot-assisted group had significantly higher postoperative American Orthopedic Foot and Ankle Society (AOFAS) scores compared to those in the traditional group, highlighting the potential benefits of robot-assisted techniques in improving patient outcomes after calcaneal fracture surgery [43]. In their study, Zhu and colleagues aimed to investigate the efficacy of AI-assisted ultrasonography-guided needle knife therapy for the treatment of chronic plantar fasciitis. The researchers discovered that patients who underwent AI-assisted therapy showed statistically significant improvements in the American Orthopedic Foot and Ankle Society (AOFAS) score. Additionally, they experienced reductions in plantar fascia elasticity and thickness compared to the control group. These results indicate that AI-assisted ultrasonography-guided needle knife therapy holds promise as an effective approach for treating chronic plantar fasciitis [44].

The advantages of 3D-based CAS are evident; however, its widespread adoption in FA surgery is hindered by its high cost, complexity, and longer operative times.

A technology that demands attention is augmented reality (AR) systems. Augmented or hybrid reality, a display technology, seamlessly blends the tangible world with the virtual realm. This innovation permits digital images from preoperative planning to merge with the surgeon's real-time view. AR enriches the surgeon's intraoperative perspective by superimposing virtual elements onto the actual patient, finding applications in diverse orthopedic procedures like tumor resection, fracture fixation, arthroscopy, and component alignment in total joint arthroplasty [45, 46]. Unlike virtual reality (VR), where users are fully immersed in a virtual environment, AR enhances the real world with additional virtual information [45]. AR modifies the user's vision through monitor-based displays, optical see-through systems, or video see-through systems. Optical see-through systems, facilitated by devices like Google Glass and Microsoft HoloLens, offer flexibility by overlaying virtual content onto the tangible world. A pivotal component of AR is the tracking system, essential for accurately placing virtual objects in the real world. Traditional systems rely on external markers, while modern marker-less systems utilize inertial measurement units (IMU), red-green-blue (RGB) cameras, and infrared sensors on head-mounted displays (HMD) for spatial mapping and real-time tracking without predetermined markers [45, 47, 48].

The applications of AR in orthopedic surgery are expanding due to its compatibility with visual data and mechanical tasks common in orthopedics, such as implant insertions and deformity corrections. AR solutions can potentially enhance surgical outcomes by providing preoperative planning directly within the surgeon's field of view or displaying correct trajectories for implant placements. For example, AR navigation has been employed in high tibial osteotomy, where parallax-free panoramic images were created using an

RGB camera setup on a C-arm. This innovative approach accurately measured the mechanical axis and misalignments, proving to be precise and a low-radiation procedure [49, 50]. Viehöfer et al. conducted a study to assess the impact of AR on the accuracy of distal osteotomy in hallux valgus surgery. Their findings suggested that AR-guided osteotomies have the potential to enhance precision during hallux valgus correction, especially for less experienced surgeons [51].

Overall, AR has the potential to save time, reduce risks and radiation exposure, and enhance accuracy in orthopedic surgery. It also serves as a valuable tool for surgical simulation and intraoperative education. With advancing computational power, the applicability of AR in orthopedic surgery is expected to grow [45, 52].

14.2.4 Total Ankle Arthroplasty

The advancements in robotic-assisted total knee arthroplasty (TKA) and total hip arthroplasty (THA) have demonstrated positive clinical outcomes, sparking discussions about their potential application in total ankle arthroplasty (TAA). However, the diverse nature of FA surgeries, combined with lower procedure volumes compared to arthroplasty, presents significant cost challenges. Consequently, the adoption of technologies like CAS and robotics in TAA is not as advanced as in TKA and THA procedures [53, 54]. The testing and investigation of biomechanics heavily depend on cadaveric studies, underscoring the crucial need for the development of dynamic robotic experimental models [1, 55, 56].

The longevity of implants is a critical factor in TAA, given that the majority of osteoarthritis cases, as indicated by several studies (over 70%), are posttraumatic in origin. These cases often affect younger patients with higher physical demands, underscoring the importance of durable implant solutions [57, 58]. Consequently, TAA has higher failure rates compared to other joints [59, 60]. Therefore, improper positioning of the implant may lead to heightened contact pressures and increased mechanical stress, resulting in postoperative pain and suboptimal function [59, 60]. Modern options such as PROPHECY™ INFINITY™, STAR ankle,[R] and VANTAGE[R], are patient-specific instrumentation (PSI) systems designed to offer precision in bony resections, assuming that the necessary anatomic landmarks for implant alignment and positioning are identifiable on preoperative patient imaging scans. These systems share the goal of improving implant positioning and alignment. They allow for a limited approach area, prioritizing soft tissue balance. This approach can significantly decrease the risk of revision surgery and enhance functional outcomes [43, 61, 62]. However, studies comparing PSI to standard referencing (SR) techniques have yielded inconsistent results. Some studies found no significant improvements in implant positioning, and the findings on operative time were inconclusive [63, 64]. For example, Adams Jr. et al. demonstrated that the accuracy of TAA tibial preparation using computer navigation was comparable to the conventional technique performed by a FA surgeon experienced in TAA [65]. Consequently, the current body of literature does not provide sufficient evidence to support the widespread adoption of PSI in TAA, particularly when considering it's additional cost [66]. However, PSI may offer significant value in complex reconstruction, where anatomical abnormalities, abnormal alignment or previous surgeries may complicate the procedure, as well as in detailed pre-operative planning to enhance surgical outcomes in these more challenging cases (Fig. 14.4).

Nevertheless, there is room for further improvement if open robotic systems are developed with capabilities for procedures that often accompany TAA. These advancements are expected to significantly improve both outcomes and patient quality of life while reducing healthcare costs. This potential revolution in the field could lead to better outcomes and an improved quality of life for patients [67]. The development of robot-assisted TAA will require surgical flexibility options, as ankle pathology and biomechanical complexity often necessitate additional procedures to enhance implant function [67, 68]. This preliminary evidence should encourage the development of more advanced computer navigation applications specific to TAA, with the potential to improve accuracy.

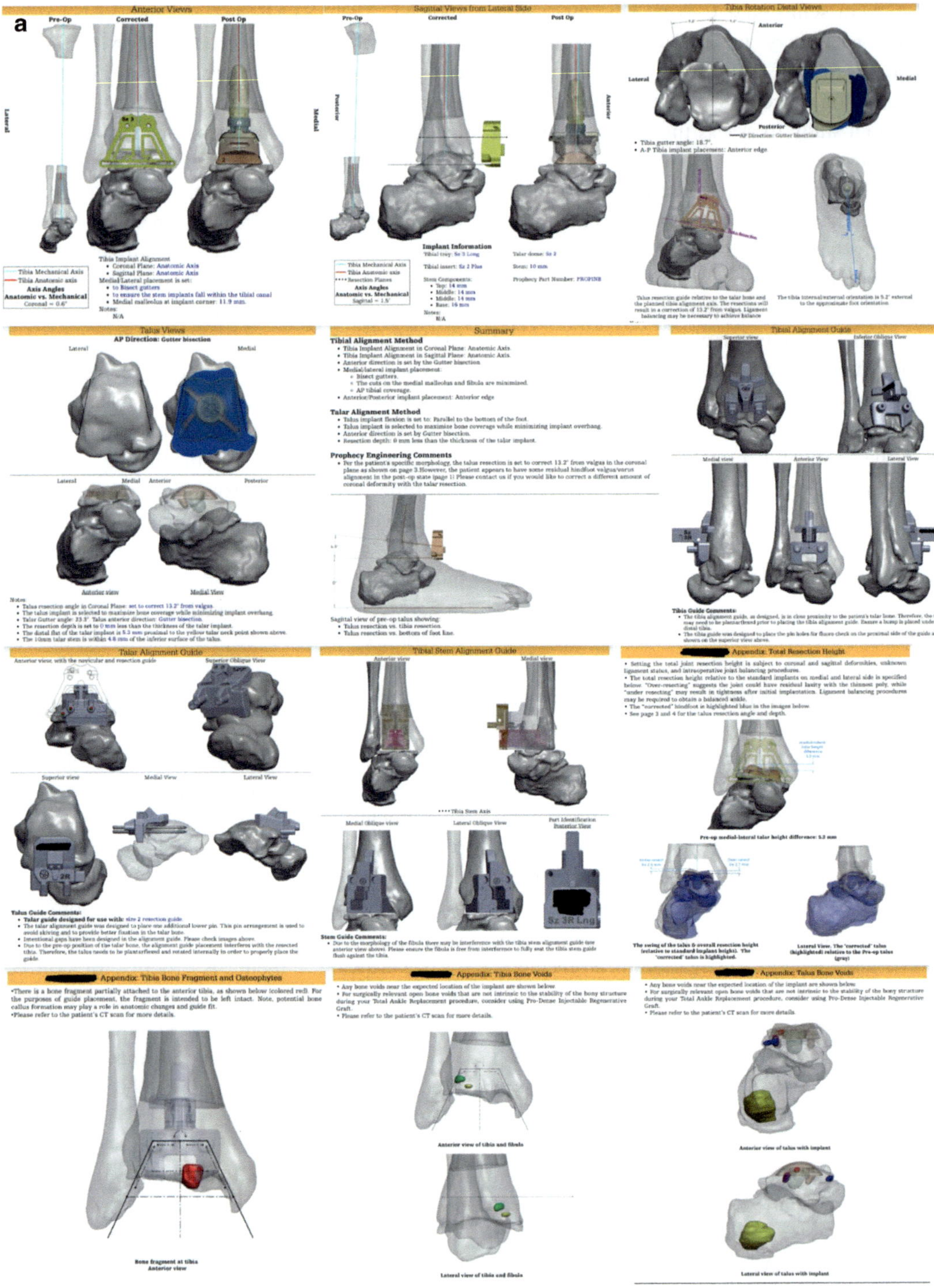

Fig. 14.4 Example of a 3D surgical alignment navigation report (**a**) utilizing PROPHECY™ and intraoperative views of the resection osteotomy blocks (**b**), in a case of total ankle arthroplasty. Of note that modern systems can give information and localize bone voids, osteophytes, and potential difficulties that may arise intraoperatively while performing the procedure, as shown in the photos. (Courtesy of Dr. Scott Ellis)

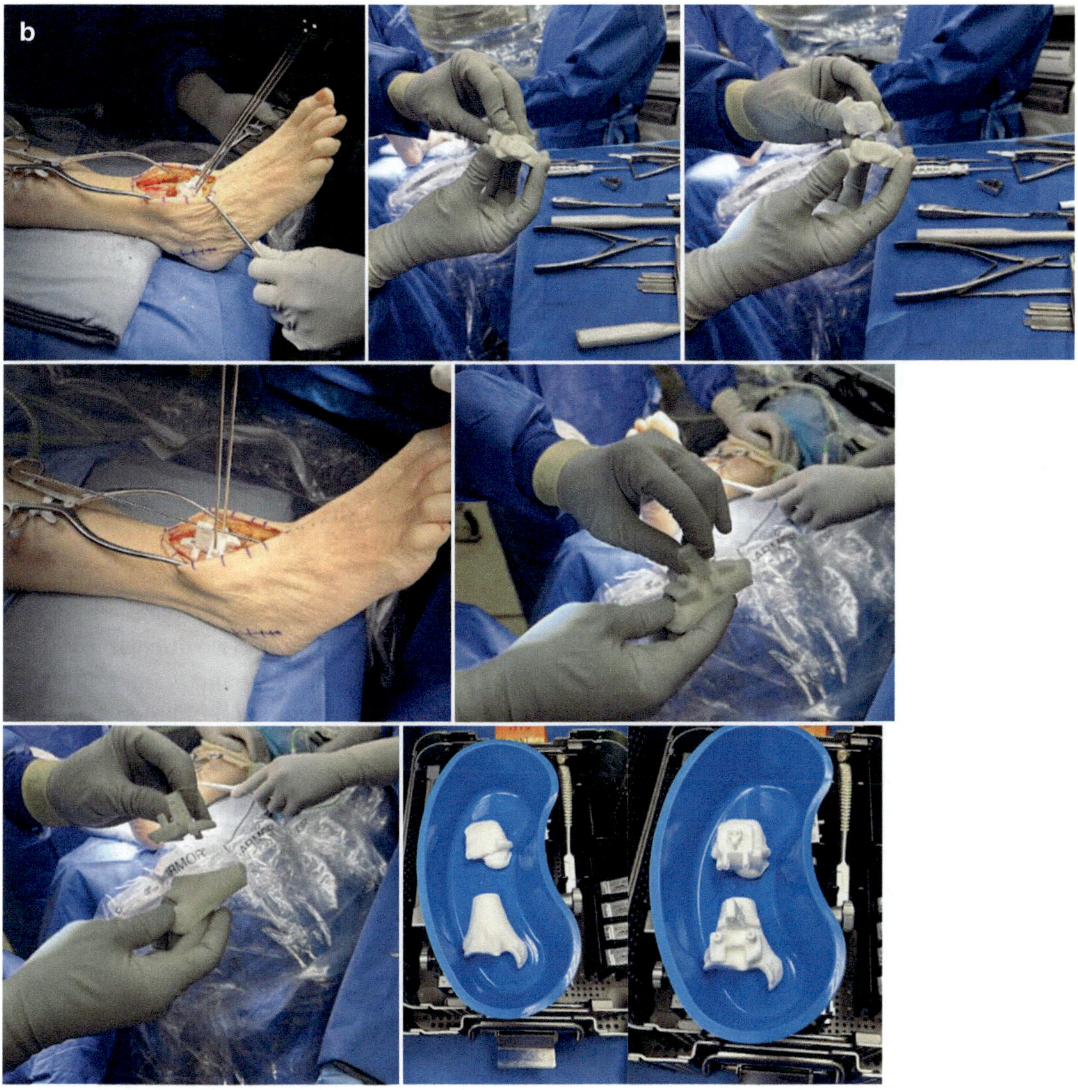

Fig. 14.4 (continued)

14.2.5 Rehabilitation, Prosthetics, and Orthotics

When it comes to prosthetics, there are numerous options available. However, the ability for patients to try a prosthesis before prescription is limited. Emulators that mimic commercially available products (using AI) could provide prosthetists and patients the opportunity to find a custom fit before a potentially costly erroneous prescription. This not only improves the functional outcome but also completes the cycle of personalized surgery with a personalized recovery. Artificial intelligence and robotic systems have been extensively researched for their applications in the field of rehabilitation and prosthetics [69, 70]. Recently, Prasanna and colleagues utilized DL to construct a dynamic system model capable of accurately estimating and predicting prosthetic ankle torque. This innovation aims to optimize prosthetic ankle torque, showcasing the potential of artificial intelligence in enhancing prosthetic design and functionality [71]. Suda and colleagues conducted an internal validation study of various support vector machine (SVM) models created to classify levels of running experience based on foot-ankle kinematic and kinetic patterns. The study's objective was to offer potential support for running rehabilitation and training. The study yielded highly promising results, with the SVM models achieving classification accuracies of 88.5%, 87.2%, and 84.6% for less experienced, moderately experienced, and experienced runners, respectively [72]. The findings of this study carry significant implications for the realm of rehabilitation and training. Accurate classification of running experience levels represents a pivotal step toward developing customized training and rehabilitation programs tailored to individual runner's needs. The SVM models employed in this study hold the potential to revolutionize running rehabilitation and training, offering a more precise and personalized approach to these practices. These studies underscore the importance of integrating advanced ML techniques into sports medicine, showcasing the potential of SVM models in delivering tailored and effective training and rehabilitation programs for runners. Additionally, the availability of robotic foot braces, emulators, and assistive limb devices with adaptive functions and real-time patient feedback further enhances personalized patient rehabilitation, particularly following injury or surgery.

14.3 Robotics

These advancements have paved the way for applications in various orthopedic specialties, including FA surgery. Robotics in orthopedics serves a multifaceted purpose, assisting in preclinical and translational research, facilitating clinical evaluations, aiding in preoperative planning, and enhancing CAS. Over time, orthopedic robotic systems have undergone significant developments, building upon the foundation laid by the initial use of the da Vinci robot. These advancements signify a promising future for robotics in orthopedic surgery, enabling more precise and efficient procedures in various specialties, including FA surgery [67]. In the realm of robotic surgery, systems can be categorized into haptic systems, where the surgeon's tactile feedback guides the operation, and autonomous robots, which function independently without direct human intervention. An example from the 1990s includes ROBODOC, utilized for total hip arthroplasty (THA) [73–75]. The distinction between image-based and imageless robots lies in their approach to operative planning. Image-based robots utilize CT or MRI scans to meticulously plan surgeries, relying on detailed preoperative anatomical information. In contrast, imageless robots perform surgeries based on real-time perioperative anatomic mapping, adapting their actions according to the patient's current anatomy during the operation [76]. Robots can be further classified based on their versatility to use different manufacturers' devices or implants for the same task. Closed-platform robots are specifically designed to work with a particular manufacturer's devices or implants, limiting their compatibility to a specific set of products. On the other hand, open-platform robots are more versatile, allowing the surgeon to use a variety of devices or implants from different manufacturers for the same task. This flexibility enhances the surgeon's options and can lead to more personalized and optimized surgical procedures [77].

It is crucial to differentiate between CAS and robotic technology in the context of surgical assistance. CAS offers the surgeon passive feedback and guidance during the perioperative process, primarily through navigation guidance. In contrast, robots are engineered to execute direct actions, varying from semi-active movements to complete autonomy. This distinction holds significant importance as it ensures the selection of the right technology for a specific surgical scenario, ultimately aiming for the best possible surgical outcomes. Therefore, a thorough comprehension of these two technologies is essential to provide high-quality healthcare services and guide the future development of medical technologies [78]. At present, various advanced robotic devices are in use across different orthopedic specialties, primarily in the context of knee arthroplasty and assisting percutaneous procedures [67]. However, in FA surgery, there are currently no autonomous systems available that offer dependable intraoperative solutions.

In research, custom cadaveric gait simulators have been employed in numerous in vitro studies focusing on foot bone and ligamentous kinematics. The utilization of dynamic robotic simulators, which offer greater degrees of freedom compared to static simulators, holds the potential to accurately position specimens and enhance our understanding of joint loading and strain. Recent simulators can replicate joint kinematics during various activities, including walking, lunging, and pivoting. They have been instrumental, for instance, in examining peak joint pressures in diabetic Charcot neuroarthropathy and measuring osseous kinematics after subtalar arthrodesis in cadavers with total ankle arthroplasty implants [79, 80]. Furthermore, other studies have showcased the replicability and correspondence with in vivo values, underscoring the advantages of robotic gait simulators in offering realistic descriptions of joint motion and bony as well as ligamentous characteristics [67, 81–83] (Fig. 14.5).

Robots equipped with force sensors can control all degrees of freedom in position, allowing for the precise repetition of actions while simultaneously recording biometric data [55, 56, 84, 85]. These simulators have the potential to enhance reduction accuracy, ensure optimal implant fixation, achieve anatomically precise positioning, and improve the precision of procedures like osteotomies. They can also reduce the necessity for surgeon intervention and limit exposure to fluoroscopy. Moreover, robotic simulators might decrease the need for extensive and time-consuming ethics board evaluations typically associated with more invasive, in vivo gait studies [67].

Richter et al. evaluated load-bearing ankle motion in cadaver specimens after total ankle replacement. The study concluded that the robot outperformed standard testing systems due to its ability to execute intricate motions under predefined, constant, or varying force or motion commands. Additionally, it could perform a broader range of movements with varying velocity magnitudes, regardless of the specimen's position [86]. The application of this technology

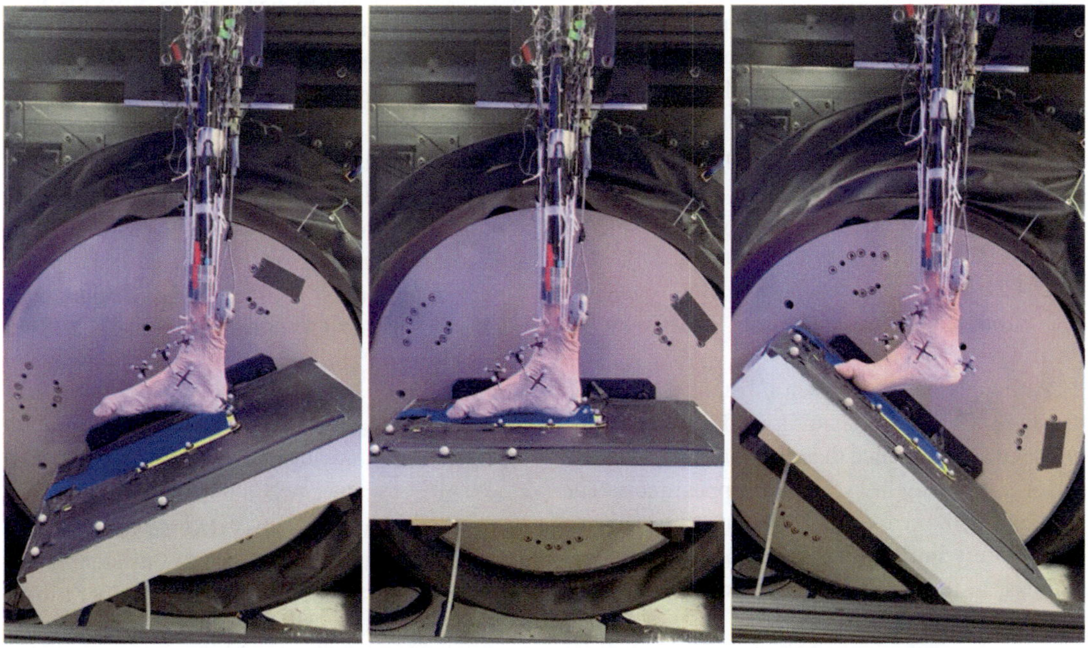

Fig. 14.5 Robotic gait simulator, displayed with specimen cadaver foot attached to robot for simulated gait and motion analysis system. (From [79], courtesy of Dr. Brett Steineman)

was showcased in a recent study by Sakakibara et al. They utilized a robotic testing simulator to study 3D kinematics and determine the optimal ankle fixation position for anterior tibiofibular ligament reconstruction. Their conclusion highlighted that fixing the reconstructed tendon graft at 30 degrees of plantarflexion provided the most accurate representation of 3D kinematics and contact pressures [87]. In another study, Hernigou et al. employed ML techniques to identify the optimal and patient-specific motion axes of the tibiotalar joint. This research aimed to enhance the effectiveness of robotic-assisted TAA. Through the application of ML, the scientists devised a more accurate and personalized approach to determine the motion axes, potentially resulting in improved outcomes for individuals undergoing TAA [88].

In the field of rehabilitation, a wide array of systems is available today. These include exoskeletons, prosthetics, and robotic rehabilitation instruments like feedback-controlled and programmed stretching devices, as well as virtual reality robots [69, 70, 89]. Rehabilitation devices typically fall into two categories: orthoses or exoskeletons, which facilitate joint mobility during daily activities and are considered dynamic systems, and platform-based systems, which are used while patients are seated and offer limited flexion-extension capabilities. The former provides more natural kinematics for the FA, while the latter is less adapted to natural movements [90, 91]. Both of these options facilitate joint movement by using either healthy reference values or AI algorithms to adjust the range and assistance based on patient feedback, including factors like effort, pain, disability level, and capability [92].

Although there have been substantial advancements in available technology, additional efforts are needed to enhance these systems, particularly in terms of weight, size, and appearance. The goal is to minimize the energy expenditure of the user, closely imitate natural gait and motion, and address aesthetic concerns linked to the use of orthotics and prosthetics [1, 92].

14.4 Cost Implications, Healthcare Management, and Limitations

While significant investments have been made in AI technologies, their full potential has yet to be fully realized, and cost-effectiveness remains a critical concern. Optimizing existing technology requires substantial investment, but immediate returns are not always expected, especially in the prototype phase. Currently, AI is costly in the medical field due to research and development investments. However, as the AI industry advances and more companies offer competitive AI technology, costs are anticipated to decrease. In the interim, it is crucial to clearly define the benefits of using AI-based solutions in specific contexts and assess various factors to make informed evaluations [67, 74, 77]. The development of AI algorithms demands meticulous consideration of their intended applications to ensure their suitability for specific tasks. Understanding the precise needs of potential users is paramount, necessitating a deep comprehension of their specific requirements. Consequently, a comprehensive understanding of the problem that the algorithm seeks to address, along with the data used for its training, is imperative. This holistic approach guarantees that AI-based solutions are precisely tailored to the challenges at hand, maximizing their effectiveness and relevance [67]. Indeed, the variability of FA surgeries, each characterized by relatively lower procedural volumes compared to more common surgeries like total joint arthroplasty, presents a barrier to the widespread adoption of pertinent technologies. The hurdle lies in the substantial costs associated with acquiring and implementing these advanced solutions.

A crucial factor in evaluating the value of AI-based solutions is their global applicability. It is essential for these models to demonstrate the ability to generalize across diverse datasets and environments while maintaining consistent levels of effectiveness, accuracy, reliability, operational cost, maintenance, and safety. A notable limitation in existing image interpretation AI models is their reliance on data from a single institution, often with uniform slice thickness and pixel dimensions. This restricted data source might constrain the adaptability of DL models when deployed in different contexts and institutions. This regional bias is further compounded by the prevalence of research papers that primarily conduct internal validation and rely solely on images from a single institution, limiting the models' broader applicability [2]. Diversifying the dataset used to train AI models is a crucial step toward addressing the regional biases and limitations observed in many current systems. Utilizing a worldwide image bank with varying qualities, resolutions, and imaging techniques can significantly enhance the robustness and adaptability of AI algorithms. Training models on a more diverse dataset ensures that they can effectively handle the inherent variability present in real-world clinical images from different institutions and geographical locations. This approach not only enhances the models' ability to generalize but also makes them more reliable and applicable across a wide range of healthcare settings. Collaboration between institutions globally to create and share such diverse datasets can significantly contribute to the development of more effective and universally applicable AI solutions in the field of FA surgeries.

When considering AI-assisted rehabilitation, allowing patients to regain mobility and functionality, the rehabilitation team can focus on more complex tasks or serve as consultants overseeing multiple patients. Improved patient outcomes can reduce healthcare costs by shortening hospital stays and enabling earlier return to work or daily activities, thereby reducing lost workdays and compensation claims. Integrating AI can also help identify cases that would benefit from specialized observation, reducing the time spent interpreting radiographic images and optimizing the tasks of surgeons and their teams.

The use of robotic technology and AI for image interpretation raises ethical questions about responsibility in the event of machine malfunction. If a patient is adversely affected due to such malfunction or AI failure to detect a pathology, determining who bears responsibility becomes crucial. Patients may also express concerns about diagnoses and rehabilitation relying solely on machines.

In the realm of augmented reality (AR), meticulous design of realistic perceptual cues is vital for effectively visualizing medical data. Incorrect perceptions can lead to confusion and hinder the integration of real and virtual information. Additionally, user-friendly interfaces and human-centered design are essential for the successful adoption of AR technology in clinical settings. Future studies must assess the clinical impact of AR in terms of cost reduction and enhancements in patient care [52].

AI-based solutions should be developed and implemented in ways that are ethically, morally, and socially responsible. Careful analysis of potential risks and hazards should be performed to ensure that the technology is safe, accurate, and reliable. Therefore, it is imperative to undertake a comprehensive evaluation of the safety and value of AI-based solutions, for their effective development and implementation.

14.5 Conclusion

The integration of AI technology in FA surgery is becoming increasingly prevalent, particularly in the interpretation of medical images. While these AI models have demonstrated impressive performance, external validation remains essential. Developing more robust models with external validation is crucial to enhancing the effectiveness of AI in FA surgery, necessitating further research in various relevant areas. Research efforts should concentrate on integrating robotic technologies into surgical procedures, research initiatives, and clinical practices. Dynamic gait simulators, both in vitro and in vivo, can transition to human subjects, facilitated by the development of less invasive versions through robotic emulators. However, a comprehensive investigation and quantification of FA biomechanics during normal human activities are necessary prerequisites.

Given the experimental nature of AI, providing detailed descriptions of the materials and methods used in research is essential to facilitate replication and further advancements. Accessibility to data, code, and protocols associated with publications is crucial, with any availability restrictions clearly stated.

The utilization of robotics in FA surgery has been explored, primarily in the development of orthotic and prosthetic devices. These systems have been evaluated for their impact on patient outcomes, especially in aiding recovery and improving functionality. Although specific protocols for ankle pathologies are lacking, multiple options for customized rehab protocols tailored to individual patient needs exist. Looking ahead, advancements in ankle prostheses, orthotics, and therapeutics will optimize these systems, creating lightweight devices that closely mimic natural motion. Patients will benefit from customizable products that support individualized recovery, guiding them through personalized, monitored routines to optimize rehabilitation post-surgery.

In terms of future directions, AI-powered simulators could offer a risk-free environment for surgeons to practice and enhance their skills. These simulators can replicate various intraoperative scenarios and complications, assisting surgeons in preparing for complex surgeries. Additionally, AR and VR can provide immersive 3D anatomy visualizations, aiding in more effective surgery planning or intraoperative magnification and AI analysis of the surgical field. This technology proves especially valuable in FA surgery, where most neurovascular structures are small compared to other fields. Future AI has the potential to provide personalized treatment plans for each patient by processing extensive patient data, leading to improved outcomes.

In summary, the integration of AI in FA surgery has the potential to enhance the technical aspects of procedures while improving patient care, safety, and overall surgical outcomes. This integration could set new standards for patient satisfaction and recovery.

Acknowledgments The authors would like to thank and give credit to: Leon Root MD, Motion Analysis Laboratory (LRMALab), Dr. Scott Ellis, Dr. Howard Hillstrom, Dr. Grace DiGiovanni, and Dr. Seif El Masry, Dr. Manuel Cassiano Neves, and Dr. Brett Steineman for their invaluable contribution of media and images to this chapter.

References

1. Vaish A, Migliorini F, Vaishya R. Artificial intelligence in foot and ankle surgery: current concepts. Die Orthop. 2023; https://doi.org/10.1007/s00132-023-04426-x.
2. Gupta P, Kingston KA, O'Malley M, Williams RJ, Ramkumar PN. Advancements in artificial intelligence for foot and ankle surgery: a systematic review. Foot Ankle Orthop. 2023;8:247301142211510. https://doi.org/10.1177/24730114221151079.
3. Anderson PG, Baum GL, Keathley N, Sicular S, Venkatesh S, Sharma A, et al. Deep learning assistance closes the accuracy gap in fracture detection across clinician types. Clin Orthop Relat Res. 2023;481:580–8. https://doi.org/10.1097/CORR.0000000000002385.
4. Guermazi A, Tannoury C, Kompel AJ, Murakami AM, Ducarouge A, Gillibert A, et al. Improving radiographic fracture recognition performance and efficiency using artificial intelligence. Radiology. 2022;302:627–36. https://doi.org/10.1148/radiol.210937.
5. Ashkani-Esfahani S, Mojahed Yazdi R, Bhimani R, Kerkhoffs GM, Maas M, DiGiovanni CW, et al. Detection of ankle fractures using deep learning algorithms. Foot Ankle Surg. 2022;28:1259–65. https://doi.org/10.1016/j.fas.2022.05.005.
6. Kitamura G, Chung CY, Moore BE. Ankle fracture detection utilizing a convolutional neural network ensemble implemented with a small sample, de novo training, and multiview incorporation. J Digit Imaging. 2019;32:672–7. https://doi.org/10.1007/s10278-018-0167-7.
7. Pinto Dos Santos D, Brodehl S, Baeßler B, Arnhold G, Dratsch T, Chon S-H, et al. Structured report data can be used to develop deep learning algorithms: a proof of concept in ankle radiographs. Insights Imaging. 2019;10:93. https://doi.org/10.1186/s13244-019-0777-8.
8. Ashkani-Esfahani S, Mojahed-Yazdi R, Bhimani R, Kerkhoffs GM, Maas M, DiGiovanni CW, et al. Deep learning algorithms improve the detection of subtle Lisfranc malalignments on weightbearing radiographs. Foot Ankle Int. 2022;43:1118–26. https://doi.org/10.1177/10711007221093574.
9. Wang Y, Li Y, Lin G, Zhang Q, Zhong J, Zhang Y, et al. Lower-extremity fatigue fracture detection and grading based on deep learning models of radiographs. Eur Radiol. 2022;33:555–65. https://doi.org/10.1007/s00330-022-08950-w.

10. Shin H, Park D, Kim JK, Choi GS, Chang MC. Development of convolutional neural network model for diagnosing osteochondral lesions of the talus using anteroposterior ankle radiographs. Medicine. 2023;102:e33796. https://doi.org/10.1097/MD.0000000000033796.
11. Hida M, Eto S, Wada C, Kitagawa K, Imaoka M, Nakamura M, et al. Development of hallux valgus classification using digital foot images with machine learning. Life (Basel). 2023:13. https://doi.org/10.3390/life13051146.
12. Li T, Wang Y, Qu Y, Dong R, Kang M, Zhao J. Feasibility study of hallux valgus measurement with a deep convolutional neural network based on landmark detection. Skeletal Radiol. 2022;51:1235–47. https://doi.org/10.1007/s00256-021-03939-w.
13. Day J, de Cesar NC, Richter M, Mansur NS, Fernando C, Deland JT, et al. Evaluation of a weightbearing CT artificial intelligence-based automatic measurement for the M1–M2 intermetatarsal angle in hallux valgus. Foot Ankle Int. 2021;42:1502–9. https://doi.org/10.1177/10711007211015177.
14. Wang C, Li C, Zhang R, Li Z, Zhang H, Zhang Y, et al. Identification of radiographic characteristics associated with pain in hallux valgus patients: a preliminary machine learning study. Front Public Health. 2022;10:943026. https://doi.org/10.3389/fpubh.2022.943026.
15. Ryu SM, Shin K, Shin SW, Lee SH, Seo SM, Cheon S-U, et al. Automated diagnosis of flatfoot using cascaded convolutional neural network for angle measurements in weight-bearing lateral radiographs. Eur Radiol. 2023;33:4822–32. https://doi.org/10.1007/s00330-023-09442-1.
16. Olczak J, Emilson F, Razavian A, Antonsson T, Stark A, Gordon M. Ankle fracture classification using deep learning: automating detailed AO Foundation/Orthopedic Trauma Association (AO/OTA) 2018 malleolar fracture identification reaches a high degree of correct classification. Acta Orthop. 2021;92:102–8. https://doi.org/10.1080/17453674.2020.1837420.
17. Prijs J, Liao Z, To M-S, Verjans J, Jutte PC, Stirler V, et al. Development and external validation of automated detection, classification, and localization of ankle fractures: inside the black box of a convolutional neural network (CNN). Eur J Trauma Emerg Surg. 2023;49:1057–69. https://doi.org/10.1007/s00068-022-02136-1.
18. Pranata YD, Wang K-C, Wang J-C, Idram I, Lai J-Y, Liu J-W, et al. Deep learning and SURF for automated classification and detection of calcaneus fractures in CT images. Comput Methods Prog Biomed. 2019;171:27–37. https://doi.org/10.1016/j.cmpb.2019.02.006.
19. Aghnia Farda N, Lai J-Y, Wang J-C, Lee P-Y, Liu J-W, Hsieh I-H. Sanders classification of calcaneal fractures in CT images with deep learning and differential data augmentation techniques. Injury. 2021;52:616–24. https://doi.org/10.1016/j.injury.2020.09.010.
20. Wang L, Wen D, Yin Y, Zhang P, Wen W, Gao J, et al. Musculoskeletal ultrasound image-based radiomics for the diagnosis of Achilles tendinopathy in skiers. J Ultrasound Med. 2023;42:363–71. https://doi.org/10.1002/jum.16059.
21. Kawanishi K, Kakimoto A, Anegawa K, Tsutsumi M, Yamaguchi I, Kudo S. Automatic identification of ultrasound images of the tibial nerve in different ankle positions using deep learning. Sensors (Basel). 2023:23. https://doi.org/10.3390/s23104855.
22. Kapiński N, Zieliński J, Borucki BA, Trzciński T, Ciszkowska-Łysoń B, Zdanowicz U, et al. Monitoring of the Achilles tendon healing process: can artificial intelligence be helpful? Acta Bioeng Biomech. 2019;21:103–11.
23. Hendrickx LAM, Sobol GL, Langerhuizen DWG, Bulstra AEJ, Hreha J, Sprague S, et al. A machine learning algorithm to predict the probability of (occult) posterior malleolar fractures associated with tibial shaft fractures to guide "malleolus first" fixation. J Orthop Trauma. 2020;34:131–8. https://doi.org/10.1097/BOT.0000000000001663.
24. Oosterhoff JHF, Gravesteijn BY, Karhade AV, Jaarsma RL, Kerkhoffs GMMJ, Ring D, et al. Feasibility of machine learning and logistic regression algorithms to predict outcome in orthopaedic trauma surgery. J Bone Joint Surg. 2022;104:544–51. https://doi.org/10.2106/JBJS.21.00341.
25. Keijsers NLW, Stolwijk NM, Louwerens JWK, Duysens J. Classification of forefoot pain based on plantar pressure measurements. Clin Biomech. 2013;28:350–6. https://doi.org/10.1016/j.clinbiomech.2013.01.012.
26. Ardhianto P, Subiakto RBR, Lin C-Y, Jan Y-K, Liau B-Y, Tsai J-Y, et al. A deep learning method for foot progression angle detection in plantar pressure images. Sensors. 2022;22:2786. https://doi.org/10.3390/s22072786.
27. Merrill RK, Ferrandino RM, Hoffman R, Shaffer GW, Ndu A. Machine learning accurately predicts short-term outcomes following open reduction and internal fixation of ankle fractures. J Foot Ankle Surg. 2019;58:410–6. https://doi.org/10.1053/j.jfas.2018.09.004.
28. Lu Y, Pareek A, Lavoie-Gagne OZ, Forlenza EM, Patel BH, Reinholz AK, et al. Machine learning for predicting lower extremity muscle strain in national basketball association athletes. Orthop J Sports Med. 2022;10:232596712211117. https://doi.org/10.1177/23259671221111742.
29. Jauhiainen S, Kauppi J-P, Leppänen M, Pasanen K, Parkkari J, Vasankari T, et al. New machine learning approach for detection of injury risk factors in young team sport athletes. Int J Sports Med. 2021;42:175–82. https://doi.org/10.1055/a-1231-5304.
30. Ruiz-Pérez I, López-Valenciano A, Hernández-Sánchez S, Puerta-Callejón JM, De Ste Croix M, Sainz de Baranda P, et al. A field-based approach to determine soft tissue injury risk in elite futsal using

novel machine learning techniques. Front Psychol. 2021:12. https://doi.org/10.3389/fpsyg.2021.610210.
31. Kwon MP, Hullfish TJ, Humbyrd CJ, Boakye LAT, Baxter JR. Wearable sensor and machine learning accurately estimate tendon load and walking speed during immobilizing boot ambulation. MedRxiv. 2023; https://doi.org/10.1101/2023.06.03.23290612.
32. Zhao Y, Zhou J, Qiu F, Liao X, Jiang J, Chen H, et al. A deep learning method for foot-type classification using plantar pressure images. Front Bioeng Biotechnol. 2023;11:1239246. https://doi.org/10.3389/fbioe.2023.1239246.
33. Diniz P, Abreu M, Lacerda D, Martins A, Pereira H, Ferreira FC, et al. Pre-injury performance is most important for predicting the level of match participation after Achilles tendon ruptures in elite soccer players: a study using a machine learning classifier. Knee Surg Sports Traumatol Arthrosc. 2022;30:4225–37. https://doi.org/10.1007/s00167-022-07082-4.
34. Yin M, Ma J, Xu J, Li L, Chen G, Sun Z, et al. Use of artificial neural networks to identify the predictive factors of extracorporeal shock wave therapy treating patients with chronic plantar fasciitis. Sci Rep. 2019;9:4207. https://doi.org/10.1038/s41598-019-39026-3.
35. Mousa KM, Mousa FA, Mohamed HS, Elsawy MM. Prediction of foot ulcers using artificial intelligence for diabetic patients at Cairo university hospital, Egypt. SAGE Open Nurs. 2023;9:23779608231185870. https://doi.org/10.1177/23779608231185873.
36. Chauhan AS, Varre MS, Izuora K, Trabia MB, Dufek JS. Prediction of diabetes mellitus progression using supervised machine learning. Sensors (Basel). 2023:23. https://doi.org/10.3390/s23104658.
37. Pakhomov SVS, Hanson PL, Bjornsen SS, Smith SA. Automatic classification of foot examination findings using clinical notes and machine learning. J Am Med Inform Assoc. 2008;15:198–202. https://doi.org/10.1197/jamia.M2585.
38. Kutaish H, Acker A, Drittenbass L, Stern R, Assal M. Computer-assisted surgery and navigation in foot and ankle: state of the art and fields of application. EFORT Open Rev. 2021;6:531–8. https://doi.org/10.1302/2058-5241.6.200024.
39. Geerling J, Zech S, Kendoff D, Citak M, O'Loughlin PF, Hüfner T, et al. Initial outcomes of 3-dimensional imaging-based computer-assisted retrograde drilling of talar osteochondral lesions. Am J Sports Med. 2009;37:1351–7. https://doi.org/10.1177/0363546509332499.
40. Kendoff D, Citak M, Gardner M, Kfuri M, Thumes B, Krettek C, et al. Three-dimensional fluoroscopy for evaluation of articular reduction and screw placement in calcaneal fractures. Foot Ankle Int. 2007;28:1165–71. https://doi.org/10.3113/FAI.2007.1165.
41. Richter M, Zech S. Intraoperative 3-dimensional imaging in foot and ankle trauma-experience with a second-generation device (ARCADIS-3D). J Orthop Trauma. 2009;23:213–20. https://doi.org/10.1097/BOT.0b013e31819867f6.
42. Chowdhary A, Drittenbass L, Dubois-Ferrière V, Stern R, Assal M. Intraoperative 3-dimensional computed tomography and navigation in foot and ankle surgery. Orthopedics. 2016;39:e1005–10. https://doi.org/10.3928/01477447-20160616-01.
43. Yuan X, Tan K, Hu J, Zhang B, Zhang H. Does robot-assisted percutaneous hollow screw placement combined with tarsal sinus incision reduction in the treatment of calcaneal fracture perform better at a minimum two year follow-up compared with traditional surgical reduction and fixation? Int Orthop. 2023;47:1575–81. https://doi.org/10.1007/s00264-023-05752-7.
44. Zhu S, Niu Y, Wang J, Xu D, Li Y. Artificial intelligence technology combined with ultrasound-guided needle knife interventional treatment of PF: improvement of pain, fascia thickness, and ankle-foot function in patients. Comput Math Methods Med. 2022;2022:1–9. https://doi.org/10.1155/2022/3021320.
45. Azuma RT. A survey of augmented reality. Presence Teleop Virt. 1997;6:355–85. https://doi.org/10.1162/pres.1997.6.4.355.
46. Abdel Al S, Chaar MKA, Mustafa A, Al-Hussaini M, Barakat F, Asha W. Innovative surgical planning in resecting soft tissue sarcoma of the foot using augmented reality with a smartphone. J Foot Ankle Surg. 2020;59:1092–7. https://doi.org/10.1053/j.jfas.2020.03.011.
47. Anderson KC, Buehler KC, Markel DC. Computer assisted navigation in total knee arthroplasty. J Arthroplast. 2005;20:132–8. https://doi.org/10.1016/j.arth.2005.05.009.
48. Bäthis H, Perlick L, Tingart M, Lüring C, Zurakowski D, Grifka J. Alignment in total knee arthroplasty. J Bone Joint Surg Br. 2004;86-B:682–7. https://doi.org/10.1302/0301-620X.86B5.14927.
49. Wang L, Traub J, Weidert S, Heining SM, Euler E, Navab N. Parallax-free intra-operative X-ray image stitching. Med Image Anal. 2010;14:674–86. https://doi.org/10.1016/j.media.2010.05.007.
50. Fallavollita P, Brand A, Wang L, Euler E, Thaller P, Navab N, et al. An augmented reality C-arm for intraoperative assessment of the mechanical axis: a preclinical study. Int J Comput Assist Radiol Surg. 2016;11:2111–7. https://doi.org/10.1007/s11548-016-1426-z.
51. Viehöfer AF, Wirth SH, Zimmermann SM, Jaberg L, Dennler C, Fürnstahl P, et al. Augmented reality guided osteotomy in hallux Valgus correction. BMC Musculoskelet Disord. 2020;21:438. https://doi.org/10.1186/s12891-020-03373-4.
52. Jud L, Fotouhi J, Andronic O, Aichmair A, Osgood G, Navab N, et al. Applicability of augmented reality in orthopedic surgery – a systematic review. BMC Musculoskelet Disord. 2020;21:103. https://doi.org/10.1186/s12891-020-3110-2.
53. Zeitlin J, Henry J, Ellis S. Preoperative guidance with weight-bearing computed tomography

and patient-specific instrumentation in foot and ankle surgery. HSS J. 2021;17:326–32. https://doi.org/10.1177/15563316211026325.
54. Siddiqi A, Horan T, Molloy RM, Bloomfield MR, Patel PD, Piuzzi NS. A clinical review of robotic navigation in total knee arthroplasty: historical systems to modern design. EFORT Open Rev. 2021;6:252–69. https://doi.org/10.1302/2058-5241.6.200071.
55. EL Daou H, Ng KCG, Van Arkel R, Jeffers JRT, Rodriguez y Baena F. Robotic hip joint testing: development and experimental protocols. Med Eng Phys. 2019;63:57–62. https://doi.org/10.1016/j.medengphy.2018.10.006.
56. El Daou H, Lord B, Amis A, Rodriguez y Baena F. Assessment of pose repeatability and specimen repositioning of a robotic joint testing platform. Med Eng Phys. 2017;47:210–3. https://doi.org/10.1016/j.medengphy.2017.06.012.
57. Barg A, Pagenstert GI, Hügle T, Gloyer M, Wiewiorski M, Henninger HB, et al. Ankle osteoarthritis. Foot Ankle Clin. 2013;18:411–26. https://doi.org/10.1016/j.fcl.2013.06.001.
58. Valderrabano V, Horisberger M, Russell I, Dougall H, Hintermann B. Etiology of ankle osteoarthritis. Clin Orthop Relat Res. 2009;467:1800–6. https://doi.org/10.1007/s11999-008-0543-6.
59. Kakkar R, Siddique MS. Stresses in the ankle joint and total ankle replacement design. Foot Ankle Surg. 2011;17:58–63. https://doi.org/10.1016/j.fas.2011.02.002.
60. Espinosa N, Walti M, Favre P, Snedeker JG. Misalignment of total ankle components can induce high joint contact pressures. J Bone Joint Surg-Am. 2010;92:1179–87. https://doi.org/10.2106/JBJS.I.00287.
61. Rajan PV, Khlopas A, Klika A, Molloy R, Krebs V, Piuzzi NS. The cost-effectiveness of robotic-assisted versus manual total knee arthroplasty: a Markov model-based evaluation. J Am Acad Orthop Surg. 2022;30:168–76. https://doi.org/10.5435/JAAOS-D-21-00309.
62. Agrawal VO, Gadekar AP, Vaidya N. Does robotic technology successfully restore the joint line after total knee arthroplasty? A retrospective analysis. Arthroplasty. 2022;4:6. https://doi.org/10.1186/s42836-021-00103-6.
63. Heisler L, Vach W, Katz G, Egelhof T, Knupp M. Patient-specific instrumentation vs standard referencing in total ankle arthroplasty: a comparison of the radiologic outcome. Foot Ankle Int. 2022;43:741–9. https://doi.org/10.1177/10711007221077100.
64. Mazzotti A, Arceri A, Zielli S, Bonelli S, Viglione V, Faldini C. Patient-specific instrumentation in total ankle arthroplasty. World J Orthop. 2022;13:230–7. https://doi.org/10.5312/wjo.v13.i3.230.
65. Adams SB, Spritzer CE, Hofstaetter SG, Jakoi AM, Pietrobon R, Nunley JA, et al. Computer-assisted tibia preparation for total ankle arthroplasty: a cadaveric study. Int J Med Robot. 2007;3:336–40. https://doi.org/10.1002/rcs.163.
66. Reb CW, Berlet GC. Experience with navigation in total ankle arthroplasty. Is it worth the cost? Foot Ankle Clin. 2017;22:455–63. https://doi.org/10.1016/j.fcl.2017.01.011.
67. Stauffer TP, Kim BI, Grant C, Adams SB, Anastasio AT. Robotic technology in foot and ankle surgery: a comprehensive review. Sensors (Basel). 2023:23. https://doi.org/10.3390/s23020686.
68. Sandomirski A, Johanshon J, Lohmann C, Lietz J. Endoprothetik des oberen Sprunggelenks. Z Rheumatol. 2023; https://doi.org/10.1007/s00393-023-01422-6.
69. Kubota S, Kadone H, Shimizu Y, Koda M, Noguchi H, Takahashi H, et al. Development of a new ankle joint hybrid assistive limb. Medicina (B Aires). 2022;58:395. https://doi.org/10.3390/medicina58030395.
70. Yeung L-F, Ockenfeld C, Pang M-K, Wai H-W, Soo O-Y, Li S-W, et al. Randomized controlled trial of robot-assisted gait training with dorsiflexion assistance on chronic stroke patients wearing ankle-foot-orthosis. J Neuroeng Rehabil. 2018;15:51. https://doi.org/10.1186/s12984-018-0394-7.
71. Prasanna C, Realmuto J, Anderson A, Rombokas E, Klute G. Using deep learning models to predict prosthetic ankle torque. Sensors (Basel). 2023:23. https://doi.org/10.3390/s23187712.
72. Suda EY, Watari R, Matias AB, Sacco ICN. Recognition of foot-ankle movement patterns in long-distance runners with different experience levels using support vector machines. Front Bioeng Biotechnol. 2020:8. https://doi.org/10.3389/fbioe.2020.00576.
73. Netravali NA, Shen F, Park Y, Bargar WL. A perspective on robotic assistance for knee arthroplasty. Adv Orthop. 2013;2013:1–9. https://doi.org/10.1155/2013/970703.
74. Lang JE, Mannava S, Floyd AJ, Goddard MS, Smith BP, Mofidi A, et al. Robotic systems in orthopaedic surgery. J Bone Joint Surg Br. 2011;93-B:1296–9. https://doi.org/10.1302/0301-620X.93B10.27418.
75. Schulz AP, Seide K, Queitsch C, von Haugwitz A, Meiners J, Kienast B, et al. Results of total hip replacement using the Robodoc surgical assistant system: clinical outcome and evaluation of complications for 97 procedures. Int J Med Robot Comput Assist Surg. 2007;3:301–6. https://doi.org/10.1002/rcs.161.
76. Smith-Bindman R. Radiation dose associated with common computed tomography examinations and the associated lifetime attributable risk of cancer. Arch Intern Med. 2009;169:2078. https://doi.org/10.1001/archinternmed.2009.427.
77. Jacofsky DJ, Allen M. Robotics in arthroplasty: a comprehensive review. J Arthroplast. 2016;31:2353–63. https://doi.org/10.1016/j.arth.2016.05.026.
78. Hernandez D, Garimella R, Eltorai AEM, Daniels AH. Computer-assisted orthopaedic surgery. Orthop Surg. 2017;9:152–8. https://doi.org/10.1111/os.12323.

79. Henry JK, Sturnick D, Rosenbaum A, Saito GH, Deland J, Steineman B, et al. Cadaveric gait simulation of the effect of subtalar arthrodesis on total ankle replacement kinematics. Foot Ankle Int. 2022;43:1110–7. https://doi.org/10.1177/10711007221088821.
80. Lee DG, Davis BL. Assessment of the effects of diabetes on midfoot joint pressures using a robotic gait simulator. Foot Ankle Int. 2009;30:767–72. https://doi.org/10.3113/FAI.2009.0767.
81. Whittaker EC, Aubin PM, Ledoux WR. Foot bone kinematics as measured in a cadaveric robotic gait simulator. Gait Posture. 2011;33:645–50. https://doi.org/10.1016/j.gaitpost.2011.02.011.
82. Zhu G, Wang Z, Yuan C, Geng X, Yu J, Zhang C, et al. In vitro study of foot bone kinematics via a custom-made cadaveric gait simulator. J Orthop Surg Res. 2020;15:346. https://doi.org/10.1186/s13018-020-01830-3.
83. Jackson LT, Aubin PM, Cowley MS, Sangeorzan BJ, Ledoux WR. A robotic cadaveric flatfoot analysis of stance phase. J Biomech Eng. 2011:133. https://doi.org/10.1115/1.4003869.
84. El Daou H, Calder JD, Stephen JM. Development and validation of a robotic system for ankle joint testing. Med Eng Phys. 2018;62:53–7. https://doi.org/10.1016/j.medengphy.2018.10.002.
85. Debski RE, Yamakawa S, Musahl V, Fujie H. Use of robotic manipulators to study diarthrodial joint function. J Biomech Eng. 2017:139. https://doi.org/10.1115/1.4035644.
86. Richter M, Zech S, Westphal R, Klimesch Y, Gosling T. Robotic cadaver testing of a new total ankle prosthesis model (German ankle system). Foot Ankle Int. 2007;28:1276–86. https://doi.org/10.3113/FAI.2007.1276.
87. Sakakibara Y, Teramoto A, Takagi T, Yamakawa S, Shoji H, Okada Y, et al. Effects of the ankle flexion angle during anterior talofibular ligament reconstruction on ankle kinematics, laxity, and in situ forces of the reconstructed graft. Foot Ankle Int. 2022;43:725–32. https://doi.org/10.1177/10711007211069327.
88. Hernigou P, Olejnik R, Safar A, Martinov S, Hernigou J, Ferre B. Digital twins, artificial intelligence, and machine learning technology to identify a real personalized motion axis of the tibiotalar joint for robotics in total ankle arthroplasty. Int Orthop. 2021;45:2209–17. https://doi.org/10.1007/s00264-021-05175-2.
89. Blaya JA, Herr H. Adaptive control of a variable-impedance ankle-foot orthosis to assist drop-foot gait. IEEE Trans Neural Syst Rehabil Eng. 2004;12:24–31. https://doi.org/10.1109/TNSRE.2003.823266.
90. Jamwal PK, Hussain S, Xie SQ. Three-stage design analysis and multicriteria optimization of a parallel ankle rehabilitation robot using genetic algorithm. IEEE Trans Autom Sci Eng. 2015;12:1433–46. https://doi.org/10.1109/TASE.2014.2331241.
91. Saglia JA, Tsagarakis NG, Dai JS, Caldwell DG. A high-performance redundantly actuated parallel mechanism for ankle rehabilitation. Int J Robot Res. 2009;28:1216–27. https://doi.org/10.1177/0278364909104221.
92. Hussain S, Jamwal PK, Ghayesh MH. State-of-the-art robotic devices for ankle rehabilitation: mechanism and control review. Proc Inst Mech Eng H. 2017;231:1224–34. https://doi.org/10.1177/0954411917737584.

Artificial Intelligence in Trauma Surgery

15

Corentin Pangaud and Matthieu Ollivier

Since the advent of modern orthopedic surgery, trauma surgeons have sought to predict the results of their unlucky patients. At first, the considerations about trauma surgery were mortality, complications, and functional results for single limb trauma care but also for severe polytraumatized patients. In 1974, the injury severity score (ISS) was published in the *Journal of Trauma*. Its aim is the triage of patients based on their short-term mortality risk considering the number and the localization of traumas on a single patient. In 1998, on behalf of the British Trauma Society, T. J. Coats mentioned the early stage of artificial intelligence (AI) using artificial neural network (ANN) to predict the outcome of trauma patients using the abbreviated injury score [1]. A total of 758 patients were included to train a model based on the mechanism of injury, the body region, age, blood pressure, and respiratory rate. The model was then tested on a new set of 300 patients and the area under the curve was recorded. These were the first public steps of AI in trauma care. We will see further in this book chapter that the reflection structure remains the same in all the recently published series: an algorithm is chosen, trained on a first set of patients, and then tested on another group of patients. The key performance indicators (KPI) are most of time: area under the curve, accuracy, sensibility, and specificity.

Artificial intelligence (AI) could be defined as a computer system being able to perform tasks requiring human intelligence. This includes visual perception, speech recognition, and decision making based on data analysis. All those various applications of AI involve different algorithms, which can all be included in the AI topic. The article of Farhadi et al. [2] published in 2022 in *Frontiers of Medical Technology* illustrates well the subsections of AI. Among the general population, the most used AI are the ones involved in relationships with humans: they are called natural language processing or large language model as ChatGpt®, Siri®, or Alexa®. In orthopedic surgery, and especially in trauma surgery, the main subsection will be machine learning.

Machine learning refers to computer systems that are made of algorithms and statistical models to analyze data that can learn from themselves. The subbranches of machine learning could be separated as "supervised algorithm" based on structured data with clear inputs and outputs chosen by humans and "unsupervised algorithm" where the AI is enabled to drive conclusions based on a dataset without human interference. Supervised algorithms are usually easier to understand and control for humans, but unsupervised algorithms are probably protected from human bias. The conventional algorithms used in

C. Pangaud (✉) · M. Ollivier
Institute of Locomotion, Hôpital Sainte Marguerite, Marseille, France

F. Familiari et al. (eds.), *Artificial Intelligence in Orthopaedic Surgery Made Easy*,
https://doi.org/10.1007/978-3-031-70310-2_15

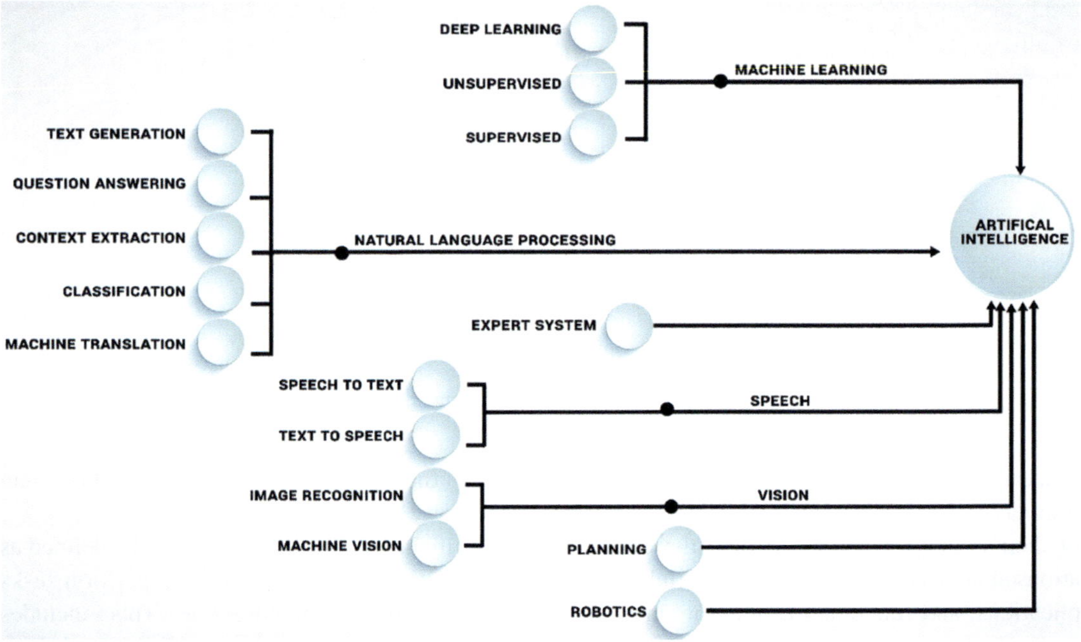

Fig. 15.1 Artificial intelligence as a global system of different algorithms (Farhadi et al. [2])

machine learning are "Decision Trees," "Random Forest," "Linear regression," and "Nearest Neighbors," Finally, "Deep Learning" is a sort of machine learning based on neural networks that permits the AI to analyze unstructured data such as texts, images, or sounds. The deep learning algorithms require multiple layers of neural networks to retrieve the data in the informatic content used as inputs (Fig. 15.1).

In this book chapter, we proposed to the reader to explore the different use cases of artificial intelligence in trauma surgery. Our plan will follow the pathway of a patient and his pathology through the healthcare system. The prediction of the risk of trauma will be the first to come, followed by the diagnosis of the pathology: clinical and image based. Then the surgical application of the recently developed algorithms will be described: surgical planning and enhanced surgical practice with robotics. A big thing in AI and trauma will be the prediction of the results after surgery and rehabilitation. We will finish this book chapter with the actual limitations of AI, a discussion about ethics, and finally some predictions for the future.

15.1 Artificial Intelligence and Prediction of the"Trauma Risk"

AI algorithms of machine learning enable clinicians to predict the risk of the occurrence of trauma. These could either occur in a young population of sports medicine patients or in a more elderly population due to osteoporosis. In order to calculate the risk of trauma, several risk factors should be included in the model. For osteoporosis, they could include gender, age, bone quality, and previous history of fracture. For the sports trauma, they would also include the training rhythm, the quality of the field, or the number of games in a championship.

Probably the first attempt to predict fracture using AI was performed by the Mayo Clinic team in 2012. Although they had a small population to train a machine learning algorithm, the concept was born. Four groups of patients were necessary for the study: 105 with forearm fracture compared to 99 without forearm fracture, 40 with vertebral deformity compared to 78 without vertebral fracture. Gradient boosting machine models were used, including age and bone density. The best results were obtained with an algorithm trained on the forearm fracture population and used on the vertebral fracture population to predict the risk of fracture: the area under the curve ranged from 0.82 to 0.95.

A paper published by Kruse et al. [3] in 2017 in *Osteoporosis International* depicts a use case of AI to predict the risk of fracture associated with osteoporosis in a female population. A total of 10, 775 women were included in the study based on the Danish National Patient Registry. The gathered data were age, Charlson's comorbidities score, bone mineral density based on dual energy X-ray absorptiometry, medication received, and the occurrence of osteoporotic fracture. An unsupervised algorithm of machine learning based on hierarchical agglomerative clustering (HAC) was then used on the database. It allowed to create nine clusters of risks of fracture based on a Z-score corresponding to a low, medium, or high risk of fracture (Fig. 15.2).

The same team published the results of 24 models of machine learning to predict fracture based on the Danish database [4]. The best models were "bagFDA" for bootstrap aggregated flexible discriminant analysis with an area under the curve of 0.92 (0.89–0.94) and "xgbTree" for eXtreme gradient boosting with AUC of 0.89 (0.82–0.95). These results are encouraging to use AI algorithm to help predict the risk of fracture in a population concerned by osteoporosis. They could help the clinicians decide whether to treat or not to prevent the next osteoporotic fracture as vertebral or femoral neck fracture.

In professional sports, athlete injuries are negative game changers among teams. When a key player is injured, it costs millions to the teams and could make a difference between losing or winning a championship. The risk factors of sports injury could be separated between internal risk factors and external risk factors. Internal risk factors are age, gender, BMI, previous history of injury, anatomy, skills level, and psychological factors. The external factors are the training pressure, protective equipment, sports equipment, the environment, and finally the game-playing situations [5].

A Spanish team reported an algorithm to predict the risk of ACL rupture [6]. Their model is based on the anatomical risk factors of ACL injury: tibial slope, meniscal height, and meniscal slope measured on MRI. Hundred patients were included: 50 ACL injury and 50 controls. The model reached 70% of validation accuracy and 92% of testing accuracy. The internal risk factors are mandatory to know which players are at risk of injury even though they are not changeable.

As mentioned previously, the external risk factors are key to prevent sports injury and luckily, they could be modified in the management of a team. The FC Barcelona Soccer Team created a forecasting model of sports injury based on GPS tracking of the players on the field [7]. Twenty-six professional players were used to train the model wearing a GPS tracker during training and games. The most important data were distance covered and acceleration. Twenty-three noncontact injuries we recorded during the study. A Decision Tree classifier algorithm was used. It was tested and the key values were: Recall 0.80 ± 0.07, F1 score 0.64 ± 0.1, and AUC 0.76 ± 0.12 in predicting the next injuries. A master risk factor of injury identified by the algorithm was the recent history of injury. This forecasting system could then be used to prevent the risk of trauma in professional athletes by identifying the players who are at risk and adapting their training workload and role on the field. Seen from the club's point of view this will help save money, players, and win championships!

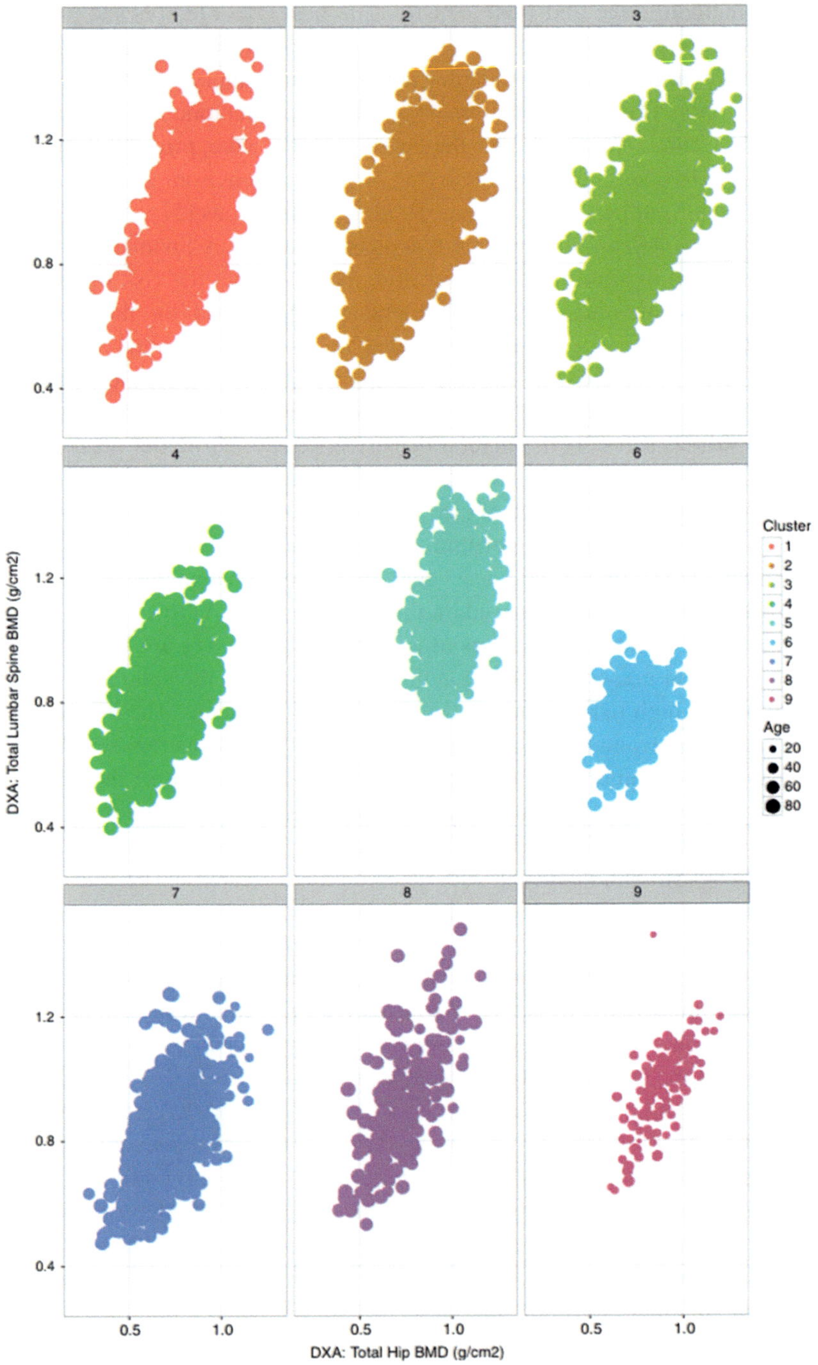

Fig. 15.2 Bone density in nine clusters of risk of osteoporotic fracture. Reproduced with permission from Kruse et al. [3]

15.2 Artificial Intelligence and Clinical Diagnosis

Bone fractures are most of the time easy to diagnose due to the major acute symptoms: recent history of trauma, noise of the bone breaking "crack," and pain-relieving posture. These suspected diagnostics are then confirmed by the X-ray. However, when it comes to sports trauma injury for example ACL injury, the clinical examination is mandatory to confirm the surgical indication. Frequently, the conclusion of the MRI will be "Partial tear of the ACL, needs to be undertaken by specialized orthopedic surgeon." The surgeon will then perform an anterior drawer test and pivot shift test to confirm knee instability and decide whether or not to perform surgery. These tests are not highly reliable according to the morphology of the patient and the experience of the surgeon. This is where AI could help us to be more accurate or deal with complex cases.

A Serbian team has created an algorithm based on linear regression to help the clinician diagnose ACL injury [8]. As we mentioned previously, the anterior translation and the rotational instability are key points in the diagnosis of ACL rupture. Thirty-five ACL-deficient patients were included in the study to undergo gait analysis measuring anterior tibial translation and rotational instability (Fig. 15.3). Three measures were done: the first before ACL reconstruction (ACLR), the second at 15 days after ACLR, and the last 6 weeks after ACLR (Fig. 15.4). The automated decision process was finally tested on three patients and compared to the clinician's opinion.

Another study was performed recently with new technologies of machine learning: Richter et al. [9] described in 2019 the use of machine learning based on gait analysis for knee instability diagnostic. Two groups of patients were included: 62 normal patients and 156 patients 9 months after ACLR. Seven exercises were done by the patients undergoing gait analysis: double leg countermovement jump, single leg jump, double leg drop jump, hurdle drop, single leg hop, planned change of direction, and unplanned change of direction. A matrix was generated including the seven exercises and three different ACL states: normal, ACL operated, and contralateral ACL operated. Eight models of machine learning were tested on the matrix: decision tree, ensemble of decision tree, discriminant analysis model, Naïve Bayesian classifier, nearest neighbor model, multi-class model for support vector machine, linear regression model, and a neural network. The study concluded that the best test to predict ACL instability was the double leg drop jump with an accuracy of 80% based on the neural network approach.

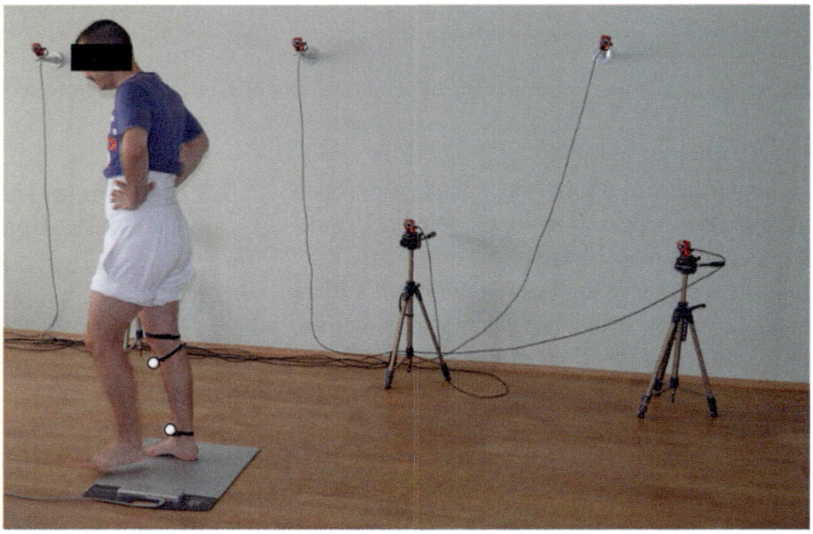

Fig. 15.3 Gait analysis before and after ACL reconstruction. Reproduced with permission from [8]

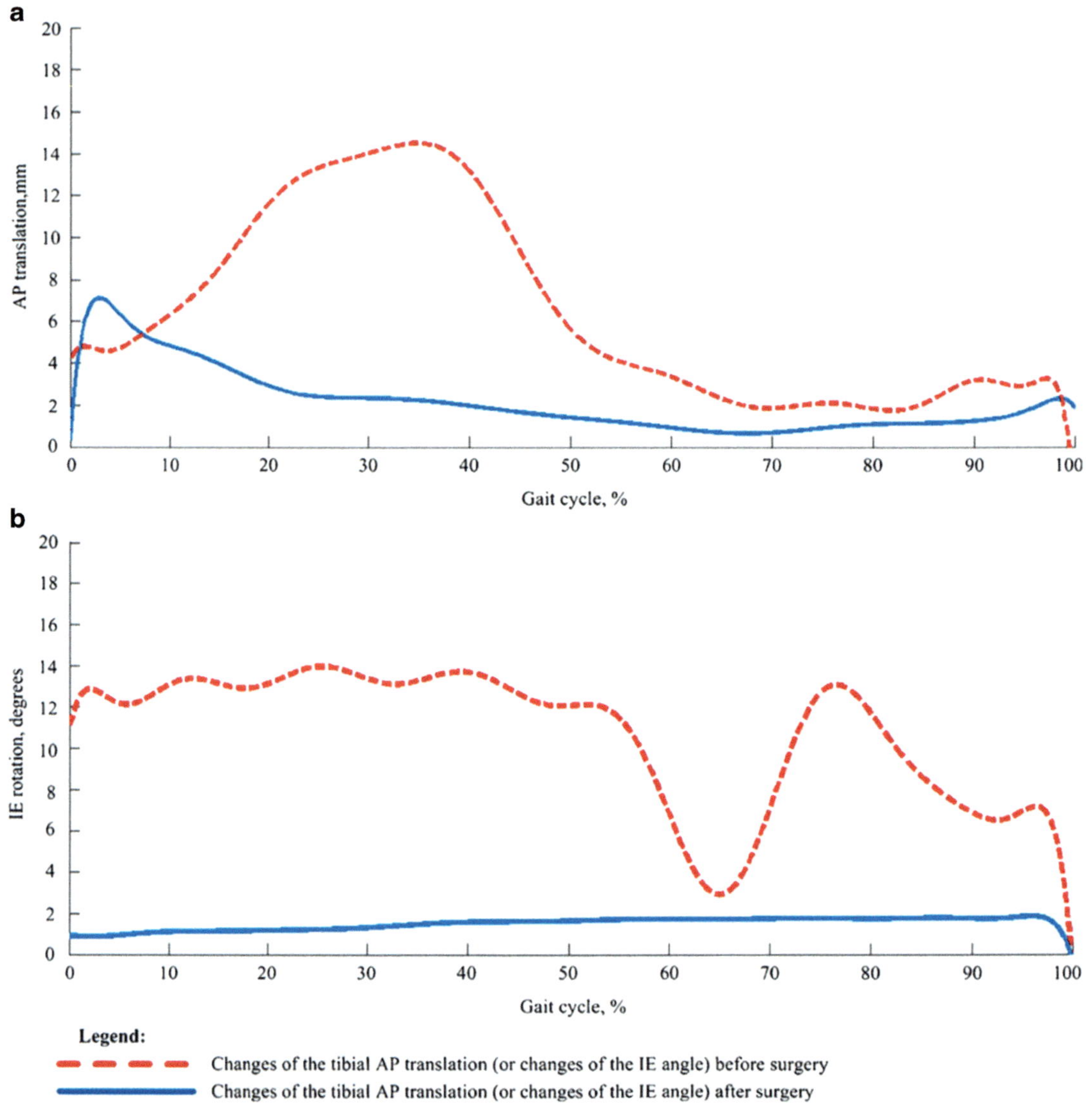

Fig. 15.4 Anterior translation and rotation before and after ACL reconstruction. Reproduced with permission from [8]

In the field of sports medicine trauma, new technologies appear to provide a reliable diagnosis of ACL-deficient knee based on gait analysis. Even though these applications are still experimental, we believe that one day every patient suffering ACL injury will undergo gait analysis with machine learning algorithm. These modern approaches could help the clinician by confirming the clinical diagnosis, deciding to perform the surgery, and evaluating the postoperative clinical results.

15.3 Artificial Intelligence and Medical Imaging

When it comes to trauma and artificial intelligence, the most advanced use cases are represented by medical imaging. Since 2014, large deep convolutional neural network has shown the ability to recognize images. These deep learning algorithms could treat unstructured data as text, sound, or images. In the case of trauma, identifying fractures on X-ray or CT scan not only

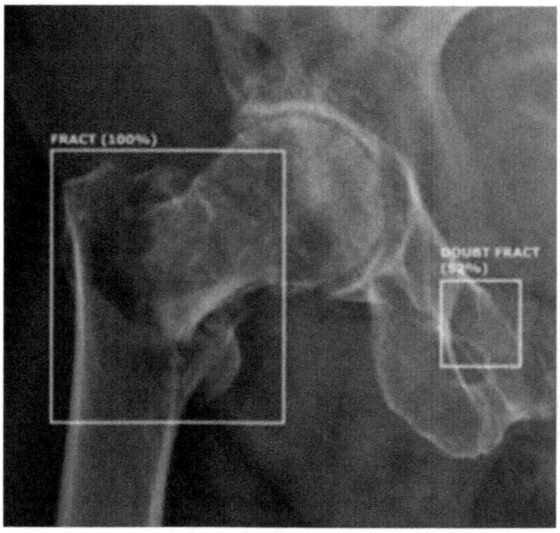

Fig. 15.5 Detection of pertrochanteric fracture by AI algorithm. Reproduced with permission from [8]

appears to be useful for the orthopedic surgeon but also for the emergency practitioner or residents.

Let us begin with X-rays, Hirschman et al. [10] published a literature review in 2019 in which they depict well the framework of deep learning for X-ray analysis. The AI feature used is the detection of abnormalities on images: the most common abnormalities will be fractures on X-ray with a trained algorithm based on normal X-ray databases (Fig. 15.5). Kriszhevsky et al. [11] reported a trained algorithm based on 1.2 million images from the ImageNet database.

The comparison of AI to orthopedic surgeons was done by Olczak et al. [12] in 2017. They included 256,458 X-rays of wrist, hand, and ankle. Five deep neural networks were trained and compared to orthopedic surgeons for the analysis of laterality, body part, exam view, and fracture detection. The 16-layers neural network called "VGG" performed best compared to the four others. The accuracy was 90% for body part and exam view while the accuracy for fracture detection was 83%. The fracture detection rate was similar to the two orthopedic surgeons compared to the algorithm.

The key performance indicators (KPI) of deep learning convolutional networks for fracture detection have been reported by Yang et al. [13] in 2020. They performed a meta-analysis of 17 studies, including 5, 434 images from various body part fractures. The average sensibility (Se) was 0.87, the average specificity (Sp) was 0.91, and the area under the curve (AUC) was 0.95.

The detection of fracture is mandatory to decide how the patient will be treated and complex fractures are usually classified to decide the treatment options. This is the case of periprosthetic fracture after hip or knee replacement. Alzaid et al. [14] trained five algorithms of deep learning to detect and classify the periprosthetic fracture based on the Vancouver classification (A, B, or C). This classification enables the surgeon to decide between three therapeutic options: orthopedic treatment and revision hip surgery of osteosynthesis. The database was made up of 1272 X-rays. The most powerful algorithm was called ResNet50; it provided 95% accuracy and an F1 score of 94% on fracture detection. The classification accuracy was 90% based on the Vancouver classification (Fig. 15.6).

The application of AI to detect fractures on X-rays appears to be useful for three main specialties of physicians: the radiologist, the emergency physician, and the orthopedic surgeon. The radiologists could reduce their time spent reading X-rays: Guermazi et al. [15] reported a reduction of 6.3 seconds per X-ray. The rate of missed fractures in the emergency could be reduced: in the same study, the sensibility gained 10% compared to the lecture on X-ray without AI by multiple physicians. Finally, the orthopedic surgeon will certainly be keen on classifying easily and rapidly the fracture before surgical treatment.

X-ray was a first step in the analysis of medical imaging as two-dimensional images were easier to treat. The next step of AI for medical imaging is the inclusion of three-dimensional images as CT scans. Hirschman et al. [10] depicted an improvement in the time of reconstruction for 3D images: sagittal, coronal, and axial. This is a time-consuming task usually done by a radio manipulator.

Al Helo et al. [16] described a computer-aided diagnosis system for vertebral compression fracture based on CT scan. Labeling and sequencing of the images were done with an active shape

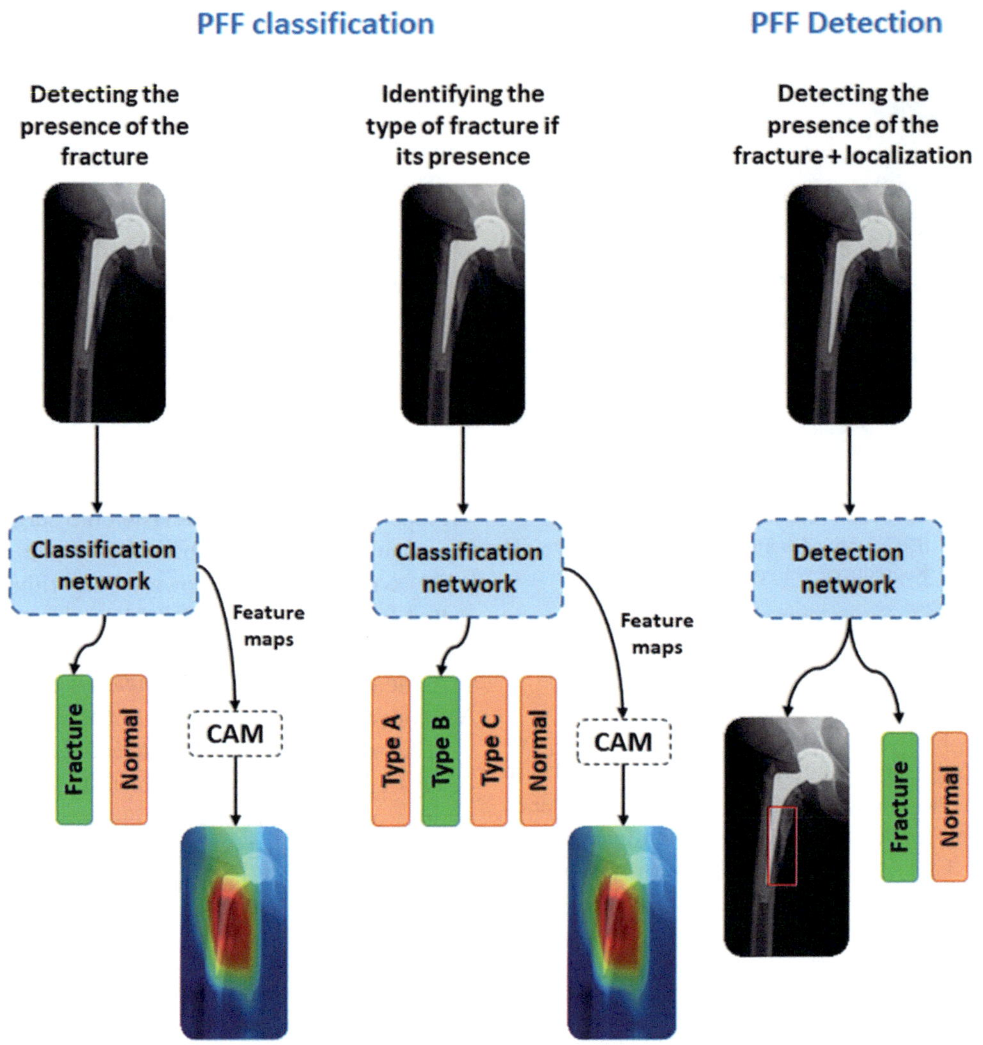

Fig. 15.6 Detection and classification of periprosthetic femoral fracture with the ResNet50 algorithm. Reproduced with permission from Alzaid et al. [14]

model and gradient vector flow active contour. Two deep learning algorithms were used: a neural network supervised learner and a K-means unsupervised learner. The algorithms were trained on 50 CT scans and the K-means learner provided 87.5% specificity and 99.0% sensibility.

In addition, the project of Alzaid et al. [14] of classifying periprosthetic femoral fracture, Aghnia Farda et al. [17] created an algorithm to analyze calcaneum fracture. The Sanders classification was chosen as it modifies the therapeutic decision. Only 14 patients were included in the database with calcaneum fracture. This resulted in a low accuracy classification system: 35%. An augmentation of the data was then performed using software to rotate, flip, and distort the images to provide better training to the neural network algorithm (Fig. 15.7). After improving the database, the accuracy of the neural network algorithm was 72% in classifying the calcaneum fracture. This value remains quite low compared to other applications, but it could probably be improved with a better database and increasing the number of layers of the algorithm.

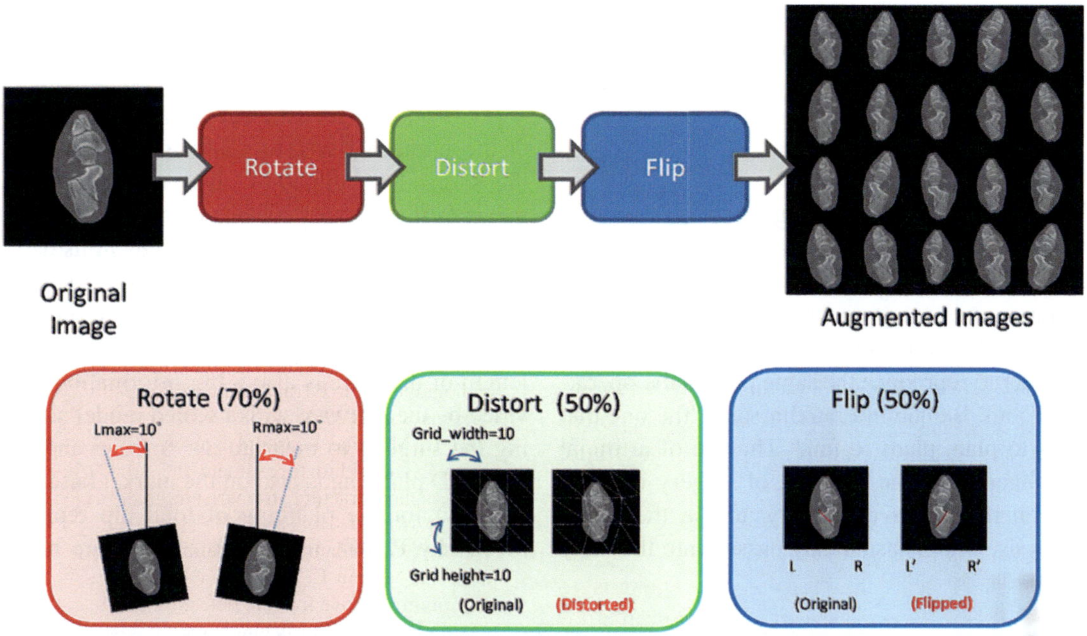

Fig. 15.7 Improving deep learning through the augmentation of image database. Reproduced with permission from Aghnia Farda et al. [17]

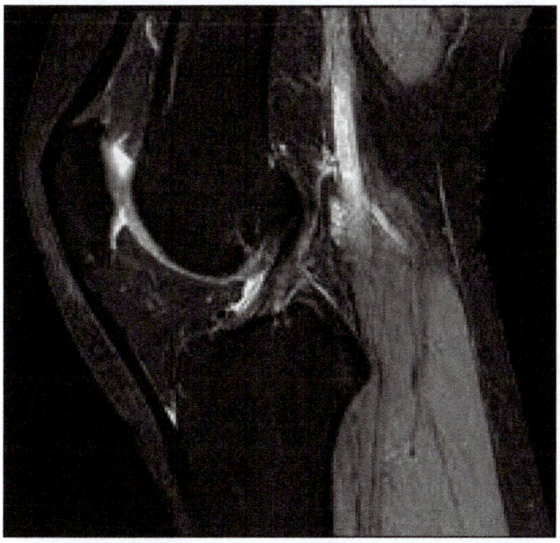

Fig. 15.8 Partial rupture of ACL on MRI. Reproduced with permission from Aghnia Farda et al. [17]

Another application of AI for three-dimensional imaging is the reading of MRI. MRIs are more used for sports trauma injuries such as ACL ruptures and meniscal tears (Fig. 15.8). A team from Stanford created a convolutional neural network called MRNet to read knee MRIs. It was trained on 1370 knee MRIs read by three musculoskeletal radiologists to establish a standard reference. The model was then tested on 120 exams to test its internal validation. The external validation was tested on 183 exams from a Croatian database. The area under the curve of the model was 0.937 (95% CI 0.895, 0.980) for detecting abnormalities, 0.965 (95% CI 0.938, 0.993) for ACL tears, and 0.847 (95% CI 0.780, 0.914) for meniscal tears. The radiologist had, however, better sensitivity for ACL ruptures and higher specificity for meniscal tears. Even though the radiologist still beats the AI in this study, the specificity of the radiologist was significantly increased when he used the AI before reading the MRI.

In the field of knee pathology and MRI, AI could have other use cases. Li et al. [18] proposed an algorithm to analyze the meniscus state: normal, torn, or degenerative. Chaudhari et al. [19] created an algorithm called DeepResolve to increase the resolution of knee MRI. Most of the time, a knee MRI is made of 25 slices of 2 to

3 mm, making it hard for the reader to see all the possible lesions. Their technique permits to generate thinner slices making the reading easier for the physician.

15.4 Artificial Intelligence and Surgical Planning

Planning a surgery consists of realizing all the steps of the future surgery, virtually or mentally in order to reproduce the same plan in the operating room. Benjamin Franklin said, "the one that fails to plan, plans to fail." The use of artificial intelligence for the planning of surgery is still a bet on the future of surgery, unlike the X-ray analysis, which has already passed into the daily habits of developed countries. However, several projects are on their way to spread AI and surgical planning (Fig. 15.9)

The software for surgical planning is already on the market and well used. TraumaCad® allows the surgeon to upload X-rays, select the fragments of the fracture, replace them, and fix them with various osteosynthesis materials in its database. The database of the trauma material includes nails and plates and permits the surgeon to choose the form tailored for the fracture. The length of the plate is also a big information provided by the software with a scaled model allowing the surgeon to measure the fracture and the plate. 3D planning is also on the market based on CT scan for the planning of total hip replacement, Hip-Plan®, for example. They are much

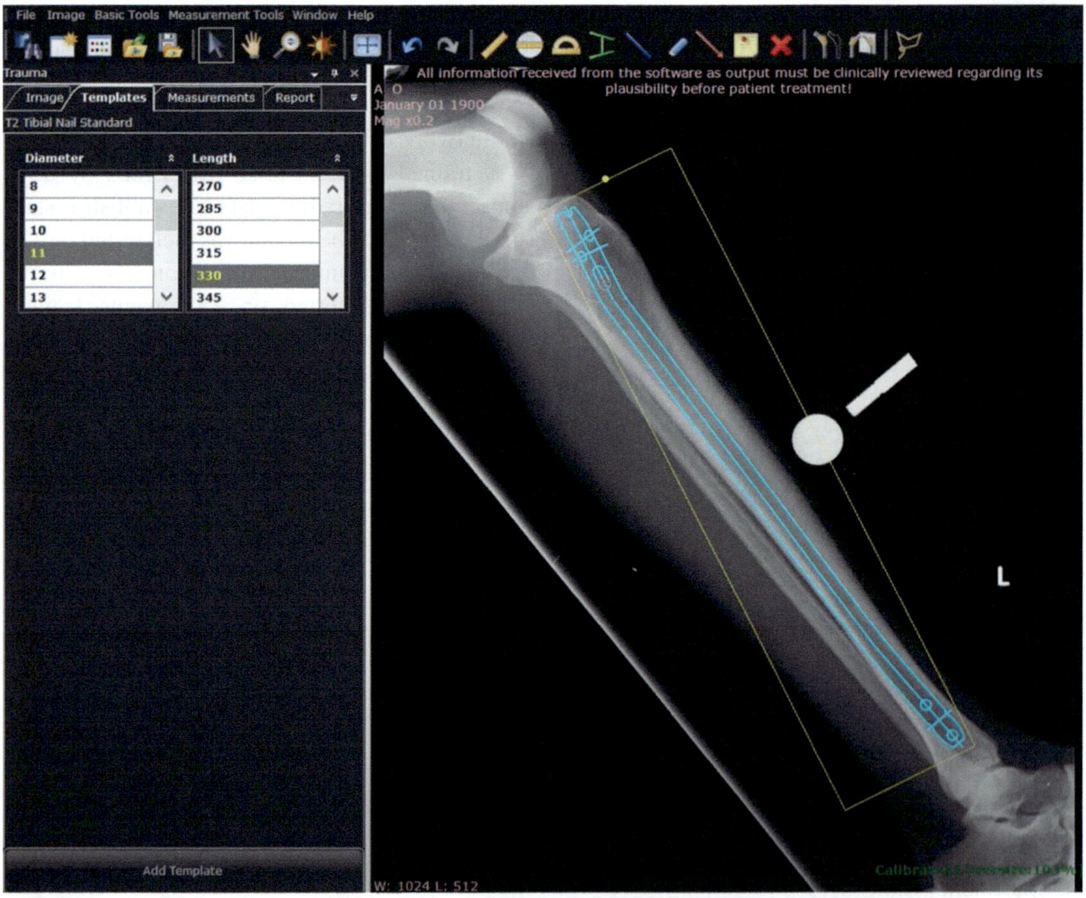

Fig. 15.9 Planning tibial osteosynthesis with nails using the software TraumaCad®. Reproduced with permission of BrainLab

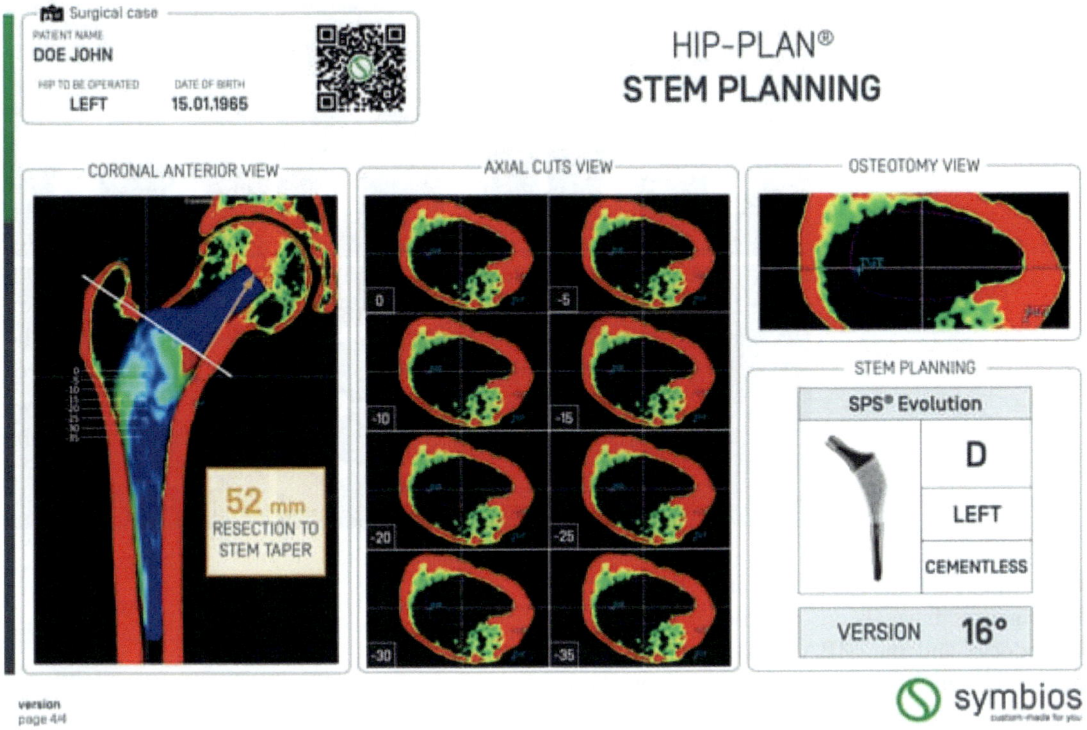

Fig. 15.10 3D planning of total hip replacement using the Hip-Plan software ®. Reproduced with permission of Symbios

more used for osteoarthritis, but they could also be used in trauma patients with femoral neck fractures undergoing total hip replacement or hemiarthroplasty. These software do not include AI for the moment and thus they still require human use. In near future, we could imagine an AI algorithm to run this software and do the planning itself (Fig. 15.10).

Baumann et al. [20] published in 2022 a model of surgical planning for pelvic fractures based on CT scan. The idea is to provide the surgeon with a 3D model of the fractured bone to allow safe sacroiliac screw placement. This is the first step of AI-assisted trauma surgery, through segmenting and modeling the bone for the surgery.

The timing between the injury and entering the operating room is also part of planning the surgery. This timing could induce complications if it is too long: skin suffering, osteonecrosis, or compartment syndrome. It could also cause other types of complications if it is too short: stiffness in ACLR or wound closing issues if the limb is too thick right after the trauma. Lu et al. [21] carried out a machine learning study of the influence of delayed ACL reconstruction on meniscus tears. The algorithm which was based on a random survival forest model identified the timing of surgery as a risk factor for meniscus tear due to instability. A delay superior to 50 days and a return to sports before 350 days appear to be risk factors for meniscal tear.

15.5 Enhancing Surgical Procedure with Artificial Intelligence

The place of artificial intelligence in the operating room is frequently associated with technologies like robotic surgery or navigation. The current trend in robotic surgery is more into haptic robotics and semi-autonomous systems that will increase the precision of the surgeon rather than replace him. However, some interesting

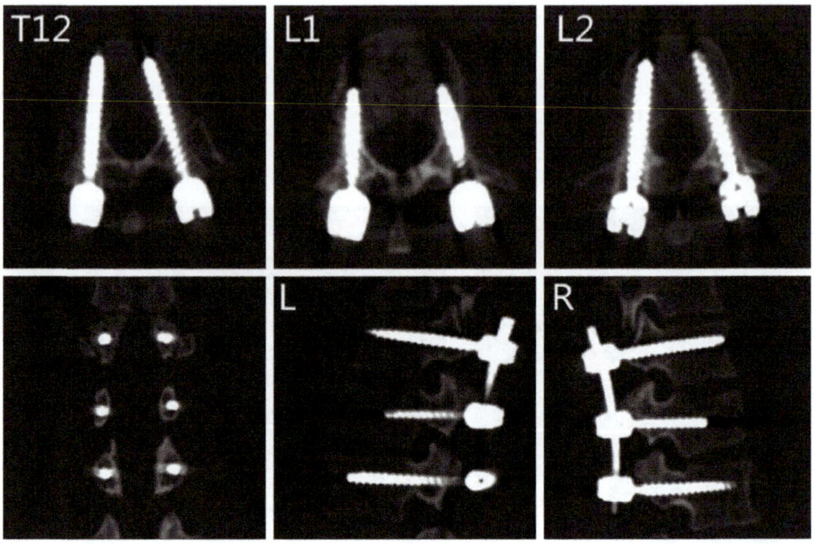

Fig. 15.11 Pedicle screw placement in spine surgery using the TiRobot system. Reproduced with permission from Tian et al. [22]

autonomous surgical robots trained by artificial intelligence have been on the market: The Robodoc® and the MBARS system® in 2005 and 2007. Due to the risk for the patient, these systems have been withdrawn from the market and left the place to the haptic systems. To enhance the surgical procedure of the trauma surgeon, artificial intelligence algorithms can be used to recognize anatomical structures for robots or increase precision placement of screws, especially in risky anatomical locations.

In 2017, Tian et al. reported a case report of pedicle screw placement using the TiRobot® from Tinavi Medical Technologies Co Ltd. The case was a burst fracture of L1 after a fall of 4 meters in a 28-year-old patient. Six screws were placed safely using the robotic system (Fig. 15.11). Two years later, Han et al. [23] realized a randomized control trial about the TiRobot® from Tinavi Medical. It is used to place pedicle screws in spine surgery based on CT scan and navigation. A total of 1116 pedicle screws were used in 234 patients separated into two groups: 119 patients in the free-hand group using fluoroscopy and 115 in the robot group. Screw placement was evaluated using the Gertzbein-Robbins scale. 95.3% of the screw placement was perfect in the robot group and 86.1% in the free-hand group. This makes us think that the precision of the trauma surgeon could be improved using AI algorithms through robotic surgery (Fig. 15.12)

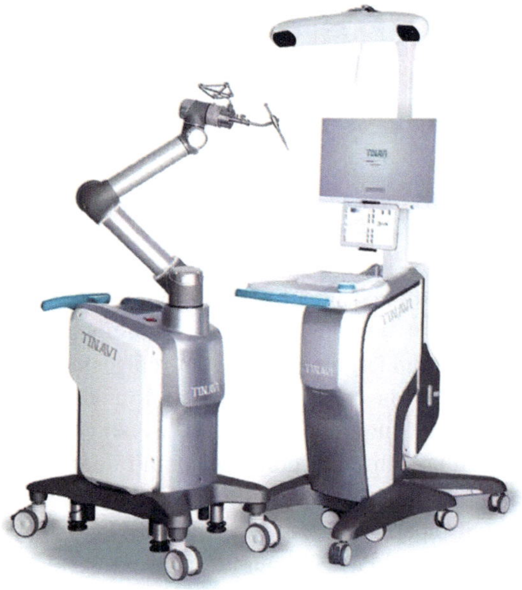

Fig. 15.12 TiRobot ® from Tinavi Medical, combining artificial intelligence and navigation for orthopedic surgery. Reproduced with permission of TinaVi

An experimental robotic system was proposed by Zhu et al. [24] for the temporary reduction of femur diaphyseal fracture during surgical fixation. The device is made of a pneumatic sleeve

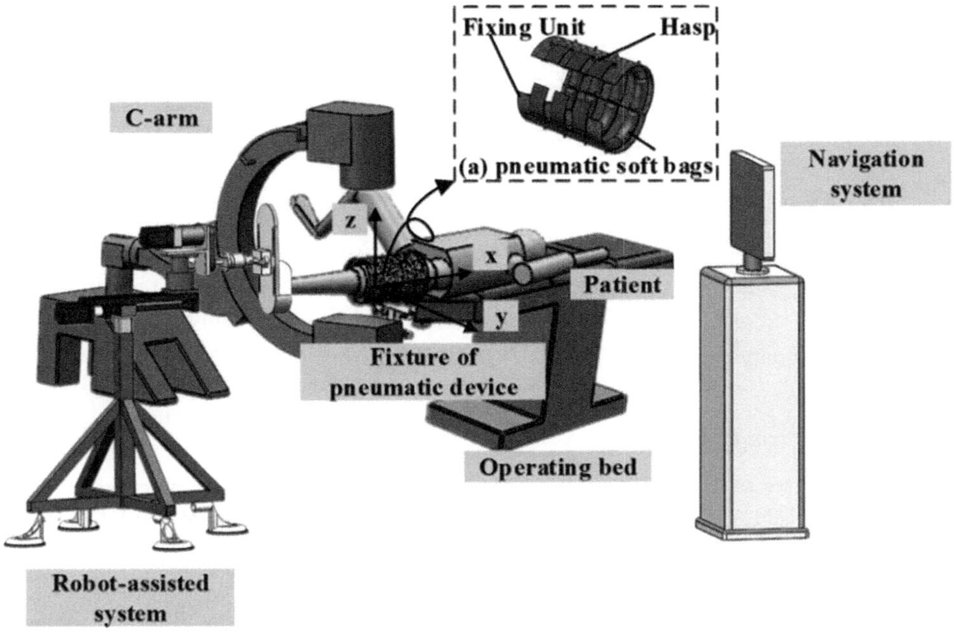

Fig. 15.13 Reduction device for femoral fracture. Reproduced with permission from Zhu et al. [25]

placed around the femur to move the part of the fractured bone and obtain reduction. It is connected to a fluoroscopic device to analyze the displacement of each fragment compared to the others. Based on this information, the device permits perfect reduction before nailing (Fig. 15.13).

Arthroscopy is more and more used in trauma surgery: tibial spine fixation, acromioclavicular disjunction, or distal radius fracture. Jonmohamadi et al. [25] proposed an algorithm of deep learning that recognizes anatomical structures on the screen of arthroscopy. A total of 3868 images of five knees based on a cadaver experiment were used to train the algorithm. A segmentation algorithm called U-Net++ was used to identify femur, tibia, ACL, and meniscus. The dice similarity coefficient for these structures was: 0.79 for the femur, 0.50 for the tibial, 0.51 for the ACL, and 0.48 for the meniscus. Although this technology has no real clinical application for the moment, two future applications appear logical. First controlling the correct placement during the reparation of an anatomical structure as the meniscal root of tibial spine avulsion. Second, training the robotic system to perform arthroscopic tasks under the control of the camera.

15.6 Predict the Results After Trauma Surgery

Since the emergence of evidence-based medicine, physicians of all specialties have sought to predict the results of their medical procedures. The main tool to predict the evolution of the patient was clinical scores. A good example is the injury severity score (ISS) published in 1974 to stratify the mortality risk of polytrauma patients. The ISS provides nine localizations of trauma (head, neck, spine, etc.) and six levels of severity (mild, severe, etc.), it is summarized on a scale ranging from 0 to 75. The score is correlated to mortality risk, morbidity, and length of stay for trauma patients. The logical evolution of these "old" scoring systems is to use artificial intelligence algorithms, including multiple KPI to predict the evolution of these severe trauma patients (Fig. 15.14).

Injury Severity Score (ISS)

Body Region
Head
Face
Neck
Thorax
Abdomen
Spine
Upper Extremity
Lower Extremity
External and other

Score	Abbreviated Injury Scale (AIS)
1	Minor
2	Moderate
3	Serious
4	Severe
5	Critical
6	Unsurviveable

All injuries are assigned from an internationally recognised dictionary that describes over 2000 injuries. Multiple injuries are scored by adding together the squares of the three highest AIS scores. The ISS can range from 1 to 75. Scores of 7 and 15 are unattainable because these figures cannot be obtained from summing squares. The maximum score is 75. By convention, a patient with an AIS of 6 in one body region is given an ISS of 75.

Fig. 15.14 Injury severity score. Reproduced with permission from Zhu et al. [24]

Ahmed et al. [26] present a deep neural network called "Deep-FLAIM" compared to multiple machine learning models: nearest neighbors, Gaussian Naïve Bayes, and linear discriminant analysis. A total of 3041 trauma patients admitted to the intensive care unit for trauma surgery were included in the dataset. The KPI associated with mortality were then identified: serum anion gap, sodium, chloride, sepsis, and systemic inflammatory response syndrome. The accuracy of the model was 92.25%, the sensitivity was 79.13%, and the specificity was 94.16%.

Cardosi et al. [27] also published an algorithm of deep learning based on a database of 2,007,485 patients to predict mortality in intensive care unit (ICU) patients. Their model included 77 variables, which is much more than the human brain could treat while deciding about one patient case. Other teams proposed to predict the length of stay based on the initial injury assessment. The multiplicity of these algorithms makes us think that they will soon be available for daily practice to predict the result of each patient entering the ICU for severe trauma.

In sports trauma surgery, already existing databases and registers make research easier in the field of artificial intelligence. For ACL reconstruction, the different outcomes to predict are ACL revision, functional results, stay overnight in case of outpatient surgery, and complications.

Martin et al. [28] published in 2022 a model of machine learning to predict ACL revision after ACLR. The model was created based on the Norwegian Knee Ligament Registry (NKLR) and tested on patients from the Danish Knee Ligament Registry to test its external validity. A total of 10,922 patients were included in the analysis. The average revision rate at 5 years of follow-up was 6.9%. The factors identified by the algorithm were graft choice, fixation device, KOOS score, years from injury to surgery, and age of the patient at surgery. The concordance of the model which corresponds to the accuracy was 0.68.

Predicting the functional outcomes of ACLR will be important for the surgeon to adapt the information given to the patients and decide whether to perform or not surgery. A team at the Hospital for Special Surgery (HSS) in New York created an algorithm whose purpose is to predict the non-achievement of minimal clinically important difference (MCID) after ACLR. A total of 442 patients were included and 39 (8.8%) did not achieve MCID. The identified risk factors by AI were BMI >27, medial collateral ligament (MCL) rupture, suspensory fixation for the femur, previous history of contralateral knee surgery, and preoperative flexion contracture.

Bone fractures are not the easiest field for predicting the results of the patients, but some teams have been working on the subject. An American military team has created an algorithm to predict the risk of amputation after calcaneus fracture due to combat injury [29]. One hundred and fifteen open wound fractures of calcaneus were included in the study with a rate of 44% of amputation. The most important factors in predicting amputation were: Gustilo-Anderson stage, plantar sensation, and associated vascular injury. The neural network evaluation showed a sensitivity of 64%, specificity of 91%, and AUC of 0.8 which was better than the logistic regression model. An Indian team created a fuzzy model based on finite element analysis to study bone healing in subtrochanteric fractures [30]. This model is a preclinical model to compare locking compression plates and dynamic compression plates. The inputs treated by the algorithm were blood perfusion bone concentration and distortional strain. The outputs were the changes in perfusion, cartilage concentration, and bone concentration.

These applications of artificial intelligence for severe trauma, sports injury, and bone fracture are still experimental but an application for daily practice might be coming soon. The surgeon could then fill in the information related to the patients in the algorithm corresponding to the pathology, which will provide the expected outcomes and recommend the best treatment option.

15.7 Artificial Intelligence and Rehabilitation

Orthopedic and trauma surgery requires most of the time rehabilitation after the surgery. Conventional rehabilitation is done by a physiotherapist at home or in his office two to three times a week for standard patients. During the COVID-19 pandemic, as patients were undergoing lockdown, a new era of rehabilitation came: patients were asked to watch videos and reproduce the movement to do their own rehabilitation. Some mobile apps have risen as Doct'Up®, MyMobility®, or Physiotrauma® to provide training programs for patients needing rehabilitation. Now that the pandemic is over, we realize that these tools will not replace physiotherapists but could significantly increase adherence to the self-rehabilitation program done in addition to the weekly session of physiotherapy.

Burns et al. [31] described an artificial intelligence tool to recognize the exercises of shoulder rehabilitation based on Apple Watch movement detection. The 20 patients undergoing rehabilitation for rotator cuff pathology were asked to do the 6 following exercises: pendulum, abduction, forward elevation, internal rotation, external rotation, and trapezius extension. A deep learning algorithm based on an activity recognition chain framework was used to identify the movement. Four common deep learning models were compared: k-nearest neighbors, random forest, support vector machine classifier, and convolutional recurrent neural network. The best model was the convolutional recurrent neuralnetwork, which provided 99.4% accuracy in recognizing the exercises.

Vélez-Guerrero et al. [32] published a literature review ranging from 2016 to 2020 concerning the use of exoskeletons for upper limb rehabilitation. Not many exoskeletons are used in daily routine for upper limb rehabilitation but lots of experiments have been done on this topic. Exoskeleton could be used for active and passive mobilization, increasing strength, and performing precise rehabilitation exercises. Furthermore, exoskeletons could be linked to AI algorithms that will enable them to learn and progress with the patients undergoing rehabilitation (Fig. 15.15).

In conclusion, artificial intelligence in the field of rehabilitation will probably be a new tool for the physiotherapist. The practitioner will be able to choose rehabilitation programs adapted to the patient's pathology and controlled by a camera or wearable device. The adherence to these programs might be improved because of their

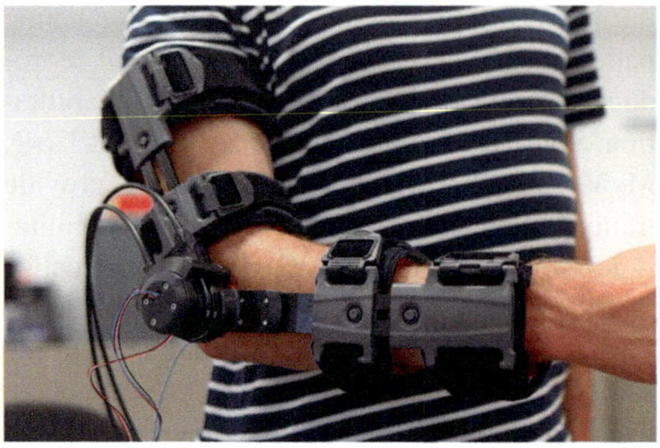

Fig. 15.15 Exoskeleton for upper limb rehabilitation

quality and interactivity. Concerning the hardware technology, the exoskeleton will surely be used in daily practice by the physiotherapist as a new tool for the recovery of joint range of motion.

15.8 Limitation of Artificial Intelligence

Artificial intelligence in trauma surgery appears to be already on the market for some applications and in its experimental way for other applications. It represents a huge progress in terms of efficiency and results prediction. However, some important limitation still exists and should be ruled out in the upcoming years.

The quality of the algorithm is not always sufficient to be used in clinical practice. Guy et al. [33], for example, reported an algorithm for fracture detection with a positive predictive value of 55%, which is not much more than flipping a coin. The key performance indicators of AI should then be carefully read before using an algorithm: sensitivity, specificity, accuracy, AUC, or F1 score. The accuracy of the deep learning algorithm is directly related to the quality of the database: too few entries or poor data quality will have consequences on the KPI of the AI. The results of internal and external validation permit the user to choose if the AI model is strong enough to be used in daily practice.

Another limitation of AI for its use in daily routine is the amount of time needed to produce and train the algorithm and the time needed to use it for every patient. The software used for X-ray analysis has mastered this issue, but this is not already the case for other applications of AI that require "user-friendly" software to gain efficiency. In the same objective to pass from experimental to daily tool, the lack of open-source algorithm is a hindrance to spreading them in other teams or other countries.

The last limitation of AI is common sense: AI algorithms need to be trained and then validated to produce good results and learn from themselves. However, AI does not have common sense and could drive foolish conclusions that would not have been made by humans. This should be understood by the users and the results provided by AI should be analyzed with critical sense. This explains why practitioners might still be reluctant to the daily use of AI when they have been facing mindless results with a previous algorithm. Furthermore, physicians are not always psychologically ready to accept their personal sensitivity and sensibility to be below the ones of an AI algorithm.

15.9 Regulation, Safety, and Ethics Around Artificial Intelligence

"With great power comes great responsibility," this famous sentence reminds us that while science progress, the new ethical debate should be done to push ahead in the right direction. The spread of AI in daily practice in all developed countries creates some new issues that should be taken into account.

As mentioned previously, the quality and the quantity of the data are mandatory to train effective algorithms. The way these data are collected must be carefully done with respect to general data protection regulation (GDPR) rules of the countries. Collection of the data must be done with the agreement of the patient and storage of these data must protect them against theft and public release. Lots of conflict of interest exists between the actors of healthcare involved in AI use: not only hospitals and insurance companies but also banks and pharmaceutical companies.

Anonymization is key to protect the patients who will give their personal information to train deep learning models.

The use of AI to decide the best treatment option for the patient implies some new ethical questions that the surgeon should be aware of. The first one is the question of responsibility in case of problem: "In case of failure, who will be responsible? The surgeon, the manufacturer, or the AI itself?". Another one is the question of treating a patient if AI predicts a 100% failure rate. We have depicted some algorithms to predict mortality after severe trauma: should a team try everything for a patient if AI predicts 100% mortality? Finally, some authors have mentioned the reimbursement of healthcare by public and private insurance. A model was created to predict the functional results of total knee arthroplasty and a new economic system was designed with proportional reimbursement of the procedure based upon AI prediction of results. No predicted improvement of the patient's health condition was associated with no reimbursement for the surgical procedure. The question is then: should the public insurance pay for healthcare if a deep learning algorithm predicts no benefits?

Obviously, these questions are new and without answers for the moment. These ethical considerations should be borne in mind while developing new AI models and spreading them across the world for daily practice.

15.10 Conclusion

In conclusion, artificial intelligence could be found in every step of the patient pathway in trauma surgery. In most of the fields, it is still experimental, whereas other applications have been spread and are used in daily practice. AI could help the surgeon predict osteoporotic fractures or sports trauma injuries. The most developed domain is radiology with algorithms to analyze X-rays and detect fractures, which are already used in emergency services. The place of AI in the operating room is still at the beginning stage and is most of the time related to robotic surgery. The prediction of results of severe trauma care, osteosynthesis, and ACL reconstruction have been widely studied and we could presume that clinical application will soon be available.

In the future, we believe that AI will not replace the surgeon, the radiologist, or the emergency practitioner. Instead, some time-consuming tasks might be done more efficiently, and some tasks might be done more accurately. It will improve diagnostic accuracy, realize some better predictions based on the patient's personal information, and perform highly precise surgery. One thing is undeniable, deep learning is starting a revolution in trauma surgery and it is time to get on board!

References

1. Coats TJ. Prediction of outcome following injury using an artifical neural network. Injury. 1998;29(2):163.
2. Farhadi F, Barnes MR, Sugito HR, Sin JM, Henderson ER, Levy JJ. Applications of artificial intelligence in orthopaedic surgery. Front Med Technol. 2022;4:995526.
3. Kruse C, Eiken P, Vestergaard P. Clinical fracture risk evaluated by hierarchical agglomerative clustering. Osteoporos Int. 2017;28(3):819–32.
4. Kruse C, Eiken P, Vestergaard P. Machine learning principles can improve hip fracture prediction. Calcif Tissue Int. 2017;100(4):348–60.
5. Bahr R, Krosshaug T. Understanding injury mechanisms: a key component of preventing injuries in sport. Br J Sports Med. 2005;39(6):324–9.
6. Tamimi I, Ballesteros J, Lara AP, Tat J, Alaqueel M, Schupbach J, et al. A prediction model for primary anterior cruciate ligament injury using artificial intelligence. Orthop J Sports Med. 2021;9(9):23259671211027544.
7. Rossi A, Pappalardo L, Cintia P, Iaia FM, Fernàndez J, Medina D. Effective injury forecasting in soccer with GPS training data and machine learning. PLoS One. 2018;13(7):e0201264.
8. Matić A, Petrović Savić S, Ristić B, Stevanović VB, Devedžić G. Infrared assessment of knee instability in ACL deficient patients. Int Orthop. 2016;40(2):385–91.
9. Richter C, King E, Strike S, Franklyn-Miller A. Objective classification and scoring of movement deficiencies in patients with anterior cruciate ligament reconstruction. PLoS One. 2019;14(7):e0206024.
10. Hirschmann A, Cyriac J, Stieltjes B, Kober T, Richiardi J, Omoumi P. Artificial intelligence in musculoskeletal imaging: review of current literature,

challenges, and trends. Semin Musculoskelet Radiol. 2019;23(3):304–11.
11. Krizhevsky A, Sutskever I, Hinton GE. ImageNet classification with deep convolutional neural networks. Commun ACM. 2017;60(6):84–90.
12. Olczak J, Fahlberg N, Maki A, Razavian AS, Jilert A, Stark A, et al. Artificial intelligence for analyzing orthopedic trauma radiographs. Acta Orthop. 2017;88(6):581–6.
13. Yang S, Yin B, Cao W, Feng C, Fan G, He S. Diagnostic accuracy of deep learning in orthopaedic fractures: a systematic review and meta-analysis. Clin Radiol. 2020;75(9):713.e17–28.
14. Alzaid A, Wignall A, Dogramadzi S, Pandit H, Xie SQ. Automatic detection and classification of periprosthetic femur fracture. Int J Comput Assist Radiol Surg. 2022;17(4):649–60.
15. Guermazi A, Tannoury C, Kompel AJ, Murakami AM, Ducarouge A, Gillibert A, et al. Improving radiographic fracture recognition performance and efficiency using artificial intelligence. Radiology. 2022;302(3):627–36.
16. Al-Helo S, Alomari RS, Ghosh S, Chaudhary V, Dhillon G, Al-Zoubi MB, et al. Compression fracture diagnosis in lumbar: a clinical CAD system. Int J Comput Assist Radiol Surg. 2013;8(3):461–9.
17. Aghnia Farda N, Lai JY, Wang JC, Lee PY, Liu JW, Hsieh IH. Sanders classification of calcaneal fractures in CT images with deep learning and differential data augmentation techniques. Injury. 2021;52(3):616–24.
18. Li J, Qian K, Liu J, Huang Z, Zhang Y, Zhao G, et al. Identification and diagnosis of meniscus tear by magnetic resonance imaging using a deep learning model. J Orthop Translat. 2022;34:91–101.
19. Chaudhari AS, Fang Z, Kogan F, Wood J, Stevens KJ, Gibbons EK, et al. Super-resolution musculoskeletal MRI using deep learning. Magn Reson Med. 2018;80(5):2139–54.
20. Baumann F, Becker C, Freigang V, Alt V. Imaging, post-processing and navigation: surgical applications in pelvic fracture treatment. Injury. 2022;53:S16–22.
21. Lu Y, Jurgensmeier K, Till SE, Reinholz A, Saris DBF, Camp CL, et al. Early ACLR and risk and timing of secondary meniscal injury compared with delayed ACLR or nonoperative treatment: a time-to-event analysis using machine learning. Am J Sports Med. 2022;50(13):3544–56.
22. Tian W, Fan MX, Liu YJ. Robot-assisted percutaneous pedicle screw placement using three-dimensional fluoroscopy: a preliminary clinical study. Chin Med J. 2017;130(13):1617–8.
23. Han X, Tian W, Liu Y, Liu B, He D, Sun Y, et al. Safety and accuracy of robot-assisted versus fluoroscopy-assisted pedicle screw insertion in thoracolumbar spinal surgery: a prospective randomized controlled trial. J Neurosurg Spine 2019;1–8.
24. Zhu Q, Liang B, Wang X, Sun X, Wang L. Minimally invasive treatment of displaced femoral shaft fractures with a teleoperated robot-assisted surgical system. Injury. 2017;48(10):2253–9.
25. Jonmohamadi Y, Takeda Y, Liu F, Sasazawa F, Maicas G, Crawford R, et al. Automatic segmentation of multiple structures in knee arthroscopy using deep learning. IEEE Access. 2020;8:51853–61.
26. Ahmed FS, Ali L, Joseph BA, Ikram A, Ul Mustafa R, Bukhari SAC. A statistically rigorous deep neural network approach to predict mortality in trauma patients admitted to the intensive care unit. J Trauma Acute Care Surg. 2020;89(4):736–42.
27. Cardosi JD, Shen H, Groner JI, Armstrong M, Xiang H. Machine learning for outcome predictions of patients with trauma during emergency department care. BMJ Health Care Inform. 2021;28(1):e100407.
28. Martin RK, Wastvedt S, Pareek A, Persson A, Visnes H, Fenstad AM, et al. Machine learning algorithm to predict anterior cruciate ligament revision demonstrates external validity. Knee Surg Sports Traumatol Arthrosc. 2022;30(2):368–75.
29. Bevevino AJ, Dickens JF, Potter BK, Dworak T, Gordon W, Forsberg JA. A model to predict limb salvage in severe combat-related open calcaneus fractures. Clin Orthop Relat Res. 2014;472(10):3002–9.
30. Nag P, Chanda S. A preclinical model of post-surgery secondary bone healing for subtrochanteric femoral fracture based on fuzzy interpretations. Tang Y, éditeur. PLoS One. 2022;17(7):e0271061.
31. Burns DM, Leung N, Hardisty M, Whyne CM, Henry P, McLachlin S. Shoulder physiotherapy exercise recognition: machine learning the inertial signals from a smartwatch. Physiol Meas. 2018;39(7):075007.
32. Vélez-Guerrero MA, Callejas-Cuervo M, Mazzoleni S. Artificial intelligence-based wearable robotic exoskeletons for upper limb rehabilitation: a review. Sensors (Basel). 2021;21(6):2146.
33. Guy S, Jacquet C, Tsenkoff D, Argenson JN, Ollivier M. Deep learning for the radiographic diagnosis of proximal femur fractures: limitations and programming issues. Orthop Traumatol Surg Res. 2021;107(2):102837.

16 Artificial Intelligence in Musculoskeletal Oncology

Raffaele Vitiello, Antonio Ziranu, and Giulio Maccauro

16.1 Introduction

In recent years, oncological orthopedics has witnessed a revolutionary transformation by integrating artificial Intelligence (AI) technologies [1, 2]. AI has been investigated for various applications, such as primary bone and soft-tissue cancer and metastatic disease [3]. In the last 20 years, the number of scientific papers on the subject has increased tenfold, with a constant increase until it became exponential about 10 years ago. This demonstrates the continuous interest of the scientific community in deepening the possible applications of this branch of research in the field of oncological orthopedics; it also illustrates how the knowledge learned in other areas of artificial intelligence is then rapidly applied to this specific branch of orthopedics and oncology, with growing interest year after year. This interest is fueled by the tangible results demonstrated by the various papers in the literature. In the face of this constant increase in scientific production and interest, unfortunately, at present, the practical applications of AI in clinical practice are very limited; as far as the authors know, a single automated bone scan index is the only technology based on the study of images in musculoskeletal oncology to have been used in clinical practice since 2021. In any case, it is software not based on the most recent technologies in AI fields [3].

Regarding the different AI technologies used in orthopedic oncology, the subfield of machine learning (ML), which enables machines to learn from data and make informed decisions without explicit programming, is undoubtedly one of the most used in this field. A subset of ML, deep learning (DL), has shown exceptional promise in solving complex problems by simulating the human brain's neural networks.

In this chapter, we will explore the applications of AI, ML, DL, and others in oncological orthopedics, focusing on their potential to revolutionize radiology, histology, molecular biology, and various other aspects of clinical practice.

16.2 Radiology

Radiological imaging plays a crucial role in diagnosing and staging musculoskeletal tumors. If it is true that the interpretation of radiological images does not allow a definitive diagnosis, it is undoubtedly true that radiology can firmly guide a diagnosis of musculoskeletal cancer; this type of diagnosis turns out to be quite complex for general radiologists and an erroneous or unacknowledged diagnosis can lead to adverse out-

R. Vitiello (✉) · A. Ziranu · G. Maccauro
Fondazione Policlinico Universitario Agostino Gemelli IRCCS, Rome, Italy

Università Cattolica del Sacro Cuore, Rome, Italy
e-mail: raffaele.vitiello@policlinicogemelli.it; antonio.ziranu@policlinicogemelli.it; giulio.maccauro@policlinicogemelli.it

F. Familiari et al. (eds.), *Artificial Intelligence in Orthopaedic Surgery Made Easy*,
https://doi.org/10.1007/978-3-031-70310-2_16

comes for the patient [4, 5]. AI-powered algorithms have shown remarkable potential in revolutionizing this field.

16.2.1 Lesions Detection

Numerous studies have focused on applying AI to enhance the ability to detect cancerous lesions in radiographic, tomographic, or magnetic resonance images or nuclear medicine. Furthermore, the AI was then trained to differentiate benign from malignant lesions.

He et al. have developed a neural network model capable of analyzing standard radiographs by classifying the lesion present in benign, intermediate, or malignant with a high level of performance testified by an accuracy of 72.1%, which increases to 91% by dividing the lesions only into benign or malignant [4]. These levels are usually achieved only by subject matter-trained radiologists. The validity of this application was then confirmed by the study by Liu et al., who showed results in line with the previous ones, reaching levels of accuracy comparable to those of an expert radiologist [6].

Other AI models were instead trained to differentiate healthy radiographs from others that showed skeletal lesions. In the study by Park et al., which focused on lesions of the proximal femur, the students created a model of a convolutional neuronal network capable of differentiating normal radiographs from pathological ones; moreover, the AI demonstrated through a gradient-weighted class action mapping (Grad-CAM) analysis to be able to accurately define the exact location of the skeletal lesion [7].

In addition to traditional radiology, several papers have focused on using AI to data from CT or MRI. Yin and colleagues demonstrated how AI could help distinguish primary lesions of the sacrum, especially sacral chordomas, from giant cell tumors based on CT images [8]. Instead, Leporq and colleagues demonstrate that radiomics allows for predicting malignancy in soft-tissue lipomatous tumors with routinely used MR acquisition in clinical oncology [9]. Other studies have instead focused on differentiating benign bone lesions from secondary lesions with convincing results, demonstrating better results than those obtained by a radiologist, not an expert in the musculoskeletal field [10].

Nuclear medicine represents one of the fields of radiology that are most often used in the diagnosis and monitoring of secondary skeletal lesions [11]; AI is mainly used to automate the calculation of the bone scan index (BSI), which represents a scoring system that allows quantifying the percentage of bone affected by a metastasis [12–14]; usually, the BSI requires manual or partially automatic procedures by healthcare professionals, AI allows this process to be speeded up and has allowed the marketing of the first technology for clinical use since 2021 [3]. Other algorithms have instead been developed to facilitate the efficacy of bone metastasis detection on bone scintigraphy [15], with good results and a negative predictive value reaching 96.5%.

Finally, some papers have focused on the ultrasound study of benign and malignant soft-tissue lesions, demonstrating that AI can distinguish between benign and malignant soft-tissue tumors [16, 17].

16.2.2 Pathological Fractures

In clinical practice, the Mirels' Classification and its revisions allow the evaluate the risk of pathological fracture or impending fracture [18, 19]. Pathological fractures or impending are critical events for the cancer patient as they are linked to adverse outcomes and deterioration of general conditions or the impossibility of further accessing cancer treatment [20]. Therefore, early treatment of these fractures is essential.

Interestingly, the Mirels score mainly considers objective parameters such as the anatomical region, the local extension, and the radiological characteristics of the secondary lesion. These characteristics make AI helpful in framing this type of injury to predict fracture risk. Unfortunately, at the moment, only one paper has concentrated in this direction [21]. Still, this chapter of oncological orthopedics will likely face a progressive increase in the future.

16.3 Pathology

16.3.1 Histopathology

Histopathological evaluation is fundamental in confirming the diagnosis and guiding treatment decisions in orthopedic oncology. The integration of AI in histopathology has significantly improved the accuracy and efficiency of tumor classification. Machine learning models can analyze digitized histological slides and identify specific cellular and tissue patterns associated with different tumor types [22], particularly in bone marrow aspirates. This expedites the diagnostic process and reduces the chances of misdiagnosis, enabling oncologists to devise optimal treatment strategies for patients. In primary bone tumors, AI has been mainly used to distinguish pathological tissue from necrotic tissue in the histopathology of osteosarcoma, fundamental data for evaluating the therapeutic response [23, 24]. Finally, some studies are trying to link histological data with the possibility of predicting responses to treatments through the use of AI [25].

16.3.2 Molecular Biology

Molecular profiling has become essential in understanding tumor biology and tailoring targeted therapies. AI-driven algorithms can analyze extensive genomic and proteomic datasets to identify genetic mutations and alterations that drive tumor growth. Through pattern recognition and predictive modeling, AI can predict treatment responses and patient outcomes based on molecular profiles, enabling personalized treatment approaches. In particular, the DL has been used to study the association between lncRNAs and the prognosis of patients affected by osteosarcoma [26]. Non-DL methods have also been used to identify and characterize miRNA-based molecular subtypes of osteosarcoma or the expression of molecules related to chemoresistance in osteosarcoma [27, 28]. Other studies have also analyzed gene expression in other tumor forms, such as Ewing's sarcoma or liposarcoma [29, 30]. This integration of AI in molecular biology empowers clinicians with invaluable insights into tumor behavior and therapeutic opportunities.

16.4 Clinical Outcomes and Research

AI has many applications in orthopedic oncology beyond radiology, histology, and molecular biology. Natural language processing algorithms can extract valuable information from unstructured clinical notes, aiding data integration and research. AI can facilitate precision medicine by matching patients to clinical trials based on their unique molecular profiles. The most frequent application of AI in this field is undoubtedly the prediction of survival of patients affected by metastatic bone disease or primary bone and soft-tissue cancers [31–34]. These studies make the use of AI promising in the field of orthopedic oncologists, also predicting in some cases not only the survival but also the local response to radiation treatments or the risk of local recurrence following surgery [35, 36]. At the moment, the clinical applications of AI in orthopedic oncology are not yet clearly established as the literature is recent and limited, but we are sure that with the exponential increase in the use of these methods, it will be possible to obtain brilliant results, especially in the personalization of treatments and in personalizing follow-up (creating specific patient risk classes with detailed postoperative monitoring).

16.5 Limitation

Despite its immense potential, AI in orthopedic oncology faces certain limitations. First of all, there are limitations related to the nature of AI. Overfitting, a common challenge in machine learning, occurs when an AI model becomes too specialized in the training data and performs poorly on new data. Deep learning models' "black-box" nature hinders interpretability, making it challenging to understand the decision-making process. Furthermore, AIs need large databases of patients to be adequately trained and validated and to guarantee repeatability in similar populations but coming from different databases, databases that are currently unavailable.Moreover, in segmentation tasks, AI may need help delineating tumor boundaries accurately and need support from healthcare professionals. Second, the quality of the current scientific literature on the uses of AI in oncological orthopedics could be better [37]; there needs to be more homogeneity in a field in which the histological nature of tumors is already highly vast. Finally, most of the studies focus on the application of AI in a specific area (for example, the prognosis of the oncological patient or the evaluation of skeletal lesions). They are not instead dedicated to a fusion of radiological and clinical data to create a more complete and totalistic assessment of the patient.

16.6 Future Perspectives

The future of AI in orthopedic oncology holds tremendous promise. Techniques like transfer learning and ensemble models must be explored to overcome overfitting, and large databases are needed. Efforts to enhance the interpretability of AI models will be crucial in gaining clinicians' trust and acceptance.

In the short term, the fastest application of AI will be their introduction into clinical practice in non-interpretive tasks, thus ensuring a streamlining of work times, especially in the radiological field. AIs have been demonstrated to identify skeletal oncological lesions superior to those of a nonexpert radiologist and almost comparable to an expert one [3, 6]; this will impact the reduction of radiological work times and could have evident repercussions both in university and non-university centers. In university hospitals, AI could be used in residency programs to train medical staff; instead, in suburban hospitals, not equipped with expert radiologists in musculoskeletal oncology, AI could support diagnoses and avoid flooding in specialized structures.

In the more distant future, when the overfitting problem is solved and we will have more extensive databases available to train the AIs adequately, it will be possible to use them more routinely and helpfully in clinical practice. It will be possible to use AIs in interpretive tasks, favoring diagnoses that are not necessarily binary (cancer/healthy) but also managing to suggest more specific histological diagnoses (tumor histotypes, in case of secondary lesions, which are primary ones). Finally, by merging clinical data with laboratory and radiological data, AIs can build prediction models capable of allowing personalized medicine, both in terms of the type of treatment and follow-up that will be studied on the risks of recurrence or the molecular resistances of the patient's cancer. AIs could help draft and optimize current guidelines. Integrating AI into clinical practice could lead to more precise diagnoses, personalized treatment strategies, and improved patient outcomes, revolutionizing the landscape of orthopedic oncology.

References

1. Topol EJ. High-performance medicine: the convergence of human and artificial intelligence. Nat Med. 2019;25:44–56.
2. Farhadi F, Barnes MR, Sugito HR, Sin JM, Henderson ER, Levy JJ. Applications of artificial intelligence in orthopaedic surgery. Front Med Technol. 2022;4:995526.
3. Li MD, Ahmed SR, Choy E, Lozano-Calderon SA, Kalpathy-Cramer J, Chang CY. Artificial intelligence applied to musculoskeletal oncology: a systematic review. Skeletal Radiol. 2022;51:245–56.
4. He Y, Pan I, Bao B, et al. Deep learning-based classification of primary bone tumors on radiographs: a preliminary study. EBioMedicine. 2020;62:103121.
5. Howe BM, Broski SM, Littrell LA, Pepin KM, Wenger DE. Quantitative musculoskeletal tumor imaging. Semin Musculoskelet Radiol. 2020;24:428–40.
6. Liu R, Pan D, Xu Y, et al. A deep learning-machine learning fusion approach for the classification of benign, malignant, and intermediate bone tumors. Eur Radiol. 2022;32:1371–83.
7. Park C-W, Oh S-J, Kim K-S, Jang M-C, Kim IS, Lee Y-K, Chung MJ, Cho BH, Seo S-W. Artificial intelligence-based classification of bone tumors in the proximal femur on plain radiographs: system development and validation. PLoS One. 2022;17:e0264140.

8. Yin P, Mao N, Zhao C, Wu J, Sun C, Chen L, Hong N. Comparison of radiomics machine-learning classifiers and feature selection for differentiation of sacral chordoma and sacral giant cell tumour based on 3D computed tomography features. Eur Radiol. 2019;29:1841–7.
9. Leporq B, Bouhamama A, Pilleul F, Lame F, Bihane C, Sdika M, Blay J-Y, Beuf O. MRI-based radiomics to predict lipomatous soft tissue tumors malignancy: a pilot study. Cancer Imaging. 2020;20:78.
10. Hong JH, Jung J-Y, Jo A, Nam Y, Pak S, Lee S-Y, Park H, Lee SE, Kim S. Development and validation of a radiomics model for differentiating bone islands and osteoblastic bone metastases at abdominal CT. Radiology. 2021;299:626–32.
11. Isaac A, Dalili D, Dalili D, Weber M-A. State-of-the-art imaging for diagnosis of metastatic bone disease. Radiologe. 2020;60:1–16.
12. Xu L, Tetteh G, Lipkova J, Zhao Y, Li H, Christ P, Piraud M, Buck A, Shi K, Menze BH. Automated whole-body bone lesion detection for multiple myeloma on 68Ga-pentixafor PET/CT imaging using deep learning methods. Contrast Media Mol Imaging. 2018;2018:2391925.
13. Zhao Y, Gafita A, Tetteh G, Haupt F, Afshar-Oromieh A, Menze B, Eiber M, Rominger A, Shi K. Deep neural network for automatic characterization of lesions on 68Ga-PSMA PET/CT images. Annu Int Conf IEEE Eng Med Biol Soc. 2019;2019:951–4.
14. Moreau N, Rousseau C, Fourcade C, et al. Deep learning approaches for bone and bone lesion segmentation on 18FDG PET/CT imaging in the context of metastatic breast cancer. Annu Int Conf IEEE Eng Med Biol Soc. 2020;2020:1532–5.
15. Hsieh T-C, Liao C-W, Lai Y-C, Law K-M, Chan P-K, Kao C-H. Detection of bone metastases on bone scans through image classification with contrastive learning. J Pers Med. 2021;11:1248.
16. Chen C-Y, Chiou H-J, Chou S-Y, Chiou S-Y, Wang H-K, Chou Y-H, Chiang HK. Computer-aided diagnosis of soft-tissue tumors using sonographic morphologic and texture features. Acad Radiol. 2009;16:1531–8.
17. Wang B, Perronne L, Burke C, Adler RS. Artificial intelligence for classification of soft-tissue masses at US. Radiol Artif Intell. 2021;3:e200125.
18. Mirels H (2003) Metastatic disease in long bones: a proposed scoring system for diagnosing impending pathologic fractures. 1989. Clin Orthop Relat Res. S4–13.
19. Hoban KA, Downie S, Adamson DJA, MacLean JG, Cool P, Jariwala AC. Mirels' score for upper limb metastatic lesions: do we need a different cutoff for recommending prophylactic fixation? JSES Int. 2022;6:675–81.
20. Piccioli A, Spinelli MS, Maccauro G. Impending fracture: a difficult diagnosis. Injury. 2014;45(Suppl 6):S138–41.
21. Oh E, Seo SW, Yoon YC, Kim DW, Kwon S, Yoon S. Prediction of pathologic femoral fractures in patients with lung cancer using machine learning algorithms: comparison of computed tomography-based radiological features with clinical features versus without clinical features. J Orthop Surg (Hong Kong). 2017;25:2309499017716243.
22. Mori J, Kaji S, Kawai H, et al. Assessment of dysplasia in bone marrow smear with convolutional neural network. Sci Rep. 2020;10:14734.
23. Arunachalam HB, Mishra R, Daescu O, Cederberg K, Rakheja D, Sengupta A, Leonard D, Hallac R, Leavey P. Viable and necrotic tumor assessment from whole slide images of osteosarcoma using machine-learning and deep-learning models. PLoS One. 2019;14:e0210706.
24. Mishra R, Daescu O, Leavey P, Rakheja D, Sengupta A. Convolutional neural network for histopathological analysis of osteosarcoma. J Comput Biol. 2018;25:313–25.
25. Chaber R, Arthur CJ, Łach K, Raciborska A, Michalak E, Bilska K, Drabko K, Depciuch J, Kaznowska E, Cebulski J. Predicting ewing sarcoma treatment outcome using infrared spectroscopy and machine learning. Molecules. 2019;24:1075.
26. Xuan P, Pan S, Zhang T, Liu Y, Sun H. Graph convolutional network and convolutional neural network based method for predicting lncRNA-disease associations. Cells. 2019;8:1012.
27. Hill KE, Kelly AD, Kuijjer ML, et al. An imprinted non-coding genomic cluster at 14q32 defines clinically relevant molecular subtypes in osteosarcoma across multiple independent datasets. J Hematol Oncol. 2017;10:107.
28. Zhu K-P, Zhang C-L, Ma X-L, Hu J-P, Cai T, Zhang L. Analyzing the Interactions of mRNAs and ncRNAs to predict competing endogenous RNA networks in osteosarcoma chemo-resistance. Mol Ther. 2019;27:518–30.
29. Ren E-H, Deng Y-J, Yuan W-H, Wu Z-L, Zhang G-Z, Xie Q-Q. An immune-related gene signature for determining Ewing sarcoma prognosis based on machine learning. J Cancer Res Clin Oncol. 2021;147:153–65.
30. Liu J, Li R, Liao X, Jiang W. Comprehensive bioinformatic analysis genes associated to the prognosis of liposarcoma. Med Sci Monit. 2018;24:7329–39.
31. Huang R, Xian S, Shi T, Yan P, Hu P, Yin H, Meng T, Huang Z. Evaluating and predicting the probability of death in patients with non-metastatic osteosarcoma: a population-based study. Med Sci Monit. 2019;25:4675–90.
32. Yan P, Huang R, Hu P, Liu F, Zhu X, Hu P, Yin H, Zhang J, Meng T, Huang Z. Nomograms for predicting the overall and cause-specific survival in patients with malignant peripheral nerve sheath tumor: a population-based study. J Neuro-Oncol. 2019;143:495–503.
33. Thio QCBS, Karhade AV, Ogink PT, Raskin KA, De Amorim BK, Lozano Calderon SA, Schwab JH. Can machine-learning techniques be used for 5-year survival prediction of patients with chondrosarcoma? Clin Orthop Relat Res. 2018;476:2040–8.

34. Kamalapathy PN, Ramkumar DB, Karhade AV, Kelly S, Raskin K, Schwab J, Lozano-Calderón S. Development of machine learning model algorithm for prediction of 5-year soft tissue myxoid liposarcoma survival. J Surg Oncol. 2021;123:1610–7.
35. He Y, Guo J, Ding X, van Ooijen PMA, Zhang Y, Chen A, Oudkerk M, Xie X. Convolutional neural network to predict the local recurrence of giant cell tumor of bone after curettage based on pre-surgery magnetic resonance images. Eur Radiol. 2019;29:5441–51.
36. Gao Y, Kalbasi A, Hsu W, et al. Treatment effect prediction for sarcoma patients treated with preoperative radiotherapy using radiomics features from longitudinal diffusion-weighted MRIs. Phys Med Biol. 2020;65:175006.
37. Lacroix M, Aouad T, Feydy J, Biau D, Larousserie F, Fournier L, Feydy A. Artificial intelligence in musculoskeletal oncology imaging: a critical review of current applications. Diagn Interv Imaging. 2023;104:18–23.

Artificial Intelligence in Spine Surgery

17

Lukas Jud, Mazda Farshad, José Miguel Spirig, Jonas Widmer, Reto Sutter, and Philipp Fürnstahl

17.1 Introduction

During the last decade, great efforts have been made to implement artificial intelligence (AI) into medicine. Increasing computational power, affordability of these resources as well as the availability of large data sets have allowed developing various applications of AI in spine care and especially in spine surgery. The number of preclinical and clinical publications related to AI in spine surgery has grown exponentially during the last years. Therefore, we found it important to summarize the current achievements of AI in spine surgery from a clinical perspective. In this chapter, we highlight the current use of AI in spine surgery, which can be subdivided into preoperative, intraoperative, and postoperative field.

In the preoperative field, AI has already been applied in diagnostics such as automated recognition of spinal pathologies, prediction of their individual course or progression, patient-specific treatment selection, and preoperative planning of spinal surgeries. Its future potential seems to be even much bigger. A major aim of using AI preoperatively will be treatment outcome prediction to facilitate clinicians' decision making. Through access to large multicenter databases such as national and international registries, it is possible to optimize the training of AI models and accelerate their development.

In the intraoperative field, AI has already been recognized as a powerful tool for surgical navigation. Since the introduction of tracking systems in the 1990s, marker-based surgical navigation and surgical robotics have made only slow progress without breakthrough innovations. This trend has changed noticeably since the advent of AI in the operating room. AI paved the way for camera-based tracking of anatomy and tools eliminating the need for fiducial markers. New

L. Jud
Department of Orthopedics, Balgrist University Hospital, University of Zurich, Zürich, Switzerland
e-mail: lukas.jud@balgrist.ch

M. Farshad (✉)
Department of Orthopedics, Balgrist University Hospital, University of Zurich, Zürich, Switzerland

Department of Spine Surgery, Balgrist University Hospital, University of Zurich, Zürich, Switzerland
e-mail: mazda.farshad@balgrist.ch

J. M. Spirig
Department of Spine Surgery, Balgrist University Hospital, University of Zurich, Zürich, Switzerland
e-mail: jose.spirig@balgrist.ch

J. Widmer
Spine Biomechanics, Balgrist University Hospital, University of Zurich, Zürich, Switzerland
e-mail: jonas.widmer@balgrist.ch

R. Sutter
Department of Radiology, Balgrist University Hospital, University of Zurich, Zürich, Switzerland
e-mail: reto.sutter@balgrist.ch

P. Fürnstahl
Research in Orthopedic Computer Science, Balgrist University Hospital, University of Zurich, Zürich, Switzerland
e-mail: philipp.fuernstahl@balgrist.ch

F. Familiari et al. (eds.), *Artificial Intelligence in Orthopaedic Surgery Made Easy*,
https://doi.org/10.1007/978-3-031-70310-2_17

AI-driven surgeon-enhancing technologies have found their way into patient care, such as the FDA-approved head-mounted display from Augmedics (Chicago, Illinois, USA) for augmented reality (AR) mediated spinal navigation. Robotic spine surgery is another area that has been shaped by AI, resulting in systems with greater autonomy and efficiency. Recent research has also shown that AI can lead to entirely new approaches to computer-assisted surgery based on the fusion of sensor and image data. Overall, the intraoperative use of AI in spine surgery has the potential to improve the prevention of surgical complications, facilitate intraoperative processes and decision making, and standardize surgical steps while not disturbing the workflow of a surgeon.

In the postoperative phase, AI has been used in several studies to predict surgical outcomes. This could eventually guide postoperative care and monitoring of high-risk patients to prevent or early detect complications or neurological deterioration. Overall, AI has the capability to process large datasets and capture nonlinear relationships in a very short time compared to traditional statistical models. This has the potential to accelerate research and to analyze unsolved scientific problems in a different way.

In summary, AI offers a wide variety of new possibilities and findings that aim to enable clinicians to provide personalized treatment and counseling based on a patient's individual profile, clinical presentation, and prognosis. However, a healthy skepticism of AI in spine surgery while having the willingness to appreciate this new promising technology is needed in the future of spine surgery.

17.2 Preoperative Role of AI in Spine Surgery

The main applications of AI in the preoperative context can be subdivided into diagnoses of pathological changes affecting the spine and treatment planning in dependence on outcome prediction.

17.2.1 Diagnostics

Automated detection of degenerative changes or traumatic injuries is attainable from images of different modalities, such as magnetic resonance imaging (MRI), computed tomography (CT), and standard radiographs. For example, the generation of high-quality MR images based on low-resolution images could allow for improved radiographic analysis while limiting hardware requirements and patient discomfort. CT images are of major importance in both diagnostics and surgical planning. A major concern associated with CT acquisition is the considerable radiation exposure for the patient. AI-based generation of pseudo-CT images from MRI scans or the enhancement of low-dose CT scans through denoising could therefore contribute to limiting radiation exposure. Further, radiological assessments of degeneration, deformation, and traumatic tissue damage can be very demanding, and intra-observer and inter-observer agreements are often limited [1, 2]. Computer-aided diagnosis (CAD) systems might provide fast screening and less time-pressure-induced errors; thanks to AI support in diagnosis [3].

Already more than 10 years ago, the number of reports on machine learning (ML)-based diagnosis of disk degeneration or lesion from features observable on midsagittal MR images (after automatized labeling and segmentation) started to rapidly increase. The achievable accuracy in diagnosing disk degeneration surpassed 90% and the first deep learning (DL) approach for grading intervertebral discs achieved a specificity of 96% and a sensitivity of 87% [4, 5]. Subsequent work focused on transitioning from the prediction of a merely binary outcome (healthy/degenerated) to ordinal gradings like the one introduced by Pfirrmann et al., and the size of datasets used for training and testing was increased [1]. Various convolutional neural networks (CNN) architectures relying on sagittal T2-weighted MRI scans have demonstrated the ability to classify pathologies other than disk degeneration and herniation, such as stenosis, endplate defects, and spondylolisthesis [6, 7].

Algorithms trained to detect anomalies in the vertebral bone were trained on both CTs and MRIs. A neural network (NN)-based approach to detect low bone density from thoracic spine segmentation of chest CT scans was successfully developed, while fractures in the posterior vertebra could be determined with an area under the curve (AUC) of up to 0.86 through a CT-trained CNN [8, 9]. Also, MRI images have been used for a similar purpose, as was showcased by a network developed to detect vertebral compression fractures (including the assessment if they were benign or malign), achieving an average AUC of 0.98 [10]. Recently, a deep convolutional neural network (DCNN) was established for morphologic measurements of vertebral bodies and the detection of vertebral insufficiency fractures [11]. In clinical routine MRI, the shape of the vertebral body and a possible vertebral height loss are often not evaluated with enough detail, resulting in an underreporting of vertebral insufficiency fractures: The DCNN helps to increase diagnostic accuracy for fracture detection in routine MR imaging of the lumbar spine.

Other AI-based tools aim at assessing the spinal alignment, enabling automated measurements of spinopelvic parameters and lordosis from spine radiographs [12, 13]. Scoliosis curve type and severity were classified with an accuracy of up to 86% with support vector machines or decision trees based on trunk topology to avoid the use of X-ray imaging [14]. More recently, a CNN approach was able to successfully identify relevant structures on radiographs and from that compute coronal alignment parameters relevant for scoliosis diagnosis [15].

17.2.2 Planning Considering Predicted Outcome

The complexity of spine surgery makes accurate preoperative planning necessary to ensure successful outcomes. AI has therefore emerged as a valuable approach to improve a variety of aspects related to spine surgery to maximize patient satisfaction and efficiency. A considerable number of publications focused on the automatized labeling and segmentation of anatomical structures from clinical images with AI algorithms [16–18]. Both, soft tissues (intervertebral discs, muscles, neural structures, and facets) and vertebral bone can be segmented and labeled with varying degrees of accuracy depending on the tissue, image modality, and degree of degeneration/deformation. The most commonly used imaging modality for three-dimensional (3D) planning in spine surgery is CT, delivering a high-resolution depiction of osseous structures. The depiction of the bone with a high spatial resolution is crucial for the production of patient-specific cutting guides, which fit exactly to the osseous surface of a specific vertebral body. However, CT is only acquired in a subset of patients prior to spine surgery. Most patients undergo MRIs ahead of planned spinal surgery to assess pathologies of the vertebral bodies and also the pathologies of the intervertebral discs as well as compression of nerve roots. The majority of clinical MR sequences have a high in-plane resolution, but a limited through-plane resolution, because of slice thickness of 3 or 4 mm of standard turbo-spin echo sequences. The low through-plane resolution does not allow for generating detailed 3D models directly from the images. There are, however, image segmentation DL algorithms to extract high-resolution anatomical models from clinical two-dimensional (2D) MRI with thick slices [18]. To establish the algorithm, the detailed information available in 3D CT images in patients that underwent both, CT and MRI, was used to generate highly detailed shape priors that complemented missing information in 2D acquisitions of clinical MRI. With this approach, advanced DL algorithms were able to segment MRI of the lumbar spine for achieving a high-resolution 3D model of the vertebral bodies, which in the future can be used for 3D surgical planning. An alternative method for achieving high-resolution 3D models of bone is the use of MRI-based synthetic CT [19], which in the past has been mainly applied for guiding radiation therapy and attenuation correction for positron emission tomography-magnetic resonance imag-

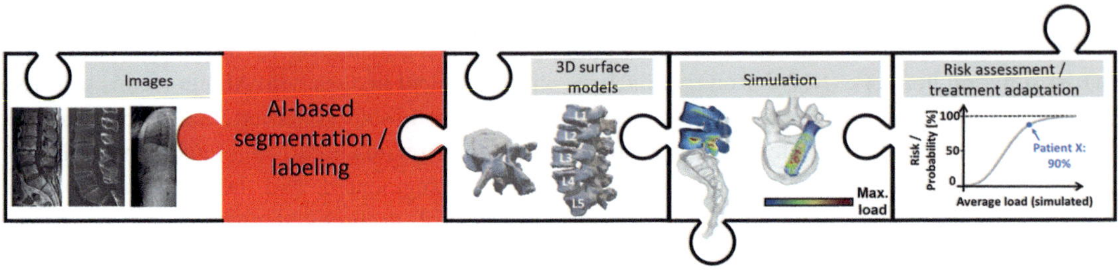

Fig. 17.1 Workflow using timesaving artificial intelligence-based algorithms

ing (PET/MRI) [20, 21]. These synthetic CT data are generated, e.g., from 3D T1-weighted radio-frequency spoiled multiple gradient-echo sequences, followed by a transformation into CT-like data with a DL-based technology based on the U-net architecture. This technology is commercially available and is now being used for planning spine surgery, but can also replace CT for diagnostic purposes [22, 23]. The surface 3D models obtained through automatized segmentation are not only relevant for the diagnosis of pathologies and direct utilization in surgical planning but can also be essential for the efficient generation of individualized biomechanical models. The latter might in turn be used to predict short-term and long-term surgical outcomes or pathology progression and therefore provide additional information to optimize surgical planning and treatment [24–26]. Avoiding manual segmentation and labeling of anatomical structures of the spine would considerably shorten the overall time-consuming task of individualized model generation and could be a major driver for the incorporation of biomechanical analysis in the clinical workflow (Fig. 17.1). Computational models (e.g., finite element and musculoskeletal models) simulating load and stress distribution in spinous biological tissues and implants can potentially also be used to generate large datasets of subject-specific or parameterized simulation results. The outcome can then be used to train predictive AI models, which can facilitate the introduction of relevant biomechanical information for preoperative planning.

Finally, AI can be used to plan surgical implant positioning. For example, decision trees were used to predict (AUC = 1.0) the biomechanical holding strength (in an experimental ex vivo setting) of pedicle screws in vertebral bone based on screw position and vertebral "bone" density [27]. Planning of pedicle screw placement after vertebral segmentation and landmark detection through NN were possible resulting in barely any pedicle breach [28, 29]. Such implant position outcomes can be used with intraoperative navigation systems to reduce surgery time and improve accuracy.

17.3 Intraoperative Role of AI in Spine Surgery

A particular goal of state-of-the-art research in surgical navigation is to replace marker-based tracking systems for anatomy tracking and instrument localization with camera-based 6 degrees-of-freedom (DoF) position estimation. To this end, depth-sensing hardware such as stereoscopic cameras, structured light systems, or time-of-flight approaches, are employed in combination with AI-powered 3D reconstruction engines capable of generating a 3D representation of the surgery. One commercial system of this kind was introduced by 7D Surgery Inc. (Toronto, ON, Canada) to provide radiation-free navigation of pedicle screw placement [30]. It features a lamp-integrated structured light system that allows the registration of a preoperatively obtained 3D surgery plan to the intraoperative anatomy. Anatomy tracking (for motion compensation) and tool localization (for surgical guidance) still relied on fiducial markers, since the registration process takes up to 20 s. In order to move toward completely marker-free navigation of spine surgeries, a major research initiative has been launched, called SURGENT, which stands for surgeon-enhancing technology (https://www.hochschulmedizin.uzh.ch/de/projekte/surgent.html). Within SURGENT, a fully fletched AR and AI navigation solution for pedicle screw placement and rod implant bending was developed. The core of the pedicle screw placement was based on an approach of Liebmann et al. [31] who proposed real-time generated 3D depth maps as the input of a deep learning pipeline for automatic vertebra-wise registration with continuous pose updates. The first stage of the pipeline relies on a segmentation network, which identifies and masks the visible bone surface in the depth map, and a regression network estimating the pose of the lumbar spine. In the second stage, the preoperatively obtained 3D surgery plan is aligned according to the predicted pose and registered 3D point cloud obtained from the masked depth maps. The validation on ex vivo data demonstrated 96% successful registrations on average, a median target registration error of 2.73 mm, a median screw trajectory error of 1.79°, and a median screw entry point error of 2.43 mm. The navigation of pedicle screw placement was complemented by a rod bending navigation approach of von Atzigen et al. [32]. The bending of rod implants is traditionally a tedious, time-consuming, and manual task that greatly benefits from the recent advances of ML. Von Atzigen et al. developed a dedicated neural network in which images of the front-facing environmental cameras of AR head-mounted devices were used to reconstruct the 3D position of the screw heads directly in the surgery. The target rod shape is calculated based on the screw positions from which a step-by-step visualization is presented as an overlay on top of the surgical bending bench to guide surgeons through the bending procedure. This approach not only displays the intended final outcome but also guides the user in effectively manipulating the tool to achieve the desired result. The integration of ML and AR has led to a considerable reduction in surgery time of more than 33%, along with a decreased need for rebending maneuvers that are often associated with inadequately contoured rods.

Given that patient registration can be seen as a main bottleneck associated with the existing surgical navigation solutions, an emerging trend for registration-free navigation alternatives using AI can be observed in recent years. In the realm of spine surgery, these registration-free surgical navigation solutions mainly operate based on sparse intraoperative data (i.e., intraoperative fluoroscopy and ultrasound) to provide up-to-date spatial feedback during the intervention without requiring preoperative imaging data or surgery plans. To that effect, more recent algorithms deliver the promise of registration-free surgical navigation through end-to-end trained convolutional neural networks capable of providing a highly accurate intraoperative 3D reconstruction of the patient's anatomy only from a few fluoroscopy shots. A pioneer in this field of spine surgery is X23D, which is the first work toward intraoperative spinal shape reconstruction based on sparse multi-view X-ray data [33]. To train X23D, a large number of digitally reconstructed radiographs (DRRs) were generated based on a finite number of patient CTs providing an annotated training dataset that consists of the input (sparse DRR images) and the associated targets (the underlying CT volume). Once trained, the authors showed that the X23D model could reconstruct an unseen patient's spine with an 88% average F1 score (Fig. 17.2).

An excellent example to showcase the impact of AI on robotic spine surgery is the European Union's Horizon 2020 research initiative functionally accurate robotic spine surgery (FAROS, https://h2020faros.eu/). FAROS develops new ways to embed physical intelligence in surgical robotics. Specifically, it constructs a functional representation of the surgical task by fusing non-visual sensing data, which is interpreted by AI to control the robotic execution (Fig. 17.3). In this context, vibroacoustic sensing has great potential to capture valuable additional information while being a noninvasive, radiation-free, and easy-to-integrate modality. The structure-borne sound generated during tissue manipulation can thereby be captured by contact microphones and evaluated to distinguish tissue structures or adverse events, such as a pedicle breach during drilling.

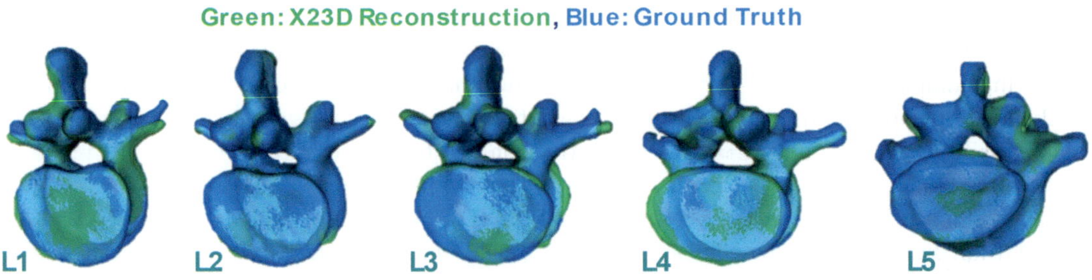

Fig. 17.2 Comparing the reconstructions achieved based on four input X-rays versus a full-resolution CT scan

Fig. 17.3 The robotic prototype of FAROS combines nonvisual sensing capabilities with artificial intelligence

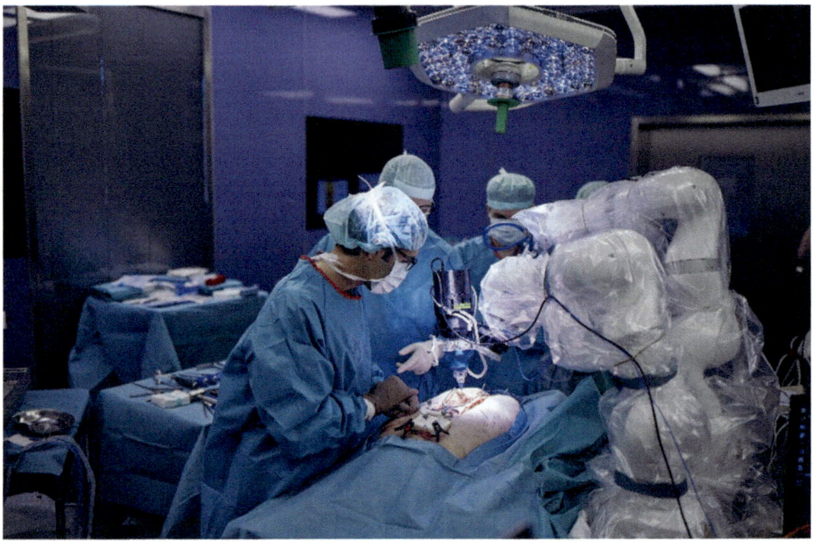

The key idea of the AI-based sensing approach of Massalimova et al. [34] was the use of Mel-Spectrograms as an image representation of acoustic signals allowing to leverage powerful CNN for detecting drill breach events. The network was trained using data from ex vivo experiments in which controlled breaches were generated along with drillings of ideal pedicle trajectories. The best-performing model used a combination of multiple sensors to achieve a breach detection rate of 98%.

A general challenge in developing intraoperative AI is the collection of large amounts of surgical training datasets, which is inherently more difficult than in the preoperative setting. Possible remedies in this regard are approaches for the generation of and augmentation by synthetic data. Hein et al. [35] showed that DL-based tool tracking purely trained on 38 k photo-realistic renderings achieved an accuracy of 2.7 mm on real data for estimating the position of a surgical drill. In the future, synthetic data generation methods should be extended to other modalities, such as vibroacoustic data. Initial promising work in this direction has shown the great potential of generative models for the synthetic generation of clinical audio data [36].

17.4 Postoperative Role of AI in Spine Surgery

Treatment expectations are a major topic of interest in daily practice of spinal surgery. From patients' point of view, it is essential to get detailed information on possible prospects to give informed consent on treatment, whereas from the surgeons' point of view, it is crucial to calculate realistic postoperative scenarios to tailor the individual offered treatments. However, due to the complexity of spinal disorders, it can be challenging to predict the actual postoperative course for every individual patient, as it depends on a wide variety of patient factors that can be difficult to take all into account in treatment planning. So far, counseling of patients is based on experience-gained knowledge and by using scientific data. However, despite broad experience and the great availability of high-level scientific evidence, this knowledge occasionally does not match the actual situation for every individual patient and therefore it still remains a major challenge to give patients a concise perspective on their situation. In these cases, AI potentially comes into play. This technology allows to process big datasets and also includes nonlinear relationships, in contrast to traditional statistical models. The superiority of ML techniques over traditional statistical models has already been recognized in the literature [37]. It offers the potential for automated processing of patient data, tailoring individual treatment strategies, and advising patients more accurately regarding their treatment expectations.

One of the most common spinal surgeries is spinal fusion, an intervention for a wide variety of spinal disorders. However, when it comes to spinal fusion, patients need to be informed about adjacent segment degeneration. Nearly 50% of patients develop radiographic signs of adjacent segment degeneration 5 years after anterior cervical discectomy and fusion (ACDF) [38]. Nevertheless, it is a major challenge to predict if a patient falls into one or the other group, and it would be favorable to have a more specific system for advising patients. Therefore, Rudisill et al. [39] developed an ML algorithm to predict early onset adjacent segment degeneration in patients undergoing ACDF. Their algorithm showed an overall good performance with an AUC of 0.794. Their predictive model identified C4/5 anterior and posterior disk bulge, C6/7 anterior disk bulge, C6 posterior superior osteophyte, and the presence of osteophytes as the most important risk factors for early onset adjacent segment degeneration. In some countries, it has become popular to perform ACDF in the ambulatory setting instead of in-patient stay. However, as complications in that kind of surgery can be life-threatening, it is necessary to properly screen patients for their suitability for ambulatory surgery. A possible tool to group patients as "safe" or "unsafe" for ambulatory surgery is the American Society of Anesthesiologists classification. However, Wang et al. [40] built an artificial neural network model to evaluate the risk of ACDF in nearly 12,500 patients. They classified patients as "unsafe" if they experienced any complications within one week after surgery. Their artificial neural network model showed an AUC of 0.740 which was significantly better than the AUC of 0.66 of the American Society of Anesthesiologists classification ($p < 0.05$).

Another complex topic in spine surgery is spinal metastases. Knowledge about life expectancy is crucial, as patients with a very short life expectancy will not experience the benefits of surgery and therefore conservative treatment should probably be considered in these cases. Different scoring systems with different accuracies have been developed in the past. Likewise, ML algorithms were developed to calculate 30-day mortality in patients undergoing surgery for spinal metastases. Karhade et al. [41] developed four ML algorithms and provided the best-performing algorithm on an open-access web application.

Surgical site infections are a devastating complication in orthopedic surgery. It may cause higher morbidity, lower patients' satisfaction, and result in higher economic costs. Therefore, many efforts have been carried out to identify risk factors for surgical site infections. Due to the vast number of factors influencing the risk of surgical site infection, it seems reasonable to process this data by AI algorithms. Hopkins et al. [42] developed a deep neural network classification model to predict the risk for postoperative spinal infection using data from 4046 posterior spinal fusion procedures. Using 35 input variables, their model showed an excellent prediction for the appearance of postoperative spinal infection with a positive predictive value of 92.6%, a negative predictive value was 98.5%, and an AUC of 0.775.

Overall, the use of AI bears high potential in supporting spine surgeons in predicting postoperative outcomes in patients undergoing spinal surgery. This seems to support clinical decision making and offers patients the possibility to get more accurate expectations of their treatment.

17.5 Discussion

Artificial intelligence is a promising new technology that will ring in a new era in orthopedic surgery. Especially in the complex field of spinal surgery, this technology likely bears an enormous potential to support diagnostics, surgical execution, and prediction of postoperative scenarios. This is also reflected by the massive increase of publications on this topic in spinal surgery in recent years. So far, diagnostics in patients with spinal disorders are based on a limited number of variables, but AI algorithms may allow to process of big data, to include a vast number of variables and therefore probably better suit the specific needs in diagnostics of individual patients. Hitherto, surgical execution mainly depends on the experience of the treating surgeon and its constitution on the day of treatment. Using newer technologies, augmented by AI systems, surgical execution can be less depending on the individual surgeon and therefore has the potential to offer more consistent treatments. Furthermore, AI may allow predicting the postoperative course that one could expect in a more detailed way, therefore potentially supporting in tailoring individual treatment strategies, and permitting for more accurate counseling of patients for their treatment expectations.

However, with the vast number of possibilities, there are also concerns rising with that new technology. AI algorithms are based on large datasets, and as a principle, the more data is imported into the algorithm during the learning phase, the more accurate the algorithm will become. However, this data contains personal clinical and imaging data. Although data is handled in an anonymized way in general, patient consent is needed for storage and transmission. Furthermore, for many healthcare providers, AI systems appear as a black box due to the complex algorithms, which often do not allow to directly control the predictions made by the model. However, diagnosis and treatment are still based on the doctors' responsibility, but in case of an error in the AI system, the problem of the responsibility is not yet solved and therefore still requires some human control [43].

References

1. Pfirrmann CWA, Metzdorf A, Zanetti M, Hodler J, Boos N. Magnetic resonance classification of lumbar intervertebral disc degeneration. Spine (Phila Pa 1976). 2001.
2. Timon SJ, Gardner MJ, Wanich T, Poynton A, Pigeon R, Widmann RF, et al. Not all spondylolisthesis grading instruments are reliable. Clin Orthop Relat Res. 2005.
3. Hao S, Jiang J, Guo Y, Li H. Active learning based intervertebral disk classification combining shape and texture similarities. Neurocomputing. 2013;
4. Castro-Mateos I, Pozo JM, Lazary A, Frangi AF. 2D segmentation of intervertebral discs and its degree of degeneration from T2-weighted magnetic resonance images. In: Medical imaging 2014: computer-aided diagnosis 2014.
5. Castro-Mateos I, Hua R, Pozo JM, Lazary A, Frangi AF. Intervertebral disc classification by its degree of degeneration from T2-weighted magnetic resonance images. Eur Spine J. 2016.
6. Balzer I, Mühlemann M, Jokeit M, Rawal IS, Snedeker JG, Farshad M, et al. A deep learning pipeline for automatized assessment of spinal MRI. Comput Methods Programs Biomed Updat. 2022.
7. Jamaludin A, Kadir T, Zisserman A. SpineNet: Automated classification and evidence visualization in spinal MRIs. Med Image Anal. 2017.
8. Breit HC, Varga-Szemes A, Schoepf UJ, Emrich T, Aldinger J, Kressig RW, et al. CNN-based evaluation of bone density improves diagnostic performance to detect osteopenia and osteoporosis in patients with non-contrast chest CT examinations. Eur J Radiol. 2023.
9. Roth HR, Wang Y, Yao J, Lu L, Burns JE, Summers RM. Deep convolutional networks for automated detection of posterior-element fractures on spine CT. In: Medical imaging 2016: computer-aided diagnosis. 2016.
10. Feng S, Liu B, Zhang Y, Zhang X, Li Y. Two-stream compare and contrast network for vertebral compression fracture diagnosis. IEEE Trans Med Imaging. 2021.
11. Germann C, Meyer AN, Staib M, Sutter R, Fritz B. Performance of a deep convolutional neural net-

work for MRI-based vertebral body measurements and insufficiency fracture detection. Eur Radiol. 2023.
12. Cho BH, Kaji D, Cheung ZB, Ye IB, Tang R, Ahn A, et al. Automated measurement of lumbar lordosis on radiographs using machine learning and computer vision. Glob Spine J. 2020.
13. Schwartz JT, Cho BH, Tang P, Schefflein J, Arvind V, Kim JS, et al. Deep learning automates measurement of spinopelvic parameters on lateral lumbar radiographs. Spine (Phila Pa 1976). 2021.
14. Komeili A, Westover L, Parent EC, El-Rich M, Adeeb S. Monitoring for idiopathic scoliosis curve progression using surface topography asymmetry analysis of the torso in adolescents. Spine J. 2015.
15. Berlin C, Adomeit S, Grover P, Dreischarf M, Halm H, Dürr O, et al. Novel AI-based algorithm for the automated computation of coronal parameters in adolescent idiopathic scoliosis patients: a validation study on 100 preoperative full spine X-rays. Glob Spine J. 2023.
16. Jokeit M, Kim JH, Snedeker JG, Farshad M, Widmer J. Mesh-based 3D Reconstruction from Bi-planar Radiographs. In: Medical Imaging with Deep Learning [Internet]. 2022. Available from: https://openreview.net/forum?id=pR6qMzFbJQX
17. Caprara S, Carrillo F, Snedeker JG, Farshad M, Senteler M. Automated pipeline to generate anatomically accurate patient-specific biomechanical models of healthy and pathological FSUs. Front Bioeng Biotechnol. 2021.
18. Turella F, Bredell G, Okupnik A, Caprara S, Graf D, Sutter R, et al. High-resolution segmentation of lumbar vertebrae from conventional thick slice MRI. In: Lecture Notes in Computer Science (including subseries Lecture Notes in Artificial Intelligence and Lecture Notes in Bioinformatics). 2021.
19. Florkow MC, Zijlstra F, Willemsen K, Maspero M, van den Berg CAT, Kerkmeijer LGW, et al. Deep learning-based MR-to-CT synthesis: the influence of varying gradient echo-based MR images as input channels. Magn Reson Med. 2020.
20. Edmund JM, Nyholm T. A review of substitute CT generation for MRI-only radiation therapy. Radiat Oncol [Internet]. 2017;12(1):28. https://doi.org/10.1186/s13014-016-0747-y.
21. Leynes AP, Yang J, Shanbhag DD, Kaushik SS, Seo Y, Hope TA, et al. Hybrid ZTE/Dixon MR-based attenuation correction for quantitative uptake estimation of pelvic lesions in PET/MRI. Med Phys. 2017.
22. Morbée L, Chen M, Herregods N, Pullens P, Jans LBO. MRI-based synthetic CT of the lumbar spine: Geometric measurements for surgery planning in comparison with CT. Eur J Radiol. 2021.
23. Morbée L, Vereecke E, Laloo F, Chen M, Herregods N, Jans LBO. Common incidental findings on sacroiliac joint MRI: added value of MRI-based synthetic CT. Eur J Radiol. 2023.
24. Widmer J, Fasser MR, Croci E, Spirig J, Snedeker JG, Farshad M. Individualized prediction of pedicle screw fixation strength with a finite element model. Comput Methods Biomech Biomed Eng. 2020.
25. Fasser MR, Jokeit M, Kalthoff M, Gomez Romero DA, Trache T, Snedeker JG, et al. Subject-specific alignment and mass distribution in musculoskeletal models of the lumbar spine. Front Bioeng Biotechnol. 2021.
26. Fasser MR, Gerber G, Passaplan C, Cornaz F, Snedeker JG, Farshad M, et al. Computational model predicts risk of spinal screw loosening in patients. Eur Spine J. 2022.
27. Varghese V, Krishnan V, Kumar GS. Evaluating pedicle-screw instrumentation using decision-tree analysis based on pullout strength. Asian Spine J. 2018.
28. Siemionow K, Forsthoefel C, Foy M, Gawel D, Luciano C. Autonomous lumbar spine pedicle screw planning using machine learning: a validation study. J Craniovertebr Junction Spine. 2021.
29. Qi X, Meng J, Li M, Yang Y, Hu Y, Li B, et al. An automatic path planning method of pedicle screw placement based on preoperative CT images. IEEE Trans Med Robot Bionics. 2022;
30. Kalfas IH. Machine vision navigation in spine surgery. Front Surg. 2021.
31. Liebmann F, von Atzigen M, Stütz D, Wolf J, Zingg L, Suter D, et al. Automatic registration with continuous pose updates for marker-less surgical navigation in spine surgery. arXiv e-prints. 2023 Aug;arXiv:2308.02917.
32. von Atzigen M, Liebmann F, Hoch A, Miguel Spirig J, Farshad M, Snedeker J, et al. Marker-free surgical navigation of rod bending using a stereo neural network and augmented reality in spinal fusion. Med Image Anal. 2022.
33. Jecklin S, Jancik C, Farshad M, Fürnstahl P, Esfandiari H. X23D—intraoperative 3D lumbar spine shape reconstruction based on sparse multi-view X-ray data. J Imaging. 2022.
34. Massalimova A, Timmermans M, Cavalcanti N, Suter D, Seibold M, Carrillo F, et al. Automatic breach detection during spine pedicle drilling based on vibroacoustic sensing. arXiv e-prints. 2023;arXiv:2303.15114.
35. Hein J, Cavalcanti N, Suter D, Zingg L, Carrillo F, Farshad M, et al. Next-generation surgical navigation: multi-view marker-less 6DoF pose estimation of surgical instruments. arXiv e-prints. 2023;arXiv:2305.03535.
36. Seibold M, Hoch A, Farshad M, Navab N, Fürnstahl P. Conditional generative data augmentation for clinical audio datasets. Lect Notes Comput Sci (including Subser Lect Notes Artif Intell Lect Notes Bioinformatics). 2022;13437 LNCS:345–54.
37. Merali ZG, Witiw CD, Badhiwala JH, Wilson JR, Fehlings MG. Using a machine learning approach to predict outcome after surgery for degenerative cervical myelopathy. PLoS One. 2019;
38. Zigler JE, Rogers RW, Ohnmeiss DD. Comparison of 1-level versus 2-level anterior cervical discectomy

and fusion: clinical and radiographic follow-up at 60 months. Spine (Phila Pa 1976). 2016.
39. Rudisill SS, Hornung AL, Barajas JN, Bridge JJ, Mallow GM, Lopez W, et al. Artificial intelligence in predicting early-onset adjacent segment degeneration following anterior cervical discectomy and fusion. Eur Spine J. 2022.
40. Wang KY, Suresh K V., Puvanesarajah V, Raad M, Margalit A, Jain A. Using predictive modeling and machine learning to identify patients appropriate for outpatient anterior cervical fusion and discectomy. Spine (Phila Pa 1976). 2021.
41. Karhade A V., Thio QCBS, Ogink PT, Shah AA, Bono CM, Oh KS, et al. Development of machine learning algorithms for prediction of 30-day mortality after surgery for spinal metastasis. Clin Neurosurg. 2019.
42. Hopkins BS, Mazmudar A, Driscoll C, Svet M, Goergen J, Kelsten M, et al. Using artificial intelligence (AI) to predict postoperative surgical site infection: a retrospective cohort of 4046 posterior spinal fusions. Clin Neurol Neurosurg. 2020;
43. Char DS, Shah NH, Magnus D. Implementing machine learning in health care—addressing ethical challenges. N Engl J Med. 2018.

Artificial Intelligence in Osteoporosis

18

Efstathios Chronopoulos, Angelos Kaspiris, Laurence Okeke, Raffaella Russo, Tiziana Montalcini, Arturo Pujia, and Edward G. McFarland

18.1 Introduction

Osteoporosis is a metabolic bone disease characterized by low mineral bone mass followed by microarchitectural changes with a subsequent decrease in bone mechanical strength (Fig. 18.1). This may result in low-energy trauma fractures, low-energy trauma being defined as a fall from standing height or less that would not normally result in a fracture [1–3]. A fracture of this nature is also called a fragility fracture and is a sign of underlying osteoporosis. Fragility fractures may occur at any skeletal site, but are most common at the spine, proximal femur, distal forearm, and shoulder in a person older than 50 years [4].

Fractures may cause chronic pain, disability, and death. Hip fractures are associated with 25%–30% increased mortality rate within 1 year, as well as a 2.5-fold increased risk of future fractures [4]. Approximately 20%–50% of hip fracture patients require long-term nursing home care and many suffer from decreased quality of life, social isolation, depression, and loss of self-esteem [5].

As life expectancy rises, osteoporosis and its clinical consequence, fragility fractures, have become a growing societal issue with regard to their medical and economic impact. The total economic burden of osteoporosis in 2019 was estimated to be €57 billion. Additionally, chang-

E. Chronopoulos
Laboratory for Research of the Musculoskeletal System, School of Medicine, National and Kapodistrian University of Athens, Athens, Greece

A. Kaspiris
Laboratory for Research of the Musculoskeletal System, School of Medicine, National and Kapodistrian University of Athens, Athens, Greece

Laboratory of Molecular Pharmacology, Group of Orthopaedic Research School of Health Sciences, University of Patras, Patras, Greece

L. Okeke · R. Russo (✉)
Department of Clinical and Experimental Medicine, University Magna Graecia of Catanzaro, Catanzaro, Italy
e-mail: lokeke1@jh.edu

T. Montalcini · A. Pujia
Department of Clinical and Experimental Medicine, University Magna Graecia of Catanzaro, Catanzaro, Italy

Research Center for the Prevention and Treatment of Metabolic Diseases (CR METDIS), University "Magna Graecia" of Catanzaro, Catanzaro, Italy
e-mail: tmontalcini@unicz.it; pujia@unicz.it

E. G. McFarland
Division of Shoulder and Elbow Surgery, Department of Orthopaedic Surgery, The Johns Hopkins University School of Medicine, Baltimore, MD, USA
e-mail: emcfarl1@jhmi.edu

F. Familiari et al. (eds.), *Artificial Intelligence in Orthopaedic Surgery Made Easy*,
https://doi.org/10.1007/978-3-031-70310-2_18

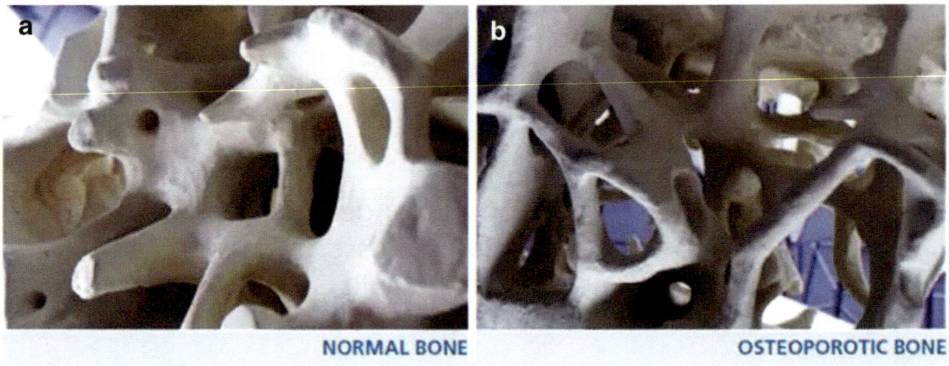

Fig. 18.1 (**a**) normal trabeculae and (**b**) osteoporotic trabeculae: decrease in cortical thickness and increase in its porosity leading to fracture. Reproduced with permission of the International Osteoporosis Foundation from https://www.osteoporosis.foundation/. All rights reserved

ing population demographics must be taken into account, as the population aged 50 years and over is expected to increase by 11.4% for both men and women between 2019 and 2034 [6]. Coinciding with this change, the annual number of osteoporotic fractures in the EU is expected to increase by 25% [6].

According to the recommendations of the World Health Organization (WHO), the diagnosis of osteoporosis measured by dual X-ray absorptiometry (DXA) scan requires a decrease in spine and/or hip bone mineral density (BMD) of at least 2.5 standard deviations (T-score) below that of a young, healthy person [7]. However, studies have shown that most fragility fractures occur at T-scores between 1.0 and 2.5 (at osteopenic BMD) or even above 1.0 (at normal BMD). This may be an indication that the sensitivity of this "gold standard" approach is insufficient and its usefulness as a screening tool is at least partially compromised [8].

It is estimated that almost 60% of osteoporotic fractures may be asymptomatic and thus undiagnosed [4]. A simple radiological examination of the thoracic and lumbar spine in the lateral projection from T4 to L4 can be useful. Using the Genant classification, a 20% reduction in vertebral height is used as the threshold for a fragility fracture diagnosis [9]. However, 25%–30% of fractures still go undiagnosed. The risk of a new osteoporotic fracture in the setting of an old one is increased threefold. This illustrates how vital it is to identify patients with this pathology [10].

Osteoporosis and the detection and prediction of fragility fractures using both clinical and imaging data have been made possible by increased recording of such data, advancements in information systems, and the integration of artificial intelligence (AI) in identifying risk factors for osteoporosis. AI has already been employed in the field of medicine through various models for identifying risk factors and population at risk groups for osteoporosis [11].

Machine-assisted knowledge acquisition, as expressed as a subset of artificial intelligence (AI), is rapidly expanding in a variety of medical science disciplines, including research related to bone metabolism. In particular, as of a few years ago, the diagnosis of osteoporosis and the detection and prediction of fragility fractures using clinical and imaging data has been made possible by the increasing recording of such data, advancements in information systems, and the integration of artificial intelligence in identifying risk factors for osteoporosis [12].

Loss of bone mineral density, characteristic of osteopenia and osteoporosis, is associated with a variety of factors that increase morbidity and mortality, including abdominal obesity, high blood pressure, dyslipidemia, and glucose metabolism abnormalities. These together constitute metabolic syndrome. Cardiovascular disease has also been linked to reduced bone mineral density, osteoporosis, and osteopenia. Studies have shown common risk factors and pathophysiological mechanisms between cardiovascular disease and osteoporosis [13, 14].

The development of specific low-cost prediction models is expected to contribute to reducing costs for both health systems and the economy as a whole [12–14]. Such models include those that aim to clarify the causal relationship between bone mineral density and metabolic syndrome. Clarification of this relationship can be achieved through a prospective study, which should not disregard factors such as gender, age, ethnicity, lifestyle, and dietary habits; these have all been demonstrated to impact the development of this syndrome.

As previously mentioned, AI has been utilized in medicine as a tool for identifying risk factors and vulnerable population groups at risk of developing osteoporosis. The development of AI models to identify high-risk populations will be particularly beneficial in developing countries, as well as in rural settlements with access to only primary care physicians. At the same time, a few studies are being conducted to develop predictive models to identify populations at risk for osteopenia, which is an early stage of osteoporosis [15]. Modern models of risk determination have been based on a sample of female and elderly patients. New prediction tools should be developed using a more diverse population, incorporating larger numbers of participants across a broader age range [14–16].

18.2 Applications in Metabolic Bone Diseases

18.2.1 Presymptomatic Screening for Osteoporosis

In the era of AI, much of the research is aimed at developing and using practical population control "tools." Consequently, the scientific community has focused on the creation of these easy-to-use and accurate diagnostic tools that will contribute to better outcomes for people at high risk of fragility fractures through early intervention, while allowing low-risk patients to optimize their relationship with the health system [17].

Most AI models have been based on predicting patients' bone mineral density through the analysis of CT images, radiographs, and certain clinical parameters [18]. The work of Fang et al. which is based on supervised learning AI, used an image analysis neural network that analyzed 1499 human CT images, with an excellent correlation of $r > 0.98$. This result holds significant importance, as it was verified through images by machines from various companies, covering different anatomical regions of the body. The model demonstrated a diagnostic accuracy for diagnosing osteoporosis ranging between 0.82 and 0.91. However, it should be noted that this study did not use dual X-ray absorptiometry (DXA) scans, which is the standard of care for measuring bone mineral density [18].

Most studies using similar convolutional neural networks (CNNs) have shown impressive results. Similarly, the results of studies that used clinical data were mostly excellent but varied depending on the type and quality of the data used [18–21]. It should be noted that in certain instances, there is a risk of overfitting [22], particularly with complex models such as the CNN, which, due to its numerous parameters, inevitably faces the possibility of such negative effects on the presentation of results. Ultimately, regardless of this risk, the development of such models in the future may provide a realistic tool for the prognosis of osteoporosis.

Rastegar et al. also developed categorization models based on features derived from radiomics, combining data from BMD images using a variety of computational algorithms. The combination of this data resulted in useful information that could be utilized as a convenient and cost-effective tool for the prediction and classification of bone metabolism disorders. At the same time, the use of radiomics, i.e., radiomic image analysis techniques, allows the acquisition of other information concerning the structural characteristics of bones. Unlike BMD, which quantifies bone strength as measured by Dual Energy X-ray Absorptiometry (DEXA) scan, radiomics allows for the prediction of mineralization disturbances with greater accuracy and contributes to a better study of human femoral loading patterns. This is essentially an attempt to classify disorders characterized by bone density loss by combining radiomics with the use of AI computer programs to categorize patients as osteoporotic, osteopenic, or normal [23, 24].

18.2.2 Presymptomatic Screening for Fragility Fractures

Artificial intelligence systems, such as OsteoDetect, have been used to diagnose and predict fractures [25]. These systems primarily use radiographs and CT scans. Areeckal et al. proposed an automated low-cost tool for early diagnosis of osteoporosis using cortical radiogrammetry and cancellous texture analysis from hand and wrist radiographs [26]. This test proved to have an accuracy of 88.5% in diagnosing osteoporosis [26]. A similar study by Chung et al. [27] using radiographic images of the humerus reported that in cases of humeral and cubitocarpal fractures, its AI model performed better diagnostically than orthopedic surgeons. In contrast, the use of AI on simple radiographic examinations did not identify hip fractures accurately. It seems that the combination of clinical symptoms, scanner accuracy (manufacturer, model), and the different incidence of hip fractures in the general population (3%) compared to the case-control cohorts (50%) contributed to the inaccuracy of the model. Studies with larger sample sizes are required to increase the diagnostic accuracy of AI models for the diagnosis of hip fractures [17].

The use of these computational systems has been suggested by some studies as superior for fracture detection and already similar systems have been accepted by the FDA and South Korea to support clinicians in fracture detection. However, despite the excitement surrounding the use of various AI models in medicine, there exists skepticism regarding their application, as many lack external validation. A recent meta-analysis evaluating AI algorithms for the diagnostic analysis of medical images reported that only 6% of them performed external validation analysis [28].

18.2.3 Risk Control

In medicine, the development of fracture prediction models has been crucial for personalized patient management and the initiation of regular check-ups. One of these models tools is the FRAX® (Fig. 18.2), a computer-based algorithm that calculates the 10-year probability of a major osteoporotic fracture (hip, clinical spine, humerus, or wrist fracture) and the 10-year probability of hip fracture alone [4].

Recently, the FRAX score has been upgraded to the FRAX PLUS tool, which is a personalized combination of the FRAX score with AI in order to modify the probability result derived from the conventional FRAX's estimation of probabilities of hip fracture and major osteoporotic fracture [4]. Newly incorporated criteria include the recency of osteoporotic fracture and higher-than-average exposure to oral glucocorticoids. Another useful tool for the prediction of fractures is the trabecular bone score (TBS), which is another indirect measure of bone strength [12, 15], however, it must be underlined that TBS is not AI by itself.

Su et al. developed a methodology for fracture prediction and thus osteoporosis diagnosis based on: (a) total hip BMD, (b) age, and (c) the femoral neck, and a FRAX score and concluded that although the FRAX tool is a good clinical indicator for hip fracture risk, a simple classification by age and hip BMD may provide an alternative way to estimate a clinical risk level of 3.0% [17].

Similarly, for postmenopausal women, the use of AI based on total BMD of the hip, lumbar spine, femoral neck, joint pain scores, serum creatinine, and homocysteine levels, outperformed FRAX in terms of accuracy [18].

A study by Muehlematter et al. used a CT image analysis model to predict fractures. The result showed that the use of CT imaging coupled with AI can identify patients at high risk for vertebral fractures [27].

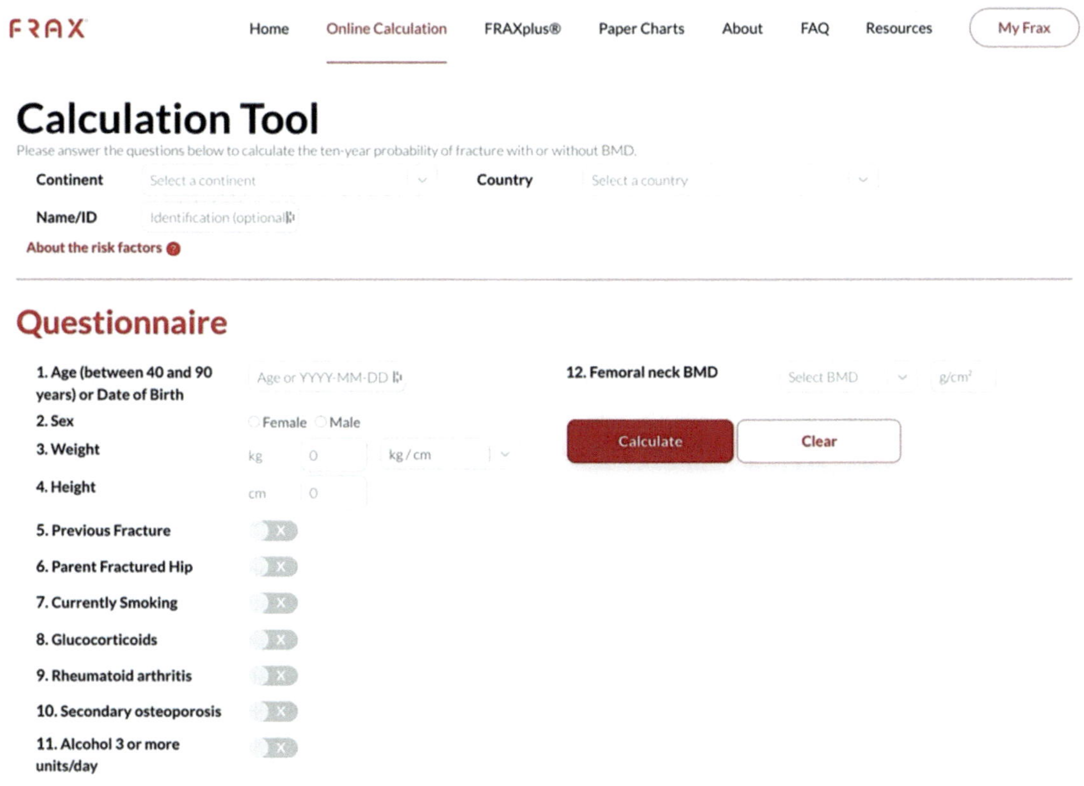

Fig. 18.2 The FRAX®. Reproduced with permission of the International Osteoporosis Foundation from https://www.fraxplus.org/calculation-tool.

In addition, several groups of scientists have attempted to predict bone loss and falls in patients using artificial intelligence models. The rate of bone mass loss over 10 years can be predicted by AI using parameters such as body mass index (BMI), age, menopause, adipose tissue measurement, and BMD. Prediction of falls was based on a combination of AI and factors such as the presence of cognitive or gait and balance disorders and Parkinson's disease, which is directly related to a difficulty in acquiring knowledge through learning.

Given the low incidence of positive results, future confirmatory studies are absolutely necessary. However, they have not been proposed for general fracture prediction, either because conventional models are well-designed and have excellent risk prediction efficiency, leaving no room for progress, or because the information obtained from imaging is not sufficient for fracture prediction. Therefore, it is necessary to explore new prediction models in the future that combine imaging information from the whole musculoskeletal system with aggregated clinical information from patients.

AI applications could also be used to predict the response to the treatment methods applied. Specifically, the response to treatment for acromegaly relies on the use of anthropometric, biochemical, and imaging characteristics of patients using a calibrated decision tree-based method. Finally, AI methods can play a role in translational research, where large amounts of genetic, epigenetic, proteomic, and molecular data can be analyzed.

18.3 Conclusions

In an era characterized by growing volumes of medical data and information, artificial intelligence presents a promising tool to provide a personalized approach to various diseases. This contributes to an enhanced understanding of such entities, including those related to bone metabolism. Indeed, the use of specific computer systems for diagnosis, classification of osteoporosis, and fracture detection seems to be continuously improving over time. Fracture prediction is an important and ever-expanding field of research that is in its infancy, but shows promise for future medical innovation.

According to the data available so far, clinicians are going to play a central role in conducting research on metabolic bone diseases, and in interpreting the results of the various models used, with an aim of enhancing the care of patients with musculoskeletal diseases. The data presented so far aims to help researchers understand the progress of AI in relation to medicine, as well as the limitations in its use.

References

1. Consensus development conference: diagnosis, prophylaxis, and treatment of osteoporosis. Am J Med. 1993;94(6):646–50.
2. Seeman E, Delmas PD. Bone quality-the material and structural basis of bone strength and fragility. N Engl J Med. 2006;354(21):2250–61.
3. Kanis JA, et al. The burden of osteoporotic fractures: a method for setting intervention thresholds. Osteoporos Int. 2001;12(5):417–27.
4. https://www.osteoporosis.foundation/Epidemiology of osteoporosis and fragility fractures.
5. Melton LJ 3rd, Achenbach SJ, Atkinson EJ, Therneau TM, Amin S. Long-term mortality following fractures at different skeletal sites: a population-based cohort study. Osteoporos Int. 2013;24:1689–96. https://doi.org/10.1007/s00198-012-2225-1.
6. Willers C, Norton N, Harvey NC, et al. Osteoporosis in Europe: a compendium of country-specific reports. Arch Osteoporos. 2022;17:23.
7. Kanis JA on behalf of the World Health Organization Scientific Group. Technical report. World Health Organization Collaborating Centre for Metabolic Bone Diseases, University of Sheffield; UK: 2007. 2007. Assessment of osteoporosis at the primary health-care level.
8. Marshall D, Johnell O, Wedel H. Meta-analysis of how well measures of bone mineral density predict occurrence of osteoporotic fractures. BMJ. 1996;312:1254e9.
9. Genant HK, Wu CY, van Kuijk C, Nevitt MC. Vertebral fracture assessment using a semiquantitative technique. J Bone Miner Res. 1993;8(9):1137–48. https://doi.org/10.1002/jbmr.5650080915.
10. Stathopoulos KD, Chronopoulos E, Galanos A, Kaskani E, Drakopoulou T, Ibro E, Tsekoura M, Kosmidis C. Prevalence of morphometric vertebral fractures in osteoporotic patients in Greece: the Vertebral Integrity Assessment (VERTINAS) study. Arch Osteoporos. 2021;16(1):165. https://doi.org/10.1007/s11657-021-01033-1.
11. Cheng C-H, Lin C-Y, Cho T-H, Lin C-M. Machine learning to predict the progression of bone mass loss associated with personal characteristics and a metabolic syndrome scoring index. Health Care. 2021;9:948. https://doi.org/10.3390/healthcare9080948.
12. Dimai HP. New horizons: artificial intelligence tools for managing osteoporosis. J Clin Endocrinol Metab. 2023;108(4):775–83. https://doi.org/10.1210/clinem/dgac702. PMID: 36477337
13. Ye C, Xu M, Wang S, Jiang S, Chen X, Zhou X, He R. Decreased bone mineral density is an independent predictor for the development of atherosclerosis: a systematic review and meta-analysis. PLoS One. 2016;11:e0154740.
14. Rodríguez AJ, Scott D, Hodge AM, English DR, Giles GG, Ebeling PR. Associations between hip bone mineral density, aortic calcification and cardiac workload in community-dwelling older Australians. Osteoporos Int. 2017;28:2239–45.
15. Smets J, Shevroja E, Hügle T, Leslie WD, Hans D. Machine learning solutions for osteoporosis—a review. J Bone Miner Res. 2021;36:833–51. https://doi.org/10.1002/jbmr.4292.
16. Cheng X, Yang Y, Schwebel DC, Liu Z, Li L, Cheng P, Ning P, Hu G. Population ageing and mortality during 1990–2017: a global decomposition analysis. PLoS Med. 2020;17(6):e1003138. https://doi.org/10.1371/journal.pmed.1003138. PMID: 32511229; PMCID: PMC7279585
17. Su Y, Kwok TC, Cummings SR, Yip BH, Cawthon PM. Can classification and regression tree analysis help identify clinically meaningful risk groups for hip fracture prediction in older American men (The MrOS Cohort Study)? JBMR Plus. 2019;3:e10207.
18. Fang Y, Li W, Chen X, Chen K, Kang H, Yu P, et al. Opportunistic osteoporosis screening in multi-detector CT images using deep convolutional neural networks. Eur Radiol. 2021;31:1831–42.
19. Ligabue G, Pollastri F, Fontana F, Leonelli M, Furci L, Giovanella S, Alfano G, Cappelli G, Testa F, Bolelli F, Grana C, Magistroni R. Evaluation of the classification accuracy of the kidney biopsy direct immunofluorescence through convolutional neural networks. Clin J Am Soc Nephrol. 2020;15(10):1445–54. https://doi.org/10.2215/CJN.03210320. Epub 2020 Sep 16. PMID: 32938617; PMCID: PMC7536749
20. Agatonovic-Kustrin S, Beresford R. Basic concepts of artificial neural network (ANN) modeling and

its application in pharmaceutical research. J Pharm Biomed Anal. 2000;22(5):717–27.
21. Liua Q, Cuia X, Chou YC, Abbodd MF, Line J, Shieh JS. Ensemble artificial neural networks applied to predict the key risk factors of hip bone fracture for elders. Biomed Signal Process Control. 2015;21:146–56.
22. Hawkins DM. The problem of overfitting. J Chem Inf Comput Sci. 2004;44:1–12.
23. Kim SK, Yoo TK, Oh E, Kim DW. Osteoporosis risk prediction using machine learning and conventional methods. Annu Int Conf IEEE Eng Med Biol Soc. 2013;2013:188–91. https://doi.org/10.1109/EMBC.2013.6609469. PMID: 24109656
24. Rastegar S, Vaziri M, Qasempour Y, Akhash MR, Abdalvand N, Shiri I, et al. Radiomics for classification of bone mineral loss: a machine learning study. Diagn Interv Imaging. 2020;101(9):599–610. https://doi.org/10.1016/j.diii.2020.01.008. Epub 2020 Feb 4
25. Voelker R. Diagnosing fractures with AI. JAMA. 2018;320(1):23. https://doi.org/10.1001/jama.2018.8565.
26. Areeckal AS, Jayasheelan N, Kamath J, Zawadynski S, Kocher M, David SS. Early diagnosis of osteoporosis using radiogrammetry and texture analysis from hand and wrist radiographs in Indian population. Osteoporos Int. 2018;29:665–73.
27. Muehlematter UJ, Mannil M, Becker AS, Vokinger KN, Finkenstaedt T, Osterhoff G, et al. Vertebral body insufficiency fractures: detection of vertebrae at risk on standard CT images using texture analysis and machine learning. Eur Radiol. 2019;29:2207–17.
28. Kim DW, Jang HY, Kim KW, Shin Y, Park SH. Design characteristics of studies reporting the performance of artificial intelligence algorithms for diagnostic analysis of medical images: results from recently published papers. Korean J Radiol. 2019;20(3):405–10.

Artificial Intelligence in Rehabilitation

19

Emily R. McDermott, Mikalyn T. DeFoor, Travis J. Dekker, and Nicholas N. DePhillipo

19.1 Introduction

Orthopedic rehabilitation focuses on restoring optimal function and mobility to individuals suffering from musculoskeletal conditions, injuries, and/or surgeries. The field encompasses a wide range of therapeutic interventions, exercises, and strategies aimed at enhancing recovery and improving the quality of life for patients. Artificial intelligence (AI) refers to the simulation of human intelligence in machines that can perform tasks that typically require human intelligence. When these two fields converge, there is immense potential for innovation and advancement in orthopedic rehabilitation, ultimately improving patient care delivery and outcomes. However, the use of AI in orthopedic rehabilitation is still in its infancy and more research is needed to evaluate the role of AI in orthopedic rehabilitation and future considerations for adoption. Therefore, the purpose of this chapter is to explore the intersection of AI and orthopedic rehabilitation, highlighting the potential applications, benefits, and challenges associated with integrating AI into rehabilitation practices.

E. R. McDermott · M. T. DeFoor
Department of Orthopaedic Surgery, San Antonio Military Medical Center, San Antonio, TX, USA

T. J. Dekker
Department of Orthopaedic Surgery, 10th Medical Group, United States Air Force Academy, CO, USA

N. N. DePhillipo (✉)
Department of Orthopaedic Surgery, University of Pennsylvania, Philadelphia, PA, USA
e-mail: Nicholas.DePhillipo@pennmedicine.upenn.edu

19.2 The Role of AI in Orthopedic Rehabilitation

19.2.1 Virtual Assistants for Personalized Rehabilitation

AI-powered virtual assistants have the potential to revolutionize the way patients receive rehabilitation guidance and support. These virtual assistants can provide personalized exercise plans, monitor progress, offer real-time feedback, and adapt the rehabilitation program based on individual needs and progress. An effective rehabilitation program incorporates a patient's characteristics and their injury and integrates individualized exercises, intensity, frequency, duration, and progress of their protocol to achieve their goals for recovery. AI virtual assistants can assist in collecting and interpreting patient data to create patient-specific protocols [1].

Adherence to physical therapy protocols is typically low, around 50%, and even lower for home-based exercise programs [2, 3]. Remote monitoring of patients has the potential to improve adherence to physical therapy protocols

F. Familiari et al. (eds.), *Artificial Intelligence in Orthopaedic Surgery Made Easy*,
https://doi.org/10.1007/978-3-031-70310-2_19

and improve patient outcomes. Virtual assistants can be used to interpret patient progress and provide real-time feedback and adjustments to a patient's physical therapy protocol [4]. AI virtual assistants can be used in conjunction with wearable technology to track patient kinematics and activity recognition as a measure of home therapy adherence and effectiveness [3, 5, 6].

19.2.2 Automated Assessment and Diagnosis

AI algorithms can analyze medical imaging data, such as radiographs, computed tomography (CT) scans, or magnetic resonance imaging (MRI) images, to aid in the diagnosis and assessment of orthopedic conditions. Machine learning algorithms can learn from large datasets of medical images to identify patterns and assist healthcare professionals in making accurate and timely diagnoses. This tool is particularly important in prioritizing the interpretation of studies in patients whose clinical outcomes rely on prompt diagnosis [7]. An AI system can identify the injury site from MRI imaging, a skill that can improve with the self-learning capability of the system. Furthermore, identifying this level of injury within a study could prompt the system to generate a standard text report, which aids in physician workload and improves the standardization of data reporting [1].

19.2.3 Intelligent Monitoring and Feedback

Wearable devices equipped with AI algorithms can track a patient's movement patterns, joint angles, and muscle activity, providing real-time feedback and objective data to both patients and healthcare providers. This information can be used to tailor physical therapy protocols to the patient's specific needs and helps to alleviate the transportation and wait time burden associated with in-person therapy [8]. Wearable technology allows continuous monitoring, which can help detect deviations from optimal movement patterns, guide rehabilitation progress, and prevent complications. In their analysis of anterior cruciate ligament reconstruction (ACLR) rehabilitation, Richter and colleagues [9] used biomechanical data to better predict those at risk of ACLR graft failure. They concluded that AI is capable of interpreting and applying complex motion analysis for clinical use.

19.2.4 Predictive Analytics and Treatment Planning

AI algorithms can leverage large volumes of patient data, including medical records, treatment outcomes, and demographic information, to generate predictive models. These models can assist in treatment planning by identifying the most effective rehabilitation strategies for individual patients, considering their unique characteristics and prognoses. One such AI algorithm incorporated patient age, body mass, alpha angle on pelvic radiographs, Tonnis grade and angle, and preoperative hip outcome scores to predict clinically meaningful improvement after hip arthroscopy with good-to-excellent discrimination [10]. Farhadi and colleagues [11] describe decision tools in AI used to incorporate predictive analytics into clinical practice to provide personalized treatment suggestions. Decision tools such as these can be used in creating patient-specific rehabilitation plans.

19.2.5 Robotics and Assistive Devices

AI-driven robotic systems and assistive devices are revolutionizing the field of orthopedic rehabilitation. Robotic exoskeletons, for instance, can provide support and assistance during rehabilitation exercises, enabling patients to regain motor function and mobility. Intelligent prosthetics and orthotics can adapt to a patient's movements, enhancing comfort and functionality. Albanese and colleagues [12] performed a randomized controlled trial on robotic-assisted rehabilitation (RAR) in those who sustained a wrist injury and compared this with a control group. They found that both groups were comparable and deemed that RAR was an effective option in post-injury rehabilitation. RAR has also been proposed in the total joint arthroplasty literature with promising results for both total knee and hip replacement [13, 14].

19.3 Benefits of AI in Orthopedic Rehabilitation

19.3.1 Enhanced Precision and Accuracy

AI technologies can offer precise and accurate assessments, diagnoses, and treatment plans, minimizing errors and optimizing outcomes. The ability of AI algorithms to process vast amounts of data and identify patterns beyond human capacity can lead to more accurate predictions and personalized interventions. Three-dimensional gait kinematics have been evaluated in total hip arthroplasty patients using an inertial sensor paired with an AI model to differentiate impaired and non-impaired gait and compare them to a healthy control. The authors found that their method of assessing gait with this technology was highly accurate [15].

19.3.2 Personalized and Adaptive Treatment Plans

By analyzing individual patient data and considering various factors such as age, injury type, comorbidities, and recovery progress, AI algorithms can generate personalized treatment plans that adapt and evolve with the patient's changing needs. This personalized approach improves the efficiency and effectiveness of rehabilitation programs [4, 5].

19.3.3 Improved Patient Engagement and Compliance

AI-powered virtual assistants and wearable devices can enhance patient engagement and motivation by providing real-time feedback, reminders, and interactive exercises. By making rehabilitation more interactive and enjoyable, AI technologies can improve patient compliance and long-term adherence to treatment plans. A cohort of 25 patients undergoing primary total knee arthroplasty were enrolled in a remote monitoring system in which subjects wore a knee sleeve that communicated with a smartphone application (app). The study highlighted that this method of acquiring continuous patient data was possible and allowed for monitoring of rehabilitation compliance and that study participants found the app to be engaging [16]. Another proof-of-concept study demonstrated that a smartwatch combined with AI was effective in assessing adherence to a home shoulder rehabilitation program [5].

19.3.4 Streamlined Workflow and Efficiency

AI algorithms can automate time-consuming tasks such as data analysis, documentation, and administrative processes. This automation can free up healthcare professionals' time, allowing them to focus more on direct patient care and decision-making, ultimately improving the efficiency of rehabilitation practices. AI recognition of injury patterns of rehabilitation progress can result in prompt diagnosis and even trigger automated texts, orders, or alerts to physicians and therapists to make changes in the patient's treatment course [1].

19.3.5 Long-term Data Analysis and Insights

AI algorithms can analyze large datasets over extended periods, providing valuable insights into treatment outcomes, patient progress, and population health trends. These insights can inform evidence-based practices, contribute to research and development, and drive continuous improvement in orthopedic rehabilitation. The automatization of standardized text can improve research efforts by providing consistent, uniform data [1].

19.4 Challenges and Considerations

19.4.1 Ethical and Privacy Concerns

The integration of AI in orthopedic rehabilitation raises ethical questions regarding patient privacy, informed consent, data security, data misuse, algorithm bias, and the responsible use of AI technologies. Clear guidelines and regulations must be established to address these concerns and ensure patient rights and safety are protected [1, 7]. The risk of a patient confidentiality breach is inherent with large datasets, and therefore, should be one of the most prominent ethical considerations. Developers need access to sensitive medical information, and collecting personal health data requires careful management and security [16, 17]. In addition to concerns of patient privacy, to retain trust in the surgeon-patient relationship and provide equitable care, physician oversight is required.

Similar to human decision-making, machine learning algorithms can develop a bias in their analysis. Bias has the potential to lead to less accurate predictions which may have more serious detriments to patient care and safety from the widespread dissemination of information and analysis from the implementation of AI software. Relying on AI may diminish human interaction and empathy, as machine learning does not possess the human traits of morality and intuition, which are important aspects of successful rehabilitation from the treatment team [17, 18]. These vulnerabilities of machine learning are often the target of exploitation for financial or political motivations.

19.4.2 Regulatory and Legal Implications

The use of AI in healthcare, including orthopedic rehabilitation, introduces new regulatory challenges. As AI and machine learning are defined as medical devices, the regulatory process falls under the advisory of the US Food and Drug Administration [18]. It is crucial to develop regulatory frameworks that govern the development, deployment, and evaluation of AI technologies to ensure patient safety, efficacy, and accountability. There is debate as to the ideal timing of addressing potential adversarial problems in AI advancement—now in the early, uncertain days to guard against unmaterialized threats in their infancy or later when the algorithms and governing protocols are better established [18]. Regardless of timing, it should be expected that perceivable threats through exploitation in the cyber world will continue to exist, which could impact rehabilitation protocols and guidelines, medical insurance claims, and device approval.

The degree of autonomy of machine learning may necessitate a change in how liability in clinical practice is conceptualized [17, 19]. Medicolegal concerns may arise when there is "disagreement" in the rehabilitation needs assessment or treatment algorithm, and as a result, it is imperative to understand that these support tools carry limitations and require constant iterative feedback and improvement by healthcare providers.

19.4.3 Data Quality and Integration

AI algorithms heavily rely on high-quality data for accurate predictions and optimal performance. The availability, interoperability, and integration of diverse datasets from different sources pose challenges that need to be addressed to fully leverage AI's potential in orthopedic rehabilitation. For instance, if there are multiple variables to a given outcome, AI might establish false correlations [7]. Additionally, AI learning algorithms are trained on data that reflects human thinking and, therefore, data that reflects second-order effects of social or historical inequities [17, 18]. User-generated data can act as a feedback loop propagating bias, which can lead to widespread systematic analytical mistakes, specifically for underrepresented groups.

Machine learning has the potential to make decisions on data that is presumed to be reliable but without the appropriate clinical context, generating incorrect conclusions that negatively affect patient recovery [18]. To ensure safety in the implementation of AI technology, the proper resources must be invested in training, evaluation, validation, and quality control of machine learning.

19.4.4 Training and Adoption by Healthcare Professionals

Healthcare professionals need to be adequately trained and educated to effectively utilize AI technologies in orthopedic rehabilitation. Training programs should encompass technical skills, ethical considerations, and the ability to interpret AI-generated insights, fostering a culture of collaboration between AI and healthcare professionals. Integration of machine learning with the clinical guidance and intuition of the medical team is imperative to avoid overreliance and clinical skill degradation.

Proper training requires direct collaboration and feedback from the development engineers and rehabilitation specialists.

19.5 Case Studies and Real-world Applications

19.5.1 Virtual Reality Rehabilitation

Virtual reality (VR) technology combined with AI algorithms offers immersive environments for rehabilitation exercises, providing sensory feedback, gamification elements, and realistic simulations to enhance patient engagement and motor learning. Telerehabilitation integrates remote patient monitoring through a VR platform to increase participation, engagement, and motivation, as well as provide real-time visual feedback and instruction on exercise techniques with home-based rehabilitation exercises [6].

There is no consensus yet on the platform with superior clinical outcomes and there are likely certain rehabilitation protocols that are better suited for a virtual platform compared to in-person sessions. However, patient perception may be a barrier to widespread acceptance of telerehabilitation. Sabesan and colleagues [20] found over half of their postoperative patients did not think they would achieve successful outcomes from virtual rehabilitation and nearly 70% stated they would not consider transitioning to virtual sessions after in-person rehabilitation after shoulder surgery.

19.5.2 Wearable Devices for Movement Analysis

Wearable devices equipped with sensors in which AI algorithms can accurately analyze movement patterns, detect abnormal kinematics, and provide real-time feedback, similar to a mobile gait lab. These devices enable remote monitoring, telerehabilitation, and objective assessment of progress. Data collected from wearable devices can be used to predict postoperative clinical measures as there are associations with changes in sensor-collected data and patient-reported outcomes over time. Furthermore, Iovanel and colleagues [21] found that step counts in patients who received feedback from a wearable device improved over time during their rehabilitation process compared to those patients who did not receive feedback after total joint arthroplasty. Wearable devices can decrease human therapist's required effort, increase repeatability, and accuracy of assessment and promote patient engagement.

19.5.3 AI-enabled Robotic Exoskeletons

Robotic exoskeletons, driven by AI algorithms, enable individuals with mobility impairments to engage in active rehabilitation by providing assistance, resistance, and real-time feedback. These devices promote motor recovery and functional independence. AI improvement of mobile robotic exoskeletons has most notably been studied in upper extremity motor rehabilitation. Robotic exoskeletons have multiple applications in rehabilitation in the upper limb including active movement assistance, neuromotor rehabilitation, and motor rehabilitation through the emphasis on ergonomic design and muscle tone assessment [22]. Artificial neural networks are at the center of processing and control of wearable robotic exoskeletons which are operated by a brain-machine interface. Adaptive algorithms provide dynamic optimization and improve machine learning by retropropagation of nonlinear optimization theory, as well as better accounting for unpredictable environmental changes and accuracy flaws in numerical computation [22].

19.5.4 Intelligent Prosthetics and Orthotics

AI-powered prosthetics and orthotics utilize sensors and AI algorithms to adapt to users' movements, optimize fit and comfort, and improve functionality. These intelligent devices enhance mobility and quality of life for individuals with limb loss or musculoskeletal disorders. High costs are a potential barrier to accessing this innovative technology. In addition to the upper extremity robotic exoskeletons discussed earlier, a hybrid AI-implemented gait orthosis has been developed for amputees and spinal cord injury patients. Machine learning lower extremity orthoses range from a microprocessor that controls the hydraulic mechanics of the knee joint for an amputee to achieve a closer approximation of natural gait to a powered ankle foot orthosis with electrodes that interface between an electrical stimulator and the nervous system [23].

Wheelchairs and walking aids reduce the amount of energy expenditure and improve mobility with ease in performance. An AI-based robotic wheelchair has been developed, which implements virtual stimulation to employ a visual joystick through recurrent neural networks that combat the problems with standard joystick maneuvers for those with reduced mobility [24].

19.6 Future Directions and Implications

19.6.1 Advancements in Machine Learning and Deep Learning

Continued advancements in machine learning and deep learning techniques hold the potential to enhance AI's capabilities in orthopedic rehabilitation, enabling more accurate predictions, improved data analysis, and refined personalized treatment approaches to restore function and mobility. Additionally, machine learning has the opportunity to remove factors contributing to burnout in medical professionals and medical mistakes, as well as improve access to affordable and timely rehabilitation care [18]. In addition to providing postoperative care and predicting changes in patient outcomes, advancement in deep learning will also improve rehabilitation efforts that include injury prevention and performance maximization.

19.6.2 Integration with Internet of Things (IoT) and Big Data Analytics

Integrating AI with IoT devices and big data analytics can provide real-time remote monitoring, seamless data exchange, and comprehensive insights for rehabilitation practices. IoT is the interconnection of data collected from smart devices and delivered to the internet to connect people with information [18]. This integration enables remote rehabilitation, data-driven decision-making, and proactive intervention. The integration of AI with IoT has been compared to the relationship of the brain with the human body, making AI an indispensable component of the future of orthopedic rehabilitation [18]. This data may include patient-reported outcome measures, steps, opioid usage, range of motion, compliance with home exercise program, and pain score. The collection of large volumes of data in real time can help develop algorithms for prediction of which patients may struggle with their rehabilitation and when patients may safely progress to the next level of their rehabilitation program [25].

19.6.3 Telerehabilitation and Remote Monitoring

AI technologies can facilitate telerehabilitation programs, enabling patients to receive rehabilitation services remotely. Real-time monitoring, video consultations, and AI-driven feedback systems can bridge the gap between patients and healthcare providers, expanding access to care. Telerehabilitation has been shown to be effective and comparable to conventional methods with lower associated costs for the improvement of physical function and pain relief, specifically after knee and hip arthroplasty [26, 27].

19.6.4 Collaborative AI-assisted Rehabilitation

AI technologies can support collaborative decision-making between patients, healthcare professionals, and AI systems. Human-AI collaboration can lead to shared decision-making, enhanced patient empowerment, and improved rehabilitation outcomes. As machine learning is an imperfect system without human decision-making capability, AI systems must be interactive and explainable. By combining machine learning algorithms with rule-based models from therapists to support decision-making on rehabilitation assessment and progress, healthcare experts and AI systems can both learn from each other to generate collective, hybrid decision-making with improved accuracy, transparency, and use acceptance [28]. While machine learning can generate abundant quantitative data, a feedback loop to refine machine learning requires collaboration among development experts, therapists, and an interactive AI system.

19.7 Conclusion

Artificial intelligence has the potential to revolutionize orthopedic rehabilitation by offering personalized treatment plans, intelligent monitoring, predictive analytics, and value-conscious care. The integration of AI technologies such as virtual assistants, robotics, and machine learning algorithms can enhance patient outcomes, streamline workflows, and drive evidence-based practices. However, ethical considerations, regulatory frameworks, data quality, and professional training are critical to ensure responsible and effective deployment of AI in orthopedic rehabilitation. Challenges regarding ethical deployment, quality control and regulation, and clinical superiority of AI over traditional platforms remain unsolved and require the effort of future research. With continued advancements and collaborative efforts, AI will undoubtedly continue to shape the future of orthopedic rehabilitation, ultimately improving the quality of life of both operative and nonoperative patients.

References

1. Cheng K, Guo Q, He Y, Lu Y, Xie R, Li C, et al. Artificial intelligence in sports medicine: could GPT-4 make human doctors obsolete? Ann Biomed Eng. 2023;51(8):1658–62. https://link.springer.com/10.1007/s10439-023-03213-1
2. Holden MA, Haywood KL, Potia TA, Gee M, McLean S. Recommendations for exercise adherence measures in musculoskeletal settings: a systematic review and consensus meeting (protocol). Syst Rev. 2014;3(1):10. https://doi.org/10.1186/2046-4053-3-10.
3. Familiari F, Galasso O, Massazza F, Mercurio M, Fox H, Srikumaran U, et al. Artificial intelligence in the management of rotator cuff tears. Int J Environ Res Public Health. 2022;19(24):16779. https://www.mdpi.com/1660-4601/19/24/16779
4. Corban J, Lorange JP, Laverdiere C, Khoury J, Rachevsky G, Burman M, et al. Artificial intelligence in the management of anterior cruciate ligament injuries. Orthop J Sports Med. 2021;9(7) http://journals.sagepub.com/doi/10.1177/23259671211014206
5. Burns DM, Leung N, Hardisty M, Whyne CM, Henry P, McLachlin S. Shoulder physiotherapy exercise recognition: machine learning the inertial signals from a smartwatch. Physiol Meas. 2018;39(7):075007.

6. Erickson BJ, Shishani Y, Gobezie R. Remote patient monitoring of postoperative rehabilitation. Phys Med Rehabil Clin N Am. 2023;34(2):489–97. https://linkinghub.elsevier.com/retrieve/pii/S1047965122001255
7. Román-Belmonte JM, la Corte-Rodríguez HD, Rodríguez-Merchán EC. Artificial intelligence in musculoskeletal conditions. Front Biosci Landmark Ed. 2021;26(11):1340–8.
8. Ianculescu M, Andrei B, Alexandru A. A Smart assistance solution for remotely monitoring the orthopaedic rehabilitation process using wearable technology: re.flex system. Stud Inform Control. 2019;28.
9. Richter C, King E, Strike S, Franklyn-Miller A. Objective classification and scoring of movement deficiencies in patients with anterior cruciate ligament reconstruction. PLoS One. 2019;14(7):e0206024. https://doi.org/10.1371/journal.pone.0206024.
10. Kunze KN, Kaidi A, Madjarova S, Polce EM, Ranawat AS, Nawabi DH, et al. External validation of a machine learning algorithm for predicting clinically meaningful functional improvement after arthroscopic hip preservation surgery. Am J Sports Med. 2022;50(13):3593–9. http://journals.sagepub.com/doi/10.1177/03635465221124275
11. Farhadi F, Barnes MR, Sugito HR, Sin JM, Henderson ER, Levy JJ. Applications of artificial intelligence in orthopaedic surgery. Front Med Technol. 2022;4:995526.
12. Albanese GA, Taglione E, Gasparini C, Grandi S, Pettinelli F, Sardelli C, et al. Efficacy of wrist robot-aided orthopedic rehabilitation: a randomized controlled trial. J NeuroEng Rehabil. 2021;18(1):130. https://jneuroengrehab.biomedcentral.com/articles/10.1186/s12984-021-00925-0
13. Yoo JI, Oh MK, Lee SU, Lee CH. Robot-assisted rehabilitation for total knee or hip replacement surgery patients: a systematic review and meta-analysis. Medicine (Baltimore). 2022;101(40):e30852. https://journals.lww.com/10.1097/MD.0000000000030852
14. Cai L, Liu Y, Wei Z, Liang H, Liu Y, Cui M. Robot-assisted rehabilitation training improves knee function and daily activity ability in older adults following total knee arthroplasty. Res Nurs Health. 2023;46(2):203–9.
15. Teufl W, Taetz B, Miezal M, Lorenz M, Pietschmann J, Jöllenbeck T, et al. Towards an inertial sensor-based wearable feedback system for patients after total hip arthroplasty: validity and applicability for gait classification with gait kinematics-based features. Sensors. 2019;19(22):5006.
16. Ramkumar PN, Haeberle HS, Ramanathan D, Cantrell WA, Navarro SM, Mont MA, et al. Remote patient monitoring using mobile health for total knee arthroplasty: validation of a wearable and machine learning-based surveillance platform. J Arthroplast. 2019;34(10):2253–9.
17. Santilli V, Mangone M, Diko A, Alviti F, Bernetti A, Agostini F, et al. The use of machine learning for inferencing the effectiveness of a rehabilitation program for orthopedic and neurological patients. Int J Environ Res Public Health. 2023;20(8):5575. https://www.mdpi.com/1660-4601/20/8/5575
18. Myers TG, Ramkumar PN, Ricciardi BF, Urish KL, Kipper J, Ketonis C. Artificial intelligence and orthopaedics: an introduction for clinicians. J Bone Jt Surg. 2020;102(9):830–40. https://journals.lww.com/10.2106/JBJS.19.01128
19. Ramkumar PN, Luu BC, Haeberle HS, Karnuta JM, Nwachukwu BU, Williams RJ. Sports medicine and artificial intelligence: a primer. Am J Sports Med. 2022;50(4):1166–74. http://journals.sagepub.com/doi/10.1177/03635465211008648
20. Sabesan VJ, Dawoud M, Stephens BJ, Busheme CE, Lavin AC. Patients' perception of physical therapy after shoulder surgery. JSES Int. 2022;6(2):292–6. https://linkinghub.elsevier.com/retrieve/pii/S2666638321002632
21. Iovanel G, Ayers D, Zheng H. The role of wearable technology in measuring and supporting patient outcomes following total joint replacement: review of the literature. JMIR Perioper Med. 2023;6:e39396. https://periop.jmir.org/2023/1/e39396
22. Vélez-Guerrero MA, Callejas-Cuervo M, Mazzoleni S. Artificial intelligence-based wearable robotic exoskeletons for upper limb rehabilitation: a review. Sensors. 2021;21(6):2146. https://www.mdpi.com/1424-8220/21/6/2146
23. Nandor M, Kobetic R, Audu M, Triolo R, Quinn R. A muscle-first, electromechanical hybrid gait restoration system in people with spinal cord injury. Front Robot AI. 2021;8:645588. https://www.frontiersin.org/articles/10.3389/frobt.2021.645588/full
24. Mrabet M, Rabhi Y, Fnaiech F. Development of a new intelligent joystick for people with reduced mobility. Appl Bionics Biomech. 2018;2018:1–14. https://www.hindawi.com/journals/abb/2018/2063628/
25. Dobkin BH. A rehabilitation-internet-of-things in the home to augment motor skills and exercise training. Neurorehabil Neural Repair. 2017;31(3):217–27. http://journals.sagepub.com/doi/10.1177/1545968316680490
26. Cottrell MA, Galea OA, O'Leary SP, Hill AJ, Russell TG. Real-time telerehabilitation for the treatment of musculoskeletal conditions is effective and comparable to standard practice: a systematic review and meta-analysis. Clin Rehabil. 2017;31(5):625–38. http://journals.sagepub.com/doi/10.1177/0269215516645148
27. Petersen W, Karpinski K, Backhaus L, Bierke S, Häner M. A systematic review about telemedicine in orthopedics. Arch Orthop Trauma Surg. 2021;141(10):1731–9. https://link.springer.com/10.1007/s00402-021-03788-1
28. Lee MH, Siewiorek DP, Smailagic A, Bernardino A, Bermúdez i Badia S. A human-AI collaborative approach for clinical decision making on rehabilitation assessment. In: Proceedings of the 2021 CHI Conference on Human Factors in Computing Systems. Yokohama: ACM; 2021. p. 1–14. https://dl.acm.org/doi/10.1145/3411764.3445472.

20 Potential Risks and Ethical Issues with Intelligent Technologies in Orthopedics

Seikai Toyooka, R. Kyle Martin, Lars Engebretsen, and Gilbert Moatshe

20.1 Introduction

Retrospective analysis has long been used to guide prospective medical care and represents level IV evidence for prognostic studies [1]. However, results from these studies are often applied to patients to guide care decisions in a general sense. In other words, these studies are useful for identifying factors or variables that may affect outcomes, and the results are often reported as relative or absolute risk, odds ratios, or comparisons between one treatment, intervention, or assessment tool and another. These studies represent an important part of research and have the potential of moving the profession forward and improving patient care.

Recently, artificial intelligence (AI) has been heralded as a novel approach to retrospective data that can help both clinicians and patients with more standardized and patient-specific guidance. As the use of these models increases, it is important to consider the multiple risks and ethical considerations in order to guide the responsible development and deployment of these models in clinical practice. The goals of this chapter are to review common and important risks and ethical considerations for those who seek to develop or utilize AI-based models for clinical care.

S. Toyooka
Oslo Sports Trauma Research Center, Norwegian School of Sport Sciences, Oslo, Norway

Department of Orthopedic Surgery, Teikyo University Hospital, Tokyo, Japan

R. K. Martin
Oslo Sports Trauma Research Center, Norwegian School of Sport Sciences, Oslo, Norway

Department of Orthopedic, University of Minnesota, Minneapolis, MN, USA

Department of Orthopedic Surgery, CentraCare, Saint Cloud, MN, USA

L. Engebretsen · G. Moatshe (✉)
Oslo Sports Trauma Research Center, Norwegian School of Sport Sciences, Oslo, Norway

Department of Orthopaedic Surgery, Oslo University Hospital and University of Oslo, Oslo, Norway

20.2 Potential Risks of Artificial Intelligence

20.2.1 Black Box Effect

Artificial intelligence refers to advanced statistical techniques that are capable of identifying complex interactions between variables in a dataset. This approach enables the creation of algorithms that excel at tasks such as outcome prediction or image and text interpretation. However, one of the biggest drawbacks of AI relates to the interpretability of models, which is why some models are referred to as "black box" models (especially large neural networks). In short, the "black box" moniker refers to models

F. Familiari et al. (eds.), *Artificial Intelligence in Orthopaedic Surgery Made Easy*,
https://doi.org/10.1007/978-3-031-70310-2_20

that produce an output without a corresponding clear explanation of how or why.

Much of the AI developed and applied in healthcare uses machine learning (ML) techniques, including deep learning. During model development, the criteria and relationships used by the AI model to make a prediction are constantly changing as the model "learns" in order to achieve optimal accuracy. To understand the basis for why the judgment was made, it is necessary to understand the criteria that change with learning. However, for algorithms with large structures and nonlinear relationships between variables, it can be challenging for humans to understand the model's decision-making criteria. Many ML algorithms, especially deep learning algorithms used for image analysis, are virtually impossible to interpret or explain. Therefore, there may be cases where a diagnosis or misdiagnosis occurs based on AI, but the decision criteria cannot be understood. Additionally, the scenario could be envisioned in which a patient may be diagnosed with a serious condition such as cancer by an AI model, but the physician may not be able to explain to the patient why such a diagnosis was made.

In the case of underperforming (misdiagnosing) models, the developer has to guess the cause, re-train the model, and then send it out into the world as "fixed" if no problems occur afterward. As long as the cause has not been identified, there is a possibility that the fault could recur in a different form. Even with highly accurate models, there is concern that the deployment of black box algorithms in health care could lead to patients' lives being entrusted to a technology that even doctors and developers do not fully understand.

Due to the obvious concerns with the application of black box models in health care, potential solutions to this problem have been pursued over recent years. One such example of a technique to address this limitation is SHapley Additive exPlanations (SHAP) for cluster interpretation in unsupervised learning models [2, 3]. This two-step process produces SHAP values, which can be used to explain the contributions of the input variables within each cluster and can be presented graphically. Martin et al. applied SHAP analysis to their unsupervised learning study of the combined Norwegian and Danish knee ligament registries, which aided in the interpretation of the patient clusters (Fig. 20.1). When counseling a patient that an algorithm assessment has led to a particular diagnosis or prediction, it is beneficial for the clinician and the patient to understand why. Explainable AI will continue to be a major focus over the coming years as the development of new clinically relevant models increases exponentially.

20.2.2 Bias

One of the expected roles of medical AI is to prevent diagnostic errors due to cognitive bias. It was hoped that AI would be able to prevent this from happening and provide support to humans through more objective data analysis and interpretation. However, the reality is that AI is often still exposed to cognitive bias. For example, Microsoft's chatbot Tay repeatedly made discriminatory remarks about people of Jewish descent and court support AI COMPAS was biased to predict that black people were at high risk of re-offending [5, 6]. The cause of these judgments by supposedly non-prejudiced AI lies in the data used for training and its treatment. In the case of Tay, for example, the bias was due to some users misusing the system that learns from conversations with humans. In the case of COMPAS, it was also due to the use of prejudiced training data, as was subject to some of the same prejudices as humans.

Medical AI faces similar challenges. Much of the available historic medical data in the United States is predominantly based on medical records of white men [7]. An algorithm trained on such data may make less accurate predictions about women, other races and ethnicities, or any other underrepresented group in the dataset. In the case of skin cancer, the likely site and appearance of the disease change slightly depending on skin

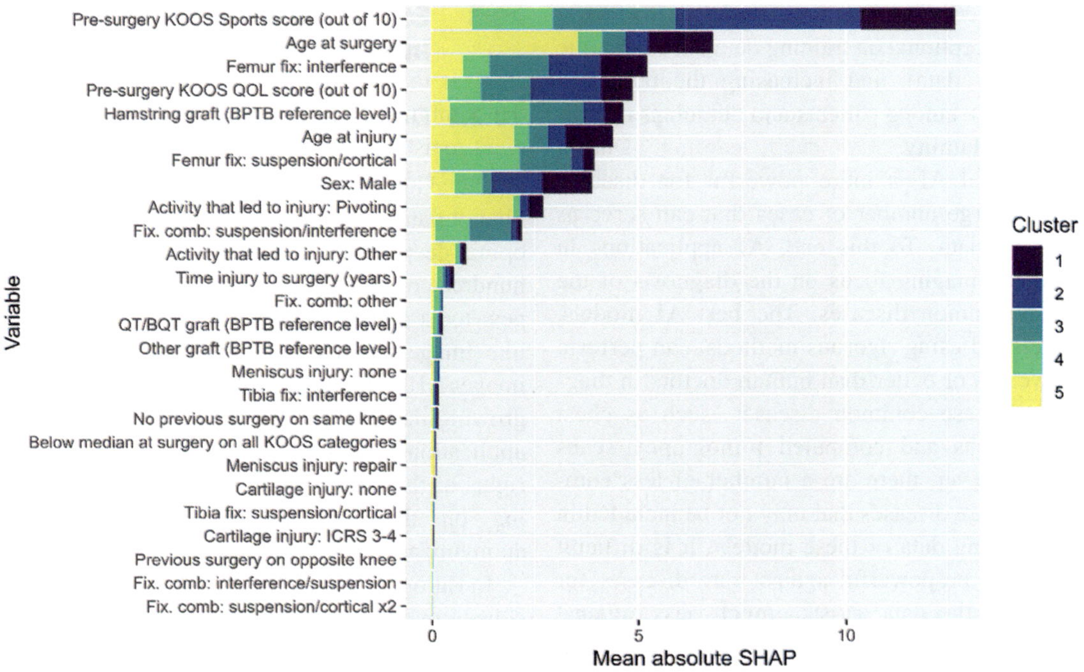

Fig. 20.1 The plot shows mean absolute SHapley Additive exPlanations (SHAP) values by variable for all clusters. Colors in the plot show the contributions from observations assigned to each cluster. *KOOS* Knee injury and osteoarthritis outcome score, *fix* fixation, *QOL* Quality of life subscale, *BPTB* Bone-patellar tendon-bone autograft, *comb* combined, *QT/BQT* Quadriceps tendon autograft, with or without bone, *ICRS* International Cartilage Regeneration & Joint Preservation Society. (Reproduced with permission from [4])

color and age [8]. Therefore, an AI that has learned from data on white people might not be able to make an accurate diagnosis if it is presented with skin cancer in non-Caucasians. This is similar to the bias of human judgment, which stems from an individual's past experiences, and in turn, can lead to inaccurate clinical decisions. However, the widespread simultaneous deployment of biased AI and its use by thousands of clinicians may have more detrimental implications for patient care and safety. Moreover, AI does not possess traits that are uniquely human like morality and intuition, and is liable to make mistakes that seem absurd to humans. The fundamental solution to AI misjudgments due to bias in training data would be to pull as much health data as possible from other facilities in as many different regions as possible, from as many diverse backgrounds as possible. However, this is subject to financial and available data constraints.

20.2.3 Generalizability and Rare Cases

Deep learning, a type of AI, has potential applications in medicine; however, there are major challenges to its widespread use in clinical practice. The first of these relates to the generalizability of clinical models. Most of the available prediction models have been developed and internally validated, without undergoing rigorous external validation. Prior to clinical application, the external validity of a model should be determined using patients that differ from the population that was used to initially train the model. The external validation should incorporate patients that differ from the original population with regard to race, ethnicity, geographic region, socioeconomic status, etc. Overall, proper external validation holds value for several reasons, which include model generalizability, bias mitigation, assessment of model overfitting (refers to model performance that is exceptional on training data but inaccurate with new data), and increasing the trust and acceptance among patients and clinicians regarding model utility.

Medical AI is more powerful for diseases with a large number of cases that can serve as training data. To this end, AI applications in medical imaging focus on the diagnosis of the most common diseases. The best AI models, developed using rigorous methods, can perform as well as or better than human doctors in diagnosing these common diseases, such as chest radiographs and computed tomography scans [9]. However, there are a number of less common or rare diseases that may not be included in the training data of these models. It is difficult for AI to be powerful against rare diseases for which little data exists, much less against unknown diseases for which no data exists, and it may not be able to accurately diagnose these rare diseases. This means that physicians need to be cautious and not rely solely on AI tools because these models may not work well in all situations. Similarly, AI models trained on certain types of images may not work well in different practices or with new patients. Training a model on data that is not representative of the population, different cases, imaging methods, or protocols may compromise its performance and reliability, especially if it is subject to overfitting. To provide the best possible care to patients, doctors need to be aware of these potential problems and use AI tools responsibly, taking into account their limitations and potential pitfalls.

While it is difficult to identify new or rare diseases, it may be possible to present doctors with a differential diagnosis. If the model can present a shortlist of diseases that are similar rather than simply reporting the correct disease name, even if the algorithm cannot make the correct decision, it can help guide the physician toward the most likely diagnoses to be considered. In addition, it is possible to efficiently derive a treatment for another disease with similar symptoms. Even if it is not possible to detect unknown diseases, it should be possible in the future to prepare the best course of action.

20.3 Ethical Issues with Aritificial Intelligence

20.3.1 Data Ownership and Sharing

Artificial intelligence systems require a large volume of data to work effectively. Scientists developing deep learning applications may require hundreds of thousands of cases to create and test new tools and often rely on available databases like ImageNet, which contains over 14 million images [10]. In the healthcare field, there is a growing demand for patient data to develop AI applications. However, the ownership and use rights of this data are complex and vary depending on the jurisdiction and the level of anonymization.

In Europe, patients have strong ownership and control over their data, while healthcare organizations in North America may own the physical records associated with patient data [11]. This variability poses several unresolved issues, especially in a global AI market where models trained on data from one country may be used and sold in another. Healthcare organizations can use de-identified patient records for research and development with patient consent or exemptions. However, questions arise regarding patient tolerance for such use under new regulations like the General Data Protection Regulation (GDPR) [12]. For example, how can companies be prevented from seeking less regulated environments with unclear data ownership rules? What recourse do European Union (EU) citizens have when their data is used in other jurisdictions like the United States of America (USA), where consent waivers may be granted? Conversely, will the GDPR discourage USA companies from working with EU companies if they have to meet the more arduous GDPR regulations? While it is unlikely that patients can claim ownership of intellectual property derived from their data, these issues may be resolved in the future through legal processes and public opinion.

Given that a large volume of data is often required for the development and validation of accurate and generalizable models, international collaboration opportunities should be encouraged. However, data transfer laws and regulations may pose a barrier to data sharing between countries. Considerable resources including personnel, time, and financial investment are often required to meet the strict demands and support international data-sharing arrangements, which may be prohibitive in many cases. Thus, it is often easiest to share AI algorithms for validation and improvement rather than patient data and requires a collaborative effort between study groups.

20.3.2 Security and Patient Privacy

Privacy protection involves regulating access to individuals and their personal information. In the context of medical AI, privacy means controlling who can access protected health information. Data security measures are used to prevent unauthorized access to this information. In AI applications, it is important for clinical and business entities to protect their data from hackers and to ensure that it is not stored on vulnerable servers. However, there can be a conflict between machine learning models that require large databases and privacy protection. Machine learning algorithms benefit from big data to learn effectively, but when data is gathered from various sources, it often becomes easier to identify individuals, which runs counter to privacy goals. Several governing bodies such as the GDPR enforced by the EU now exist and impose strict rules on how personal data is used [12]. Companies must be transparent about data usage, limit data collection to what is necessary, and allow individuals to access, modify, or delete their data upon request. Noncompliance can result in heavy fines. While data de-identification is often proposed as a privacy solution, it may not be entirely effective. Manual and automated approaches to de-identification have limitations, and some types of protected health information may not be completely removed. For example, de-identifying medical imaging data stored in the DICOM standard requires removing metadata that may contain personal information. This process requires expertise in metadata registration.

20.3.3 Responsibility for Medical Treatment and Diagnosis

Currently, the ultimate responsibility for the use of medical AI lies with the physician. However, if mistakes are made in diagnosis or treatment based on an AI model, which is a type of medical device, and patients are harmed as a result, the developers of the AI could conceivably be held responsible. For a medical AI model to acquire capabilities equal to or exceeding those of a physician, it requires a rigorous process of learning from data, including from its own mistakes. Developers must, therefore, collect sufficient training data and then create models that perform with an acceptably low frequency of mistakes, or they will not be able to bring it to the market. This creates a delicate balance that must be struck between developers and users regarding the responsible deployment of the models. Too much responsibility falling on the shoulders of developers would make it difficult to develop new AI models owing to the risk they incur. On the other hand, if the developers' responsibility is minimized and physicians are asked to carry the burden, it may result in the development and deployment of models that are less ideal. In this scenario, the advantage would go to developers that were earlier to market, even if their models are less accurate or more prone to error. This will be an important concept moving forward and will require a constant and mature debate on the balance of responsibility between developers and users of medical AI models.

20.3.4 Ethical Implementation

Artificial intelligence advancements enable the creation of patient-specific clinical prediction tools. These may come in the form of an online calculator or other in-office tool that can estimate an individual's specific likelihood of achieving a specified outcome. Several examples of this exist in the medical literature, and model performance often matches or exceeds that of medical experts [1, 13–18]. A dilemma facing researchers who seek to develop medical AI models relates to the appropriate implementation of these tools into clinical practice. Developers have a responsibility to the entire profession—the researchers, clinicians, and patients—to provide appropriate context and honesty regarding model validity to ensure that they are not misused or misinterpreted.

There are several ways clinical prediction models may be misused. First, clinicians may inappropriately utilize the tool on a population that is different than the one used to train the model. This represents the main barrier to the widespread implementation of many AI models as most have not had rigorous external validation [19]. Researchers must be careful not to advocate for the utilization of their patient-specific prediction models by clinicians and patients in other regions of the world until the validity of the model on these different populations has been evaluated.

A second way medical AI models may be misused is through clinician overreliance on the model output. Clinicians must be careful to not accept the results as truth or fact. This is true of all AI-related tasks and has garnered significant attention recently. One example of this is the large language models like Chat Generative Pre-Trained Transformer (ChatGPT) and its propensity to hallucinate [20, 21]. Researchers and clinicians must understand that the performance of medical AI models is imperfect and should be used as an adjunct clinical tool, rather than the absolute ground truth to be accepted as fact.

Researchers must act to minimize the risk of overreliance on their models, and this can be accomplished in several ways. Honesty with respect to the performance of the models is crucial to avoid falsely elevating the expectations of clinicians. This may occasionally require a delicate balance between not overstating the utility of the model and simultaneously advocating for the positive impact the models may have among colleagues who exhibit skepticism of new technology. In the early stages of AI adoption within health care, those who are more familiar with the techniques and technology should take on leadership roles to guide the profession toward responsible research. These leaders must advocate for ethical applications and engage in peer education to empower clinicians and researchers to critically appraise and properly interpret the findings of AI-based studies.

The third way medical AI-driven models may be misused relates to the temporal nature of their creation and implementation. This is especially true of models that do not apply reinforcement learning (models that continue to learn as they receive new data). Using an example from orthopedic sports medicine, Martin et al. developed and externally validated a clinical prediction tool capable of estimating the risk of subsequent anterior cruciate ligament revision after primary reconstruction [22, 23]. The model was developed using data collected from the Norwegian Knee Ligament Register between 2004 and 2020. Over that time period, surgical techniques, implants, and instruments along with the understanding of risk factors and outcomes have advanced considerably. Given the ongoing evolution that is expected to continue, it is unreasonable to expect that the prediction model will maintain relevance far into the future.

The difficulty lies in identifying the point at which a model is no longer relevant. It is, therefore, imperative that researchers continually assess the effect that new data and knowledge can have on the prediction models. This can be achieved by evaluating the model performance prospectively and scrutinizing for deterioration over time, or through recalibration of the model with new data on an ongoing basis. Since data quantity is an important contributor to model performance, the establishment of international collaborative efforts aimed at aggregating large volumes of clinical data for this purpose could be pursued.

20.4 Conclusion

In an era increasingly being shaped by AI, the risks and ethics of these models will remain an important topic for the foreseeable future. Model interpretability, bias, generalizability, and data security concerns will certainly remain at the forefront as patient data is collected and utilized at an exponential rate. Scientists engaged in big data research and clinical care should possess a thorough understanding of these issues along with those related to the ethical dissemination and clinical application of the models. Discussions related to these ethical principles should occur frequently to ensure that patients are not forgotten amid the vast troves of data and that they are protected at every step—from data collection through to clinical care.

References

1. Choi JW, Cho YJ, Lee S, Lee J, Lee S, Choi YH, et al. Using a dual-input convolutional neural network for automated detection of pediatric supracondylar fracture on conventional radiography. Investig Radiol. 2020;55(2):101–10.
2. Chowdhury SU, Sayeed S, Rashid I, Alam MGR, Masum AKM, Dewan MAA. Shapley-additive-explanations-based factor analysis for dengue severity prediction using machine learning. J Imaging. 2022;8(9):229.
3. Lundberg S, Lee S-I. A unified approach to interpreting model predictions 2017.
4. Martin RK, Wastvedt S, Pareek A, Persson A, Visnes H, Fenstad AM, et al. Unsupervised machine learning of the combined danish and norwegian knee ligament registers: identification of 5 distinct patient groups with differing ACL revision rates. Am J Sports Med. 2024;52(4):881–91.
5. Lee D. Tay: Microsoft issues apology over racist chatbot fiasco. 2016. https://www.bbc.com/news/technology-35902104.
6. Stevenson MT, Slobogin C. Algorithmic risk assessments and the double-edged sword of youth. Behav Sci Law. 2018;36(5):638–56.
7. Martinho A, Kroesen M, Chorus C. A healthy debate: exploring the views of medical doctors on the ethics of artificial intelligence. Artif Intell Med. 2021;121:102190.
8. Apalla Z, Lallas A, Sotiriou E, Lazaridou E, Ioannides D. Epidemiological trends in skin cancer. Dermatol Pract Concept. 2017;7(2):1–6.
9. Kumar Y, Koul A, Singla R, Ijaz MF. Artificial intelligence in disease diagnosis: a systematic literature review, synthesizing framework and future research agenda. J Ambient Intell Humaniz Comput. 2023;14(7):8459–86.
10. Lin Y, Ding W, Qiang S, Deng L, Li G. ES-ImageNet: a million event-stream classification dataset for spiking neural networks. Front Neurosci. 2021;15:726582.
11. Grande D, Luna Marti X, Feuerstein-Simon R, Merchant RM, Asch DA, Lewson A, et al. Health policy and privacy challenges associated with digital technology. JAMA Netw Open. 2020;3(7):e208285.
12. Hussein R, Wurhofer D, Strumegger EM, Stainer-Hochgatterer A, Kulnik ST, Crutzen R, et al. General Data Protection Regulation (GDPR) toolkit for digital health. Stud Health Technol Inform. 2022;290:222–6.
13. Esteva A, Kuprel B, Novoa RA, Ko J, Swetter SM, Blau HM, et al. Dermatologist-level classification of skin cancer with deep neural networks. Nature. 2017;542(7639):115–8.
14. Rouzrokh P, Wyles CC, Philbrick KA, Ramazanian T, Weston AD, Cai JC, et al. A deep learning tool for automated radiographic measurement of acetabular component inclination and version after total hip arthroplasty. J Arthroplast. 2021;36(7):2510–7.e6.
15. Schock J, Truhn D, Abrar DB, Merhof D, Conrad S, Post M, et al. Automated analysis of alignment in long-leg radiographs by using a fully automated support system based on artificial intelligence. Radiol Artif Intell. 2020;3(2):e200198.
16. Senior AW, Evans R, Jumper J, Kirkpatrick J, Sifre L, Green T, et al. Improved protein structure prediction using potentials from deep learning. Nature. 2020;577(7792):706–10.
17. Urakawa T, Tanaka Y, Goto S, Matsuzawa H, Watanabe K, Endo N. Detecting intertrochanteric hip fractures with orthopedist-level accuracy using a deep convolutional neural network. Skeletal Radiol. 2019;48(2):239–44.
18. Yamada Y, Maki S, Kishida S, Nagai H, Arima J, Yamakawa N, et al. Automated classification of hip fractures using deep convolutional neural networks with orthopedic surgeon-level accuracy: ensemble decision-making with antero-posterior and lateral radiographs. Acta Orthop. 2020;91(6):699–704.
19. Collins GS, Reitsma JB, Altman DG, Moons KGM. Transparent reporting of a multivariable prediction model for individual prognosis or diagnosis (TRIPOD): the TRIPOD statement. BMC Med. 2015;13(1):1.
20. Goddard J. Hallucinations in ChatGPT: a cautionary tale for biomedical researchers. Am J Med. 2023;136(11):1059–60.
21. Sallam M. ChatGPT utility in healthcare education, research, and practice: systematic review on the promising perspectives and valid concerns. Healthcare (Basel). 2023;11(6):887.
22. Martin RK, Wastvedt S, Pareek A, Persson A, Visnes H, Fenstad AM, et al. Predicting anterior cruciate ligament reconstruction revision: a machine learning analysis utilizing the norwegian knee ligament register. J Bone Joint Surg Am. 2022;104(2):145–53.
23. Martin RK, Wastvedt S, Pareek A, Persson A, Visnes H, Fenstad AM, et al. Machine learning algorithm to predict anterior cruciate ligament revision demonstrates external validity. Knee Surg Sports Traumatol Arthrosc. 2022;30(2):368–75.